Children's Upper and Lower Limb Orthopaedic Disorders

Michael Benson • John Fixsen • Malcolm Macnicol
Klaus Parsch

Editors

Children's Upper and Lower Limb Orthopaedic Disorders

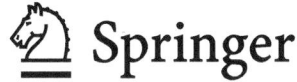 Springer

Editors
Michael Benson
Ridgway
Harberton Mead
OX3 ODB Oxford
United Kingdom
michael.benson@doctors.org.uk

John Fixsen
West Barn
Clamok Farm Barns
Wier Quay
PL20 7BU Bere Alston
United Kingdom
jafixsen@btinternet.com

Malcolm Macnicol
Red House
Gillsland Road 1
EH10 5DE Edinburgh
United Kingdom
mmacnicol@aol.com

Klaus Parsch
Weinbergweg 68
70569 Stuttgart Baden-
Württemberg
Germany
kparsch@t-online.de

ISBN 978-0-85729-560-6   e-ISBN 978-0-85729-561-3
DOI 10.1007/978-0-85729-561-3
Springer London Dordrecht Heidelberg New York

British Library Cataloguing in Publication Data
A catalogue record for this book is available from the British Library

Library of Congress Control Number: 2011929879

Cover design: eStudio Calamar S.L.

Printed on acid-free paper

Springer is part of Springer Science+Business Media (www.springer.com)

Foreword

Confirming the British genetic trait for writing and publishing (as well as acting), two English (Oxford and London) and a Scottish orthopaedic surgeon (Edinburgh) have produced a third edition of their comprehensive text, joined, as in the second edition by an editor from Germany, recognizing its part in the European community. The 62 physician contributors are drawn from pink-colored countries in our childhood geography books—the old British Empire from Australia to Zambia and two from the former colony, the USA.

The original purpose of the book was to give residents or registrars an easily accessible and concise description of diseases and conditions encountered in the practice of paediatric orthopaedic surgery and to prepare for their examinations. But the practicing orthopaedic surgeon will find an update of current practice that can be read for clarity and constraint—enough but not too much. A foreword might be a preview of things to come, but a "back word" of what was thought to be the final say on the subject is needed for a perspective in progress.

A "back word" look reveals the tremendous progress in medical diagnosis and treatment of which paediatric orthopaedics and fracture care is a component. Clubfoot treatment based on the dictums of Hiram Kite has had a revolutionary change by Ponseti. The chapter by Eastwood has the details on cast application and orthotics follow-up to obtain the 95% correction without the extensive surgery many of us thought was needed.

Paediatric fracture care has also changed from traction for fractures of the femoral shaft in the ages of 5–15 years to intramedullary fixation with elastic stable nails originated in Nancy and Metz, France—"Nancy nails." Klaus Parsch's chapter tells us that it is their preferred method of treatment in Stuttgart, Germany.

Robert Dickson's lucid writing on idiopathic scoliosis as primarily a rotation of the lordotic thoracic spine again bears study to deepen the understanding that it is a three-dimensional deformity. As in the past editions, a coat hanger helps to appreciate the distortion of curvatures in a one-dimensional radiograph. Those orthopaedists who need courage to resist pressure to encase children in casts or braces or orthoses will be heartened to know that none of these conservative measures have shown any effect in prevention or curve progression. What to do instead of "treatment"? Read on.

This is not a book to learn the details of surgical technique–other texts and only experience can do that. Even though a seasoned orthopaedic surgeon does not need this knowledge to pass an examination, he or she is expected to know something about the subject. Once identified as an orthopaedic surgeon, your opinion is often sought at social events usually standing with a drink in hand. And commonly it is advice sought by your married children about a grandchild's musculoskeletal problem. Can you answer sensibly? If, "I'll get back to you later" is your response, a quick perusal of the contents of this volume should help maintain your professional standing and as is now the fashion of school teachers, your "self-esteem." And you won't have to log on to the Internet.

Eugene E Bleck

Preface

Having considered the more generalised neuromuscular and skeletal problems of childhood we concentrate in this section on regional disorders. The upper limb chapters describe foetal development and how this may go wrong. As always, function dominates our management plans although cosmetic considerations must be borne in mind. Perinatal brachial plexus injury is analysed and a plea made for early recognition and reconstruction of both plexus lesions and peripheral nerve injuries. The lower limb chapters consider limb deficiency and deformity and how best we should manage them. Those prominent afflictions of the child's hip - dysplasia, Perthes' disease and epiphyseal slipping - are fully discussed. Chapters on the common conditions affecting the knee, foot and ankle complete this section.

Michael KD Benson, Oxford, UK   John A Fixsen, London, UK

Malcolm F Macnicol, Edinburgh, UK   Klaus Parsch, Stuttgart, Germany

June, 2011

Contents

Contributors

Michael K. d'A. Benson Nuffield Orthopaedic Centre, Oxford, UK

Rolfe Birch Peripheral Nerve Injury Unit, Royal National Orthopaedic Hospital, Stanmore, UK

Peter D. Burge Hand Surgery Unit, Nuffield Orthopaedic Centre, Oxford, UK

Anthony Catterall Catterall Unit, Royal National Orthopaedic Hospital, Stanmore, UK

Deborah M. Eastwood Department of Paediatric Orthopaedics, Great Ormond Street Hospital, London, UK

John A. Fixsen Orthopaedic Department, Great Ormond Street Hospital for Sick Children, London, UK

Alain L. Gilbert Clinique Jouvenet, Paris, France

Franz Grill Department of Pediatric Orthopaedics, Orthopaedic Hospital Vienna, Vienna, Austria

Robert A. Hill Orthopaedic Department, Great Ormond Street Hospital NHS Trust, London, UK

David M. Hunt Department of Orthopaedics, St. Mary's Hospital, London, UK

Malcolm F. Macnicol University of Edinburgh; Royal Hospital for Sick Children; Edinburgh and Murrayfield Hospital; Royal Infirmary; Edinburgh, UK

Andrew Wainwright Nuffield Orthopaedic Centre, Oxford, UK

Chapter 1

Developmental Anomalies of the Hand

Peter D. Burge

Incidence

A large study of limb reduction defects in British Columbia reported an incidence of 5.97 per 10,000 live births, with 75% affecting the upper limb [1]. Half the cases had associated abnormalities, mostly in the musculoskeletal system, but defects of other organ systems were also common.

Limb Development

The upper limb bud appears toward the end of the fourth week of intrauterine life and is fully differentiated by the end of the seventh week. Digits become separated at just over 50 days. The developing limb bud comprises a core of mesenchymal tissue covered with ectoderm and its three orthogonal axes are proximo-distal, anteroposterior (i.e., radio-ulnar), and dorso-ventral. The distal outgrowth of the limb bud requires the activity of members of the fibroblast growth factor (Fgf) family that are synthesized in the apical ectodermal ridge (AER), a signaling center at the tip of the limb bud. Removal of the AER results in truncation of the limb. Fgf signaling also maintains the expression of sonic hedgehog (Shh) which is produced by a second signaling center, the polarizing zone, in the posterior margin of the limb bud. Shh provides positional information across the anterior–posterior limb axis and also acts to maintain the expression of several Fgfs in the overlying AER [2]. Transplantation of the polarizing zone to the anterior aspect of another limb bud produces a symmetrical duplication that imitates the rare human malformation of mirror hand. The Wnt signaling pathway may control dorso-ventral development. Much work remains to characterize fully the molecular basis of limb development, which may eventually explain the wide phenotypic expression of congenital anomalies of the upper limb. For the present, the cause of most malformations is unknown.

Identification of genes associated with inherited upper limb anomalies is increasing rapidly (e.g., Holt–Oram syndrome, triphalangeal thumb) [3]. However, many anomalies that are sporadic and unilateral presumably result from vascular or other insults to the limb at a crucial stage of development. The developing limb bud is sensitive to teratogenic agents, but the variety of defects that can be produced by a single agent probably reflects the critical effects of timing and concentration upon the interactions between components of the limb bud during development. Conversely, defects that are superficially similar, such as transverse deficiencies, may have differing causes.

Classification

The classification adopted by the International Federation for Societies for Surgery of the Hand (IFSSH) is widely used [4], although some malformations do not sit easily in a system that attempts to give embryological explanations for abnormalities that at present have only morphological descriptions. The classification divides malformations into seven categories. The list below shows how the anomalies described in this chapter fit into the classification.

I. **Failure of formation of parts**

   Transverse arrest
   　Proximal forearm
   　Digital absence
   　Symbrachydactyly
   Longitudinal arrest
   　Radial dysplasia
   　Ulnar dysplasia
   　Cleft hand
   　Intercalated defects (phocomelia)

P.D. Burge (✉)
Hand Surgery Unit, Nuffield Orthopaedic Centre, Oxford, UK

II. **Failure of differentiation (separation) of parts**

Soft-tissue involvement
Syndactyly
Clasped thumb
Absent finger extensors
Windblown hand
Camptodactyly
Trigger digits
Skeletal involvement
Radio-ulnar synostosis
Radial head dislocation
Clinodactyly
Kirner deformity
Triphalangeal thumb
Congenital tumorous conditions
Neurofibromatosis
Hereditary multiple exostoses

III. **Duplication**

Thumb
Post-axial polydactyly

IV. **Overgrowth**

Macrodactyly

V. **Undergrowth**
VI. **Congenital constriction band syndrome**
VII. **Generalized abnormalities and syndromes**

Madelung's deformity

General Principles of Management

Aims of Treatment

Treatment of congenital hand anomalies is directed at achieving the best possible function. Cosmesis may be an indication for operation but it should not be achieved at the expense of function.

The main requirements for function of the hand are *control of its position* in space, *sensate skin*, and motor activity sufficient for *power grasp* and *precision handling*. The function of congenitally deficient hands is remarkable when compared with hands that have suffered anatomically similar defects as a result of trauma because the developing brain "grows up" with the anomalous hand and learns the most effective pattern of control. But the functional needs of the small child are not those of the adult. Decisions about treatment need to consider the future needs of the patient and should aim to maximize the function and options for employment in the longer term. In unilateral defects, the presence of a normal limb ensures that most daily activities can be completed without assistance, regardless of the deficiency of the anomalous limb. However, the presence of a simple pinch or grasp in the abnormal limb confers the great benefit of *bimanual* activity and should be provided if possible. Bilateral defects impair function much more severely and consequently justify more extensive procedures.

A sympathetic approach to parents and a realistic prognosis are important aspects of general management. An early consultation with the team that will be responsible for management can do much to allay anxiety and reduce feelings of guilt [5]. Genetic counseling may be required and parents should be informed about support groups that exist for patients and their families. Referral to a paediatrician for exclusion of anomalies in other organ systems may be appropriate. Parents should be helped to understand the limitations of surgical reconstruction; it is seldom possible to replace what is missing, only to rearrange what remains. Videotapes of post-operative cases or, even better, meeting a patient with a similar problem may help them to understand what surgery will achieve.

Timing

Reconstruction of congenital hand anomalies should be completed before school age, if possible, bearing in mind that more than one operation is required in some cases. There is an increasing trend to operate between the ages of 1 and 2 years. Edema distal to a constriction band may require operation during the neonatal period. Early surgery (between 6 and 12 months of age) is needed in conditions that are liable to cause progressive deformity such as radial dysplasia or syndactyly between digits of different length.

Failure of Formation

Transverse Absence

Proximal Forearm

The commonest site of terminal transverse absence is the upper third of the forearm. It is usually sporadic, not associated with other anomalies, and more common on the left side. The high prevalence of digital nubbins suggests that many transverse absences are types of symbrachydactyly [6]. A light plastic prosthesis fitted in the first few months of life improves cosmesis and accustoms the child to wearing a prosthesis. At about 18 months of age a gripping device such as a split hook operated by a motivating cord and loop from the opposite shoulder can be fitted. Training in its use by a therapist, regular review, and support of the parents are essential at this stage. At the age of 3.5 years a myoelectric prosthesis operated by electrical impulses generated in the forearm muscles may be fitted. Small children can learn to make excellent functional use of a myoelectric prosthesis.

Transverse absence at the level of the carpus is consistent with useful manipulative function using the mobile proximal carpal row which is usually present. A prosthesis interferes with sensibility and impairs function but may be worn for cosmesis on social occasions.

Digital Absence

Transverse absence of digits is seen in three situations:

1. Transverse absence
2. Symbrachydactyly
3. Congenital constriction band syndrome

The term symbrachydactyly has been used to denote a type of terminal absence characterized by digital nubbins containing rudimentary nails that may retain connections to tendons, causing the nubbins to retract with active movement (Fig. 1.1). The appearance suggests an intercalary defect in which the skeleton has failed to develop, leading to secondary failure of development of the soft tissues. Whether this anomaly is truly different to simple transverse absence is unknown. Symbrachydactyly shows a teratogenic sequence that ranges from simple shortness of the middle phalanges to absence of all phalanges with short metacarpals. The index,

middle, and ring fingers are most severely affected and the thumb least affected. Absence of the central digits gives the appearance formerly termed atypical cleft hand.

Four types of symbrachydactyly are recognized:

1. Short finger type
2. Cleft hand type
3. Monodactylous type; a hypoplastic thumb is the only digit
4. Absence of all five digital rays

Most cases are unilateral and sporadic. Tendons and arteries that are useful for reconstruction are usually present in the more distal lesions.

Absence of one or two fingers is consistent with good function. In more extensive anomalies, the aim should be the provision of a basic type of grasp. This requires a minimum of two digits, at least one of which must be mobile. Therefore, if a single digit is present, every attempt should be made to provide another digit or "post" for opposition. Lengthening of a short metacarpal or deepening of the first web may give side-to-side pinch. Short digits may be lengthened by transfer of toe phalanges, which are more likely to grow if they are transferred extraperiosteally as nonvascularized grafts before the age of 15 months. This transfer is indicated if a modest increase in length will improve function and the recipient ray has functioning tendons. Microvascular transfer of a second toe is feasible if suitable nerves and tendons can be found in the hand. Loss of the second toe is functionally and cosmetically acceptable. Transfer of one or both second toes can greatly improve function of the severely deficient hand [7].

Longitudinal Absence

Radial Dysplasia

Radial dysplasia is the commonest form of longitudinal deficiency. This ugly deformity results from complete or partial absence of the radius, but the deficiency affects other tissues in the limb. Although many cases are sporadic, there are important associations with anomalies in different organ systems, especially the hemopoietic and cardiovascular systems (Fig. 1.2), that influence decisions about surgical management (Table 1.1). The thumbs are present in the thrombocytopenia-absent radius (TAR) syndrome but often absent in other forms of severe radial dysplasia. Thrombocytopenia is usually transient in this autosomal recessive disorder. Fanconi anemia is an autosomal recessive, progressive pancytopenia of childhood in which the cells exhibit extreme chromosomal instability.

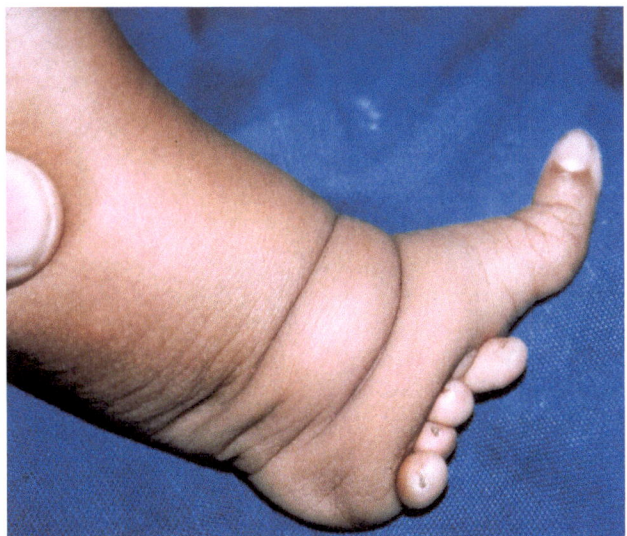

FIG. 1.1   Symbrachydactyly

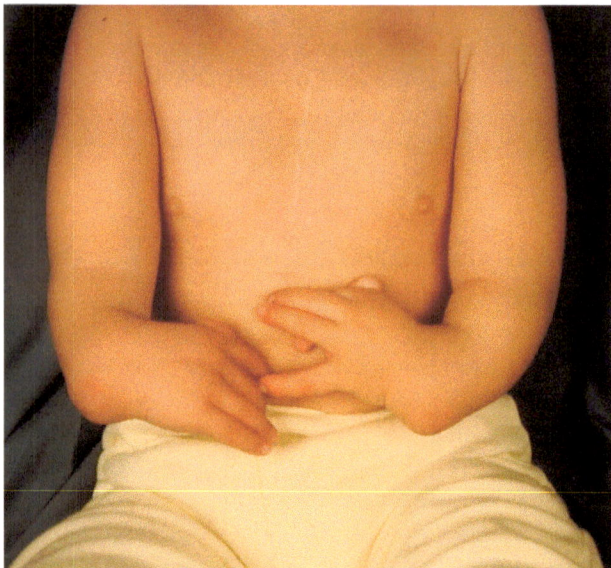

Fig. 1.2 Bilateral radial absence with floating thumbs. Note the median sternotomy scar

Table 1.1 Anomalies commonly associated with radial dysplasia

Thrombocytopenia—absent radius (TAR) syndrome
Fanconi anemia
Holt–Oram syndrome
VACTERL association

Holt–Oram syndrome is an autosomal dominant disorder that includes radial dysplasia (often comprising triphalangeal thumb) and cardiac anomalies such as septal defects and Fallot's tetralogy. VACTERL is a mnemonically useful acronym for vertebral anomalies, anal atresia, cardiac malformations, tracheoesophageal fistula, renal anomalies, and limb anomalies (humeral hypoplasia and radial aplasia). There are many rare syndromes that may be associated with radial dysplasia [8].

Skeletal deficiency ranges from mild shortening to absence of the radius (Table 1.2). In complete absence, the ulna is bowed and typically grows to 60% of the length of the normal forearm (Fig. 1.3). The carpus articulates with the radial aspect of the distal ulna. The scaphoid and trapezium may be absent. Muscle anomalies tend to be proportional to the skeletal deficiency and chiefly affect the radial side of the limb. The radial flexor and extensor muscles of the wrist are often fused and inserted into the carpus via a short tendon. Extensor tendons of the index and middle fingers may be absent or show abnormal insertions. The superficial radial nerve is absent, being represented by a radial branch of the median nerve. The median nerve itself is abnormally situated and at risk of operative injury, lying just beneath the deep fascia on the radial side of the forearm. The radial artery

Table 1.2 Classification of radial dysplasia

Type 1.	Short distal radius
Type 2.	Hypoplastic radius
Type 3.	Partial absence of radius
Type 4.	Absent radius

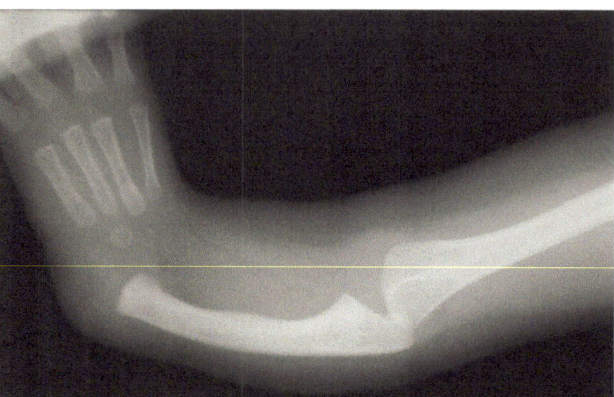

Fig. 1.3 Radiograph of radial absence. The ulna is bowed and the thumb is absent

is absent; the hand is supplied by the ulnar artery, which is usually normal, and by the anterior interosseous artery.

The thumb may be absent or hypoplastic. The index and middle fingers often show hypoplasia, contractures, and stiffness, reflecting the deficiency that extends widely across the radial side of the limb. The ring and little fingers usually have normal movement and may be preferred by the patient for manipulative activity. The elbow may lack passive flexion at birth but the range usually improves with growth. However, bilateral lack of elbow flexion is a contraindication to centralization, as the hands may then fail to reach the mouth.

The deformity of radial absence is unsightly. The power of the finger muscles is dissipated by instability at the wrist. Centralization of the carpus gives a marked esthetic improvement and also increases function [9].

The management of the newborn child comprises exclusion of other anomalies and prevention of fixed contracture until centralization can be performed at the age of 6–12 months. In most cases of radial absence, the deformity is correctable at birth. Regular passive stretching should be instituted as soon as possible. After each feed, gentle traction and ulnar deviation are applied. Splintage is difficult to maintain in the neonate but may have place in the older infant. If the deformity is not correctable, distraction lengthening may be needed prior to centralization.

The surgical treatment of radial absence has a long history but modern efforts have centered on placement of the carpus on the ulna. Two operations are in common use.

Centralization places the distal ulna in a slot cut into the carpus [9]. (Fig. 1.4a). In radialization, the carpus is mobilized extensively and the ulna is placed beneath the radial aspect of the carpus so as to maximize the moment arm of muscles on the ulnar side (Fig. 1.4b) [10]. Re-balancing of the deforming forces by shortening of the extensor carpi ulnaris tendon and transferring of the deforming radial wrist muscles to the ulnar side of the wrist are essential components of each procedure. In every case, the position is maintained by a longitudinal pin (Fig. 1.5). Osteotomy of a bowed ulna may be performed at the same time. Great care must be taken to avoid damage to the distal ulnar epiphysis and its blood supply. Radialization requires that the deformity is correctable and is best performed between 6 and 12 months of age. It retains some useful wrist motion from the neutral position into flexion (Fig. 1.6). The skeletal shortening of centralization allows correction of fixed deformities and is more applicable to older children or those with fixed deformity. Although centralization aims to maintain some motion

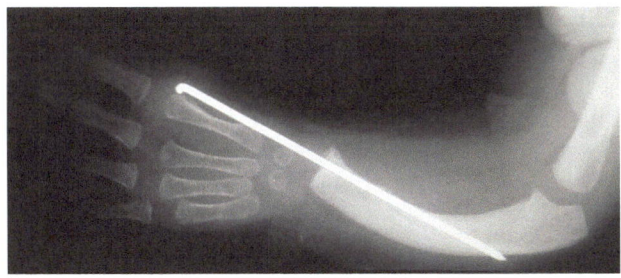

Fig. 1.5 Radiograph after radialization of the carpus

Fig. 1.6 Appearance of the forearm 3 years after radialization

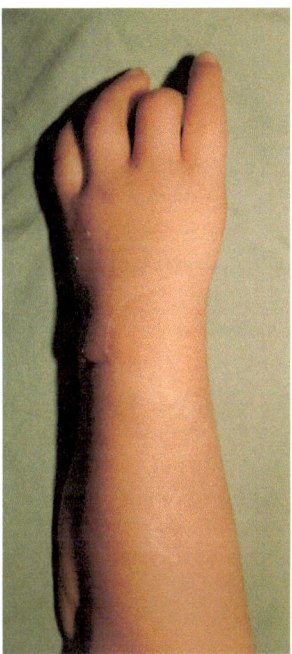

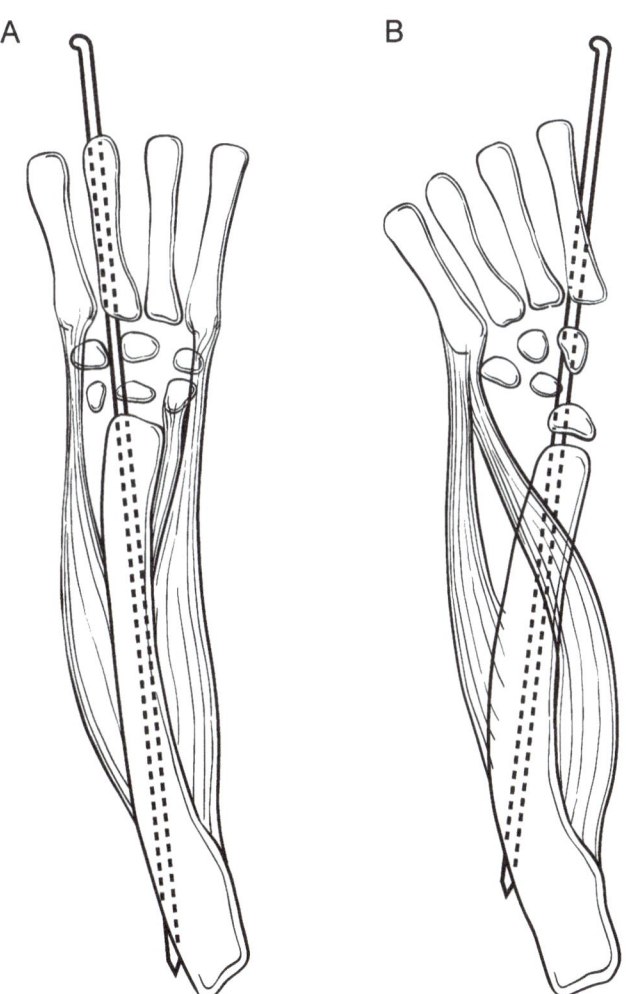

Fig. 1.4 (**a**) "Centralization" of the carpus. (**b**) "Radialization" of the carpus, preserving carpal bone

between carpus and ulna, long-term maintenance of correction is often associated with spontaneous ulno-carpal fusion. The wrist is stiff but there may be a little motion at the carpometacarpal joints. Skeletal distraction with an external fixation device is being used increasingly to correct fixed deformities prior to radialization or centralization [11].

The pin is removed some months later. If necessary, pollicization of the index finger is performed at a later stage. The wrist is splinted full time for several months and at night until skeletal maturity. There is a tendency to recurrent radial angulation in many cases [12], although seldom to the original position. Complications of centralization and radialization include premature closure of the distal ulnar epiphysis, pin breakage, and recurrent deformity.

Ulno-carpal fusion may be needed at or near skeletal maturity for persistent deformity or instability. Distraction lengthening of the ulna has been used but it is questionable whether the gain in length justifies the high-complication rate [13].

Ulnar Dysplasia

Ulnar dysplasia is several times less common than radial dysplasia. Most cases are sporadic but may be associated with lower limb anomalies such as fibular ray deficiency [14]. Absence of the ulna may be associated with radiohumeral synostosis (Table 1.3). Unlike radial dysplasia, associated anomalies in other organ systems are uncommon.

Table 1.3 Classification of ulnar dysplasia

Type 1.	Hypoplastic ulna
Type 2.	Partial absence of ulna
Type 3.	Absent ulna
Type 4.	Absent ulna and radiohumeral synostosis

Hypoplasia of the ulna is associated with bowing of the radius and dislocation of the radial head, but the carpus is supported by the radius and does not show the acute angulation that characterizes radial dysplasia (Fig. 1.7).

Deficiencies in the hand tend to be more extensive in ulnar dysplasia than in radial dysplasia [15]. Multiple digital absence, syndactyly, and camptodactyly are common, but there is no correlation between the extent of hand deformity and the degree of ulnar deficiency.

The main determinants of functional impairment are the extent of hand deformity and stiffness of the elbow rather than bowing of the forearm. Management of the hand deformities may include release of syndactyly and correction of first web space contractures. Progressive bowing of the forearm has been treated by excision of the fibrous anlage of the ulna but its value is unclear. Severe instability of the forearm can be corrected, at the expense of rotation, by creation of a one-bone forearm, fusing the ulna proximally to the radius distally. Some patients with radiohumeral synostosis have a severe internal rotation or adduction posture that may be improved by osteotomy of the humerus.

Cleft Hand

Cleft hand is characterized by a central V-shaped cleft with absence of one or more digits. Unlike radial and ulnar dysplasia, it is not accompanied by deficiency in the forearm. In the past, cleft hand has been grouped with other causes of central deficiency such as symbrachydactyly. True cleft hand is often familial, bilateral, and associated with cleft feet. Inheritance is autosomal dominant with variable penetrance. Cleft hand may be part of syndromes such as EEC (ectrodactyly, ectodermal dysplasia, and cleft lip/palate) and the split hand/split foot malformation (SHSM) [16].

The depth of the cleft varies from absence of the phalanges only to a deep cleft extending into the carpus. Syndactyly between the border digits (thumb/index and ring/little) and contracture of the thumb web are common (Fig. 1.8). Skeletal remnants of the missing rays may be aligned transversely or fused with adjacent bones. The term "lobster claw hand" is disliked by patients and their families; *cleft hand*, which is neutral and more accurate, is preferred

Flatt has stated that typical cleft hand is "a functional triumph and a social disaster" [17]. Functional impairment results more from syndactyly and thumb web contracture than from the cleft itself. Border syndactyly should be released by the age of 6 months, before unequal growth can produce angular deformity of the longer digit. Early

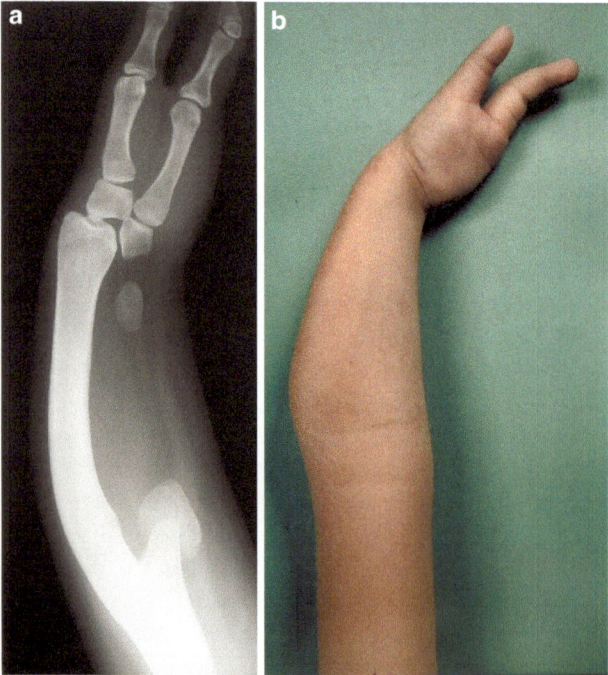

Fig. 1.7 Ulnar dysplasia. (**a**) Absent ulna and radiohumeral synostosis (type IV). (**b**) The forearm is bowed to the ulnar side in a type III case

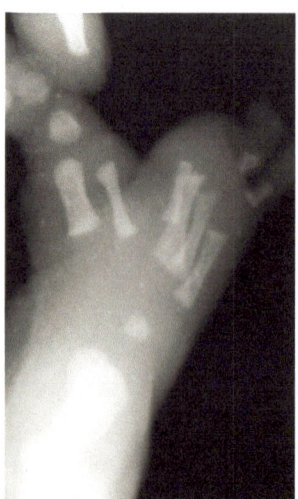

Fig. 1.8 Cleft hand with complex syndactyly

removal of transverse bones that are causing deformity may also be needed. In a typical case of first web contracture and absence of the middle ray, simultaneous closure of the cleft and widening of the thumb web are performed at around 18 months.

Failure of Differentiation

Syndactyly

Syndactyly is a common congenital anomaly of the hand. It is an example of incomplete differentiation of digital rays, which normally occurs by programmed cell death (apoptosis) of interdigital tissue. The process begins distally and proceeds proximally; its failure leads to partial or complete syndactyly.

Simple syndactyly involves skin and soft tissue; in *complex* syndactyly, the digits are also connected by bone. *Complete* syndactyly extends to the fingertips, *partial* syndactyly does not. In *acrosyndactyly,* which occurs in congenital constriction band syndrome and in association with craniofacial deformities such as Apert's syndrome, short digits are fused at the tips and are often separated proximally by fenestrations.

Syndactyly may occur in association with other hand anomalies, such as ulnar dysplasia, cleft hand, or as a feature of a syndrome (Poland's syndrome, craniofacial syndromes, constriction band syndrome). Simple syndactyly is inherited in at least 10% of cases, usually as an autosomal dominant trait. In half the cases it is bilateral. The distribution of syndactyly between the digital rays is shown in (Fig. 1.9).

Syndactyly *always* represents a shortage of skin [18]. Although it might appear that there is *additional* skin joining the digits, simple geometry shows that 22% *less* skin covers the syndactylized digits than surfaces two separate fingers. Skin is also deficient transversely in the interdigital web, as may be seen by measurement of the distance along the web from the tip of one finger to the tip of its neighbor.

Syndactyly between digits of unequal length (thumb–index, ring–little) should be released by the age of 6 months, before unequal growth deforms the longer digit. Otherwise, the timing of release is not critical but is generally before the age of 3 years. Successful release of syndactyly requires the use of acute zigzag incisions, local flap skin for reconstruction of the web, and full-thickness skin grafts. Skin grafts are taken from the groin crease, lateral to the femoral pulse (to avoid growth of hair at puberty). If a finger is joined to the digits on each side, only one surface should be released at one operation.

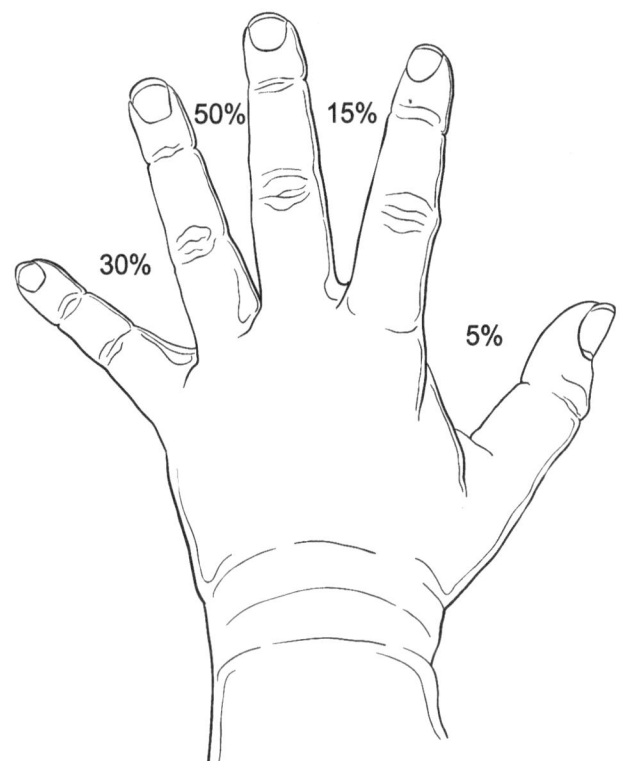

Fig. 1.9 The frequency of syndactyly of digital clefts

Congenital Clasped Thumb

A congenital clasped thumb lies flexed across the palm and cannot be extended actively. Two types of clasped thumb can be recognized [19].

Supple clasped thumb is due to isolated deficiency of the thumb extensor tendons. It is often bilateral and is more common in males. Passive extension is usually normal at birth but may be lost if the disorder is untreated. Clasped thumb may present as loss of extension at the interphalangeal (IP) joint, at the metacarpophalangeal (MP) joint, or at both joints. Differentiation from trigger thumb is straightforward if there is no loss of passive extension. In cases of clasped thumb with flexion contracture, the contracture usually affects the MP joint and other soft tissues, whereas the contracture of trigger finger is confined to the distal joint.

Supple clasped thumb frequently responds to continuous and prolonged splintage in extension if treatment is started soon after birth. A plaster cast extending to the thumb tip is changed every few weeks to accommodate growth and retained for 3–6 months. If active extension is not regained, tendon transfer is required.

Complex clasped thumb refers to disorders in which the thumb is part of a more extensive anomaly such as arthrogryposis, thumb hypoplasia, or Freeman–Sheldon (windblown hand) syndrome. The skin, thumb web, adductor pollicis, and flexor pollicis longus may require lengthening, in addition to chondrodesis of the MP joint and augmentation of extension by tendon transfer.

The Windblown Hand

Congenital flexion deformity of the fingers takes several forms and probably has several causes. Less severe types resemble the supple clasped thumb, affecting one or more fingers with deficient active extension but normal passive extension. They are probably due to congenital deficiency of the extensor mechanism and may respond to prolonged splintage in extension. Reconstruction by tendon transfer is required in some cases.

The combination of flexion contracture of the fingers, ulnar deviation at the MP joints, and a flexion/adduction contracture of the thumb is known as windblown hand. It is a feature of distal arthrogryposis and the Freeman–Sheldon (whistling face) syndrome.

Splintage can improve contractures or hold them stable until the child is fit for surgery. Correction of the thumb web contracture is valuable; surgery can improve the fingers but does not provide full movement. Each component of the deformity requires correction. Releases of skin and fascia at the base of the digits are closed with full-thickness skin grafts. Centralization of the extensor mechanism at the MP joint requires release of tight ulnar sagittal bands and plication or reconstruction of elongated radial sagittal bands, as well as crossed intrinsic transfer in some cases [20]. Release of the thumb web contracture generally creates a defect that requires a transposition flap from the dorsoradial aspect of the index. An unstable thumb MP joint may be stabilized by ligament reconstruction or by chondrodesis. Tendon transfers may augment thumb extension.

Thumb Hypoplasia

Hypoplasia of the thumb is frequently associated with radial dysplasia and may, therefore, be accompanied by visceral malformations. The classification of Blauth is widely used (Table 1.4) [21].

Type I hypoplasia is consistent with normal function and requires no treatment. In type II (Fig. 1.10), function is impaired by instability of the MP joint, contracture of the thumb web, weakness of opposition, and limited motion of the IP joint. Release of the web usually requires lengthening of the web skin by Z-plasty or by a transposition flap from the dorsum of the thumb or index finger. If the ring superficialis tendon is employed as an opposition transfer, it may be

Table 1.4 Classification of thumb hypoplasia

I	Minor hypoplasia, normal function
II	Thumb web contracture; thenar muscle hypoplasia MP joint instability; anomalous flexor tendon
III	A severe skeletal and muscle hypoplasia
B	+ deficient basal joint
IV	Floating thumb
V	Absent thumb

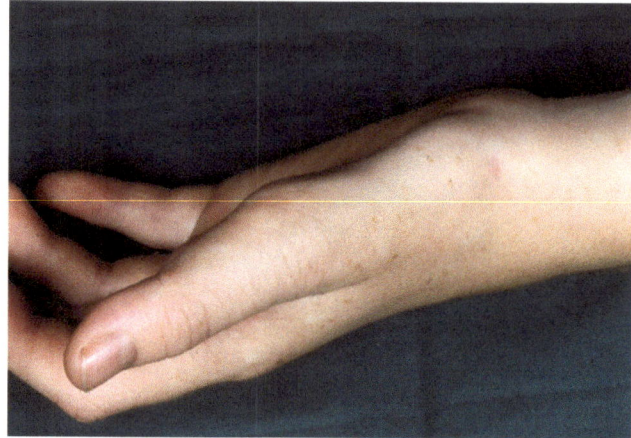

Fig. 1.10 Type II hypoplasia of thumb showing hypoplasia of the thenar muscles

passed through the metacarpal neck and used to reconstruct the ulnar collateral ligament of the MP joint. Anomalous connections between the long flexor and the extensor tendons may limit IP joint flexion or lead to abduction deformity (pollex abductus).

It may be difficult to decide whether a type III hypoplastic thumb is worthy of reconstruction (Fig. 1.11) and even more difficult to convince parents that it is not. Much depends upon the tissues that are available. However, if the basal joint is unstable, pollicization of the index finger is likely to provide better function.

Attempts at reconstruction of the floating thumb (type IV) are fruitless; the digit contains no useful skeleton or tendons and it is attached too far distally and dorsally to be functional (Fig. 1.12). Pollicization of the index finger provides much better function [22]. Pollicization is also the appropriate treatment for the absent thumb (type V) (Fig. 1.13). Current techniques of pollicization are based on the work of many surgeons over the last 50 years, notably Buck-Gramcko [22]. In essence, the index finger is mobilized on the intact digital neurovascular bundles and dorsal veins, excising the shaft of the metacarpal and placing the metacarpal head anterior to the base of the metacarpal. The metacarpal head is sutured into place with the MP joint extended, otherwise the new thumb may exhibit excessive hyperextension at its basal joint. The digit is rotated 160° into opposition. The first dorsal and first palmar interosseous muscles are sutured

Fig. 1.11 Type III hypoplasia of thumb with deficient basal joint

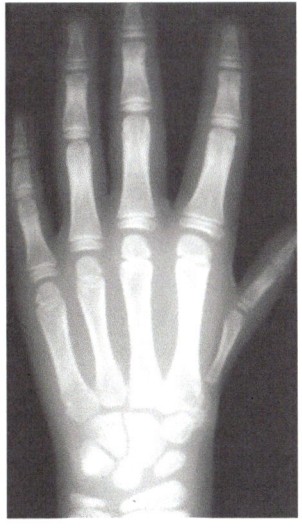

Fig. 1.12 Floating thumb (type IV hypoplasia) is not capable of useful reconstruction. It should be excised and replaced by pollicization of the index finger

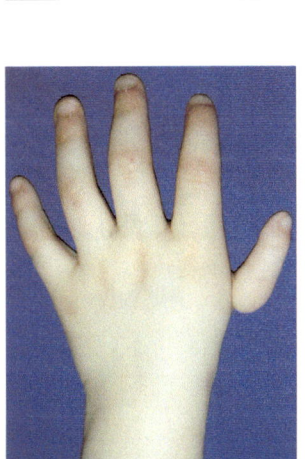

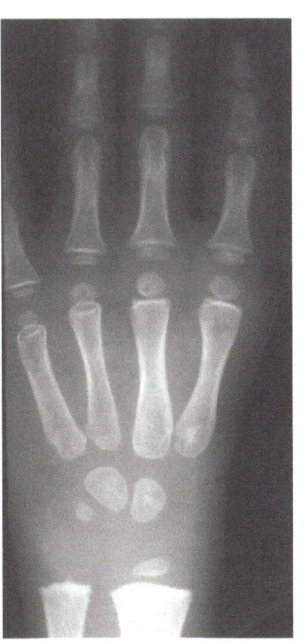

Fig. 1.13 Absent thumb

into the lateral bands at the level of the proximal interphalangeal (PIP) joint, becoming the short thumb abductor and the adductor pollicis, respectively. It is necessary to shorten the extensor tendons, but the flexor tendons will in time accommodate to the shorter skeleton. For the index finger to look like a thumb, skin flaps must be designed so that the new thumb web reaches the digit at the level of the PIP joint (the new MP joint) (Fig. 1.14). When the absent thumb is accompanied by a normal radius, the index finger usually has good musculature and supple joints; it will make a satisfactory thumb. The decision to pollicize the index finger should take into account the pattern of prehensile function that the child shows. Children who lack thumbs employ a "cigarette" grip between adjacent fingers. When the thumb is missing as part of severe radial dysplasia, the index frequently lacks good motion. Nevertheless, it may still make a satisfactory thumb provided that the child uses the index–middle cleft for prehension. If the child excludes the index finger from hand function, the digit may be ignored after pollicization.

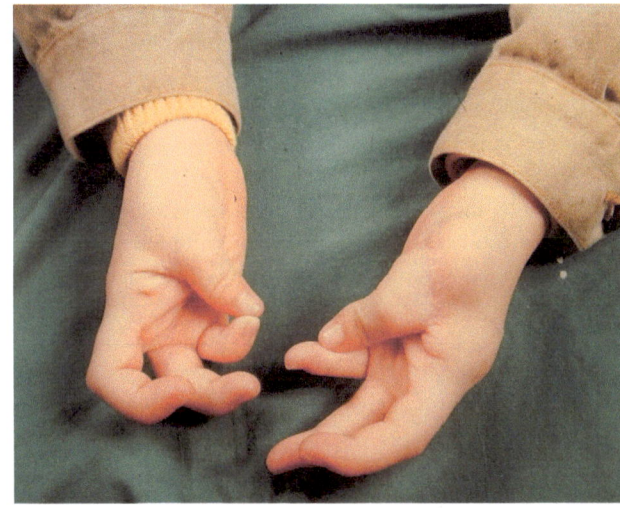

Fig. 1.14 Pollicization of the index fingers for bilateral absent thumb

Camptodactyly

Camptodactyly describes a common, painless, nontraumatic flexion deformity of the PIP joint, usually affecting the little finger. An autosomal dominant pattern of inheritance is frequently present. Camptodactyly occurs in two age groups that coincide with periods of rapid growth of the hand. In *infants,* it may affect any finger; it is equally common among males and females, and it may be associated with other anomalies. In *adolescents*, camptodactyly is more frequent in females and almost invariably affects the little finger. It

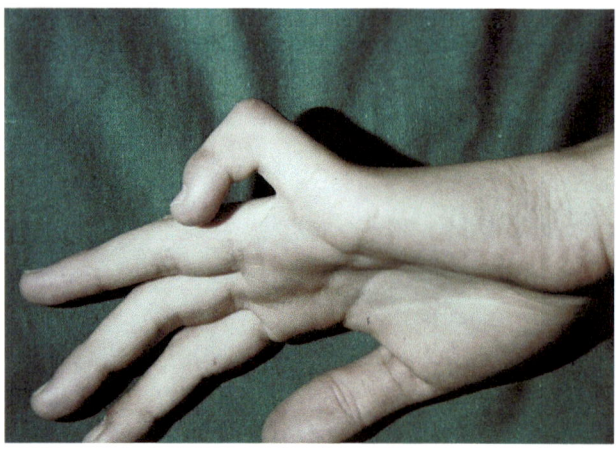

Fig. 1.15 Camptodactyly

appears as a fixed flexion contracture of the PIP joint which is usually at least 30° at the time of presentation (Fig. 1.15). The little finger may adopt the intrinsic-minus posture of hyperextension of the MP joint with increased flexion of the PIP joint when the fingers are extended actively. Involvement of more than one finger suggests one of the many syndromes associated with camptodactyly.

Camptodactyly may be distinguished from post-traumatic boutonnière deformity by the absence of swelling and by the presence of full distal joint movement. Ulnar nerve palsy is excluded by the absence of neurological signs.

In an established case of adolescent camptodactyly, examination will demonstrate tightness of the volar PIP joint capsule, the superficialis tendon, and the skin. It is not surprising, therefore, that almost every structure which crosses the palmar aspect of the PIP joint has been implicated in the etiology of camptodactyly. Imbalance between the extrinsic and intrinsic muscles of the little finger during the periods of growth is the most plausible mechanism. This explanation is consistent with recognized mechanisms of musculoskeletal deformity and is supported by the frequent finding of an abnormal insertion of the lumbrical muscle into the capsule of the MP joint, the superficialis tendon, or the extensor expansion of an adjacent finger [23]. Shortening of the superficialis muscle is a common and probably secondary feature that may be demonstrated by the effect of wrist and MP joint position on deformity of the PIP joint.

Treatment

Infancy

As much correction as possible should be obtained by splintage. Static splints such as serial plaster casts are easier to manage at this age than dynamic splints. Persistent

contractures may be managed by the release of tight volar soft tissues and tendon transfer to augment extension. However, it may be difficult to restore normal movement. Long-term extension splintage is often required.

Adolescence

It is difficult to restore full extension in adolescent camptodactyly. Static and/or dynamic splintage may produce useful improvement but splintage must be continued until skeletal maturity [24]. Since a moderate flexion deformity is consistent with good function and less disabling than loss of flexion, most patients should be advised to use a splint and accept the deformity unless it is severe or the patient has a specific requirement for good extension. The results of operative treatment of fixed contracture are unpredictable and the chief risk is loss of flexion [25]. Soft tissue release is contraindicated if there is bony deformity of the PIP joint (Fig. 1.16); dorsal angulation osteotomy through the neck of the proximal phalanx will improve extension at the expense of flexion. The rare patient who exhibits inadequate active PIP joint extension but who has full passive extension may be improved by transfer of a superficialis tendon or extensor indicis proprius into the extensor mechanism over the PIP joint.

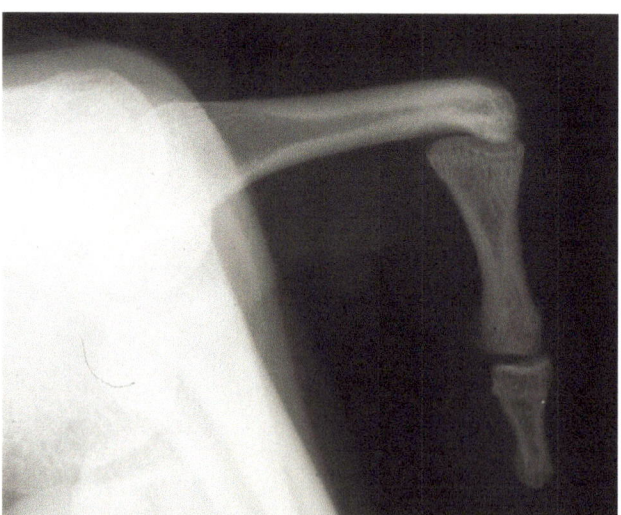

Fig. 1.16 Long-standing camptodactyly with secondary deformity of the head of the proximal phalanx, precluding soft tissue release

Clinodactyly

Clinodactyly is angulation of a digit to the radial or ulnar side. It is a manifestation of a variety of syndromes, but the common isolated form is bilateral radial angulation of the little finger with autosomal dominant inheritance. Clinodactyly is the result of abnormal growth, usually of the middle phalanx, which may have many causes.

Three types of clinodactyly are encountered:

1. Minor angulation, normal length
2. Minor angulation, short phalanx
3. Marked angulation, delta phalanx

Minor degrees of clinodactyly are common and consistent with normal function. Corrective osteotomy is indicated if the finger overlaps the adjacent digit on flexion, using a closing wedge osteotomy if the length of the phalanx is normal and an opening wedge if it is short.

Although delta phalanx is named after the triangular Greek letter, the bone is usually trapezoidal. It is a curious anomaly in which the proximal epiphysis extends beyond its normal transverse position to pass along the shorter side of the bone to its distal end (Fig. 1.17). The C-shaped epiphysis effectively constitutes a bony bridge that restricts longitudinal growth and causes progressive angulation. Delta phalanx is frequently found in association with triphalangeal thumb and with polydactyly.

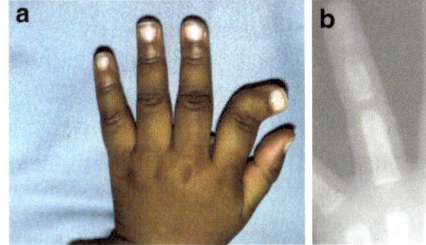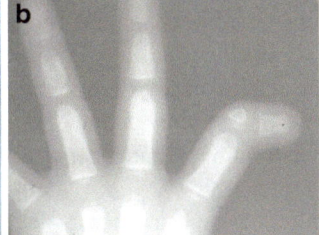

Fig. 1.17 Angular deformity of the index finger resulting from a delta phalanx

Division of the longitudinal bar and interposition of a free fat graft may permit more normal growth. For later cases, reverse wedge or opening wedge osteotomy is the best option. Great care must be taken to avoid damage to the joint surfaces and to divide the small bone cleanly. The osteotomy is transfixed with a Kirschner wire for 4–6 weeks.

Kirner Deformity

In 1927 Kirner described a curvature of the distal phalanx in a radial and palmar direction. It affects females more commonly than males and may be inherited as an autosomal dominant trait. The onset is between 8 and 12 years, beginning with painless swelling of the distal phalanx followed by progressive radio-palmar deviation of both little fingers. The age of onset, the presence of swelling, and the radiographic

appearance of lysis within the growth plate (Fig. 1.18) suggest that the disorder is acquired rather than congenital. Its nature is unknown. A similar deformity may follow epiphyseal damage by frostbite or by an infected open fracture. Severe deformity may be improved by osteotomy of the distal phalanx.

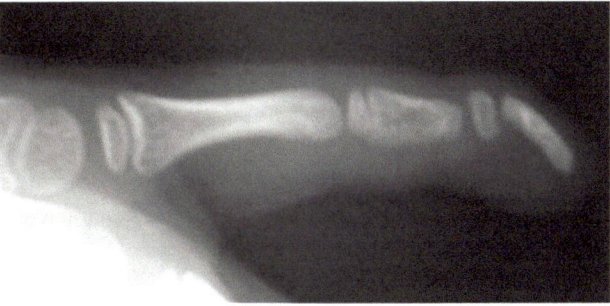

Fig. 1.18 Kirner deformity with palmar angulation in the distal phalanx

Trigger Digits

Trigger thumb is the most common hand disorder in children. It presents with painless loss of passive extension of the interphalangeal (IP) joint. The clicking which characterizes trigger thumb in adults is uncommon in children. A nodule may be palpable at the proximal (A1) flexor tendon pulley at the level of the metacarpophalangeal (MP) joint. It should be distinguished from congenital clasped thumb (see above), in which the deformity usually affects the MP joint.

Trigger thumb is seldom present at birth; no cases were found in a screening study of 1116 neonates [26]. The normal infant tends to hold the thumb flexed into the palm and it may be sometime before the problem is noticed. Approximately 30% of trigger thumbs presenting in infancy resolved spontaneously within 12 months [27]. Of those presenting between 6 and 36 months, 12% resolved within 6 months of presentation. A period of observation is appropriate in children presenting in the first year. Extension splintage appears to cure a proportion of trigger thumbs [28]. If the condition persists, division of the A1 pulley is curative. Permanent IP contracture does not seem to occur provided that the digit is released by the age of 4 years. The skin is incised transversely at the proximal MP joint crease, avoiding the digital nerves which lie immediately beneath the skin. The A1 pulley is incised longitudinally under direct vision, revealing a nodule (Notta's node) or thickening of the flexor tendon. The oblique pulley should be preserved so as to avoid bowstringing of the flexor tendon.

Trigger finger is much less common than trigger thumb in children. In contrast to adult cases, some cases in children may occur at the flexor digitorum superficialis (FDS)

decussation rather than at the A1 pulley [29]. These cases may need excision of one of the slips of the FDS tendon in addition to A1 pulley release.

Congenital Radio-ulnar Synostosis

Synostosis may be longitudinal (e.g., humeroradial synostosis in type-IV ulnar dysplasia) or transverse. Radio-ulnar synostosis is the most common form (Fig. 1.19), resulting from the failure of completion of the distal-to-proximal separation of the forearm mesenchyme. It may be unilateral or bilateral and is usually at the proximal end of the forearm. Some compensatory rotation occurs at carpal level.

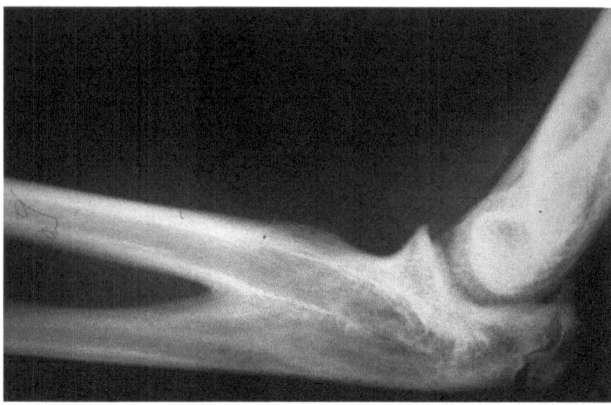

Fig. 1.19 Radiograph of congenital radio-ulnar synostosis at the typical proximal site

Disability depends upon the rotational alignment of the forearm. Internal rotation and abduction of the shoulder can bring a supinated hand into the palm-down position. Shoulder motion compensates less readily for fixed pronation. Unilateral synostosis causes little disability and seldom requires treatment. Bilateral synostoses are often fixed in marked pronation, causing difficulty with accepting coins and holding a glass.

Until recently, attempts to restore rotation had been unsuccessful and operative correction was confined to rotational osteotomy, generally through the fusion mass. The technique of Green and Mital [30] controls alignment with a longitudinal intramedullary pin and rotation with a transverse trans-ulnar pin incorporated in a cast. The method allows the correction to be undone easily in the event of neurovascular compromise post-operatively. Further experience is required to determine if rotation can be restored reliably by excision of the synostosis, interposition of a vascularized fat-fascia flap, and relocation of the dislocated radial head by radial shortening osteotomy [31].

Congenital Radial Head Dislocation

Dislocation of the radial head may be congenital, traumatic, or secondary to diminished growth of the ulna (e.g., ulnar dysplasia, multiple hereditary exostoses). Congenital dislocation is posterior in two-thirds of cases; the remainder is lateral or anterior. Differentiation between traumatic and congenital dislocation is sometimes difficult since deformity of the radial head and hypoplasia of the capitellum are features of both types. Dislocation is likely to be congenital if it is bilateral, familial, associated with other malformations, or present in infancy. A healed fracture of the ulna or heterotopic ossification suggests that dislocation was the result of injury.

Congenital dislocation of the radial head is a feature of numerous malformation syndromes, which should be sought during examination. The dislocation causes remarkably little loss of function during childhood, although radial head excision after skeletal maturity may be indicated for pain and prominence of the radial head if these symptoms are clearly attributable to the dislocation.

Dislocation of the radial head is liable to occur whenever growth of the ulna is diminished and radial growth continues. It may be possible to prevent dislocation if the length of the ulna can be maintained by distraction lengthening, with or without radial shortening or epiphyseal stapling. Parents may ask that the radial head be relocated. However, the indication for operative reduction of established congenital radial head dislocation has not been defined. The procedure may involve osteotomy of a bowed ulna and radial shortening in addition to reconstruction of the annular ligament. Considering the minimal symptoms experienced by most patients, such surgery is seldom justified.

Duplication

Duplication may be *radial* (preaxial), *ulnar* (post-axial), or, rarely, *central*. It is probably the commonest congenital anomaly in the hand. Ulnar polydactyly is common as an autosomal recessive condition in African-Americans, in whom it is seldom associated with other abnormalities. It is 8–10 times less common in Caucasians but is more likely to be part of a syndrome.

Radial polydactyly is usually sporadic. Wassel [32] described a logical classification based upon the level of duplication (Fig. 1.20). Almost half the cases are type IV (Fig. 1.21). In types I and II, where the duplication is symmetrical, a central wedge may be excised and the defect closed by apposition of the outer halves of the distal phalanges (Bilhaut–Cloquet procedure). Nail bed deformity

Fig. 1.20 Wassel classification of thumb duplication. Type IV accounts for almost 50% of cases

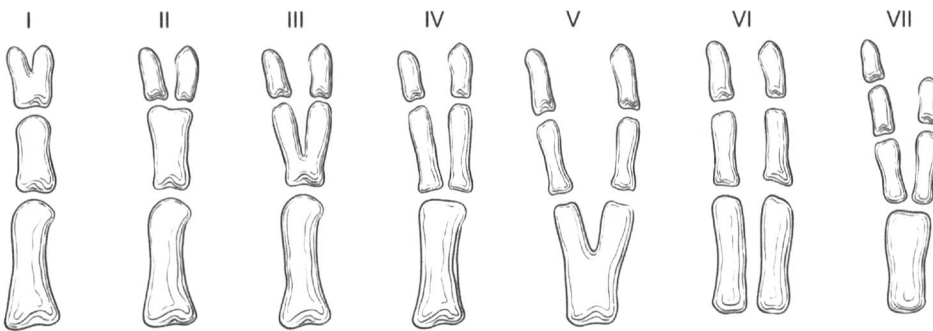

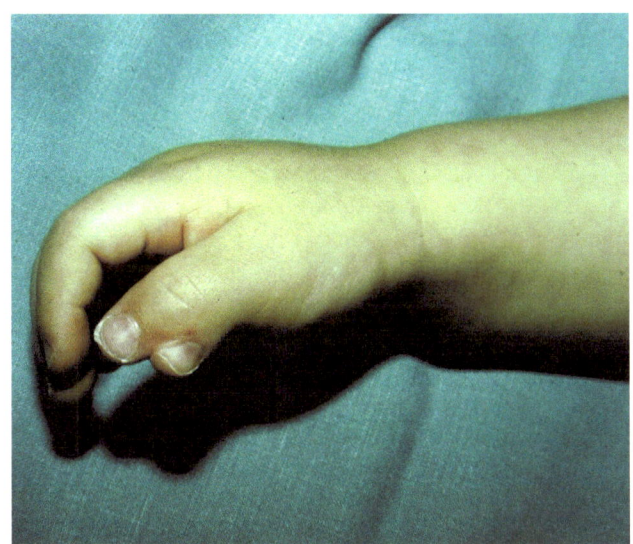

Fig. 1.21 Wassel type IV duplication of the thumb

and premature epiphyseal closure may mar the final result. Instead of splitting the nail, the entire nail bed may be taken from one thumb and the nail bed of the other discarded.

In considering operative treatment of types III–VII, it is vital to regard the procedure as a reconstruction of a split thumb and not excision of an extra thumb. A decision on which thumb should be discarded is based upon size, deviation, passive joint mobility, stability, and anomalous tendon insertions of the parts. The principles of reconstruction include zigzag incisions (to avoid later scar contracture), preservation or reconstruction of ligaments, alignment of the skeleton, and alignment of tendon insertions. It may be necessary to augment the remaining thumb with tissues from the excised segment.

Triphalangeal Thumb

Triphalangeal thumb may be part of type VII duplication, when it is an autosomal dominant condition, or an isolated anomaly. The additional bone is interposed between the distal and proximal phalanges. It may be a normal phalanx, a

short phalanx, or a delta phalanx; as a result, the thumb may be too long, angulated, or both. The metacarpal may also be too long.

Triphalangeal thumb is consistent with good function but many fine precision activities are hampered by excessive length. Excision of a delta phalanx should be performed as early as possible and the soft tissues of the IP joint reconstructed. For cases presenting later in childhood it may be necessary to fuse the distal phalanx to the proximal phalanx after excision of the intervening delta phalanx. Correction of thumb web narrowing and thenar muscle hypoplasia may also be required.

Overgrowth

Macrodactyly

Macrodactyly is congenital enlargement of a digit. It is very rare and is not inherited; 90% of cases are unilateral. In 70% of patients, more than one digit is affected and the involvement corresponds with the territory of one or more peripheral nerves, most frequently the median. The enlargement may be present at birth and grow in proportion with other digits but more commonly it progresses during childhood. Macrodactyly affects all tissues in a digit and should be distinguished from other causes of enlargement such as hemangioma, arteriovenous malformations, and lymphedema.

Three types of macrodactyly are seen. *Nerve territory orientated macrodactyly* is associated with enlargement or lipofibromatous hamartoma of a peripheral nerve. The peripheral nerve is thickened by infiltration with fat and fibrous tissue; these changes may extend well proximal to the enlargement of other tissues and, in the case of the median nerve, may lead to its compression within the carpal canal. Skin, nerve, and bone are affected more than tendon or blood vessels. Less frequently, macrodactyly is associated with *neurofibromatosis*. In the rare *hyperostotic macrodactyly,* osteocartilaginous protuberances arise around the digital joints and limit motion. In addition to the serious cosmetic impairment, these large digits are likely to be stiff, deformed, and prone to ulceration.

Treatment of macrodactyly is difficult. Amputation may be appropriate for digits that are severely deformed, stiff, painful, or ulcerated. In childhood, cosmetic considerations often demand attempts at reduction procedures, which should be staged to avoid vascular impairment [33]. The blood supply of the skin is relatively poor and necrosis of skin flaps is a common complication. Longitudinal growth may be controlled by fusion of the phalangeal epiphyses when the digit has reached its expected adult length; however, circumferential growth may continue.

Constriction Band Syndrome

Constriction band syndrome (also known as amniotic band syndrome and Streeter's dysplasia) occurs sporadically at the rate of around 1:15,000 live births. Amniotic disruption leading to constricting intrauterine amniotic bands is currently thought to be the mechanism. The abnormalities are asymmetrical and present at birth. Four types of lesion occur.

1. Simple constriction bands
2. Constriction rings with distal deformity and/or lymphedema
3. Soft tissue fusion of distal parts (acrosyndactyly)
4. Amputation

Constriction band syndrome is distinguished from other types of congenital deformity and amputation by the presence of constriction bands, by the multiple asymmetrical defects, and by the normality of the part proximal to the band. Deep constriction bands may seriously impair vascular supply and innervation; a temperature gradient across the band and distal lymphedema are signs of vascular impairment.

Circular constricting bands are excised and the circular scar broken up by Z-plasties. Bands that produce severe distal lymphedema in the neonate may require urgent release. Syndactyly and intrauterine amputations may also need treatment. The normality of proximal nerves, vessels, and tendons is a distinct advantage during reconstruction.

Miscellaneous Abnormalities and Syndromes

Madelung's Deformity

Madelung's deformity is a congenital disorder that affects growth of the distal radius. It is seldom evident before the age of 8 years. Females are affected more often than males and it

is usually bilateral. The primary abnormality is failure of normal growth of the ulnar and palmar halves of the distal radial physis, leading to curvature in an ulnar and palmar direction (Fig. 1.22). A localized area of radiolucency may appear on the ulnar edge of the distal radius and the ulnar part of the physis fuses prematurely. The ulna is relatively long and becomes prominent dorsally. The carpus sinks, along with the ulnar half of the distal radial articular surface, into the gap between the two forearm bones. Rotation of the forearm is limited by incongruity of the distal radio-ulnar joint.

The cause of Madelung's deformity is unknown. It may be inherited as part of dyschondrosteosis (Leri–Weill disease). Similar deformities may occur in multiple hereditary exostoses, multiple epiphyseal dysplasia, and dyschondroplasia (Ollier's disease), or after damage of the distal radial physis by trauma or infection.

Many patients with Madelung's deformity function well and the problem is chiefly cosmetic. Pain may develop at the wrist or distal radio-ulnar joint as the patient approaches skeletal maturity. Pain may improve after skeletal maturity.

During growth, deformity may be controlled or reduced by physiolysis of the volar/ulnar part of the distal radial physis [34]. Unfortunately, patients tend to present at an age when there is little possibility for correction with further growth. Excision of the volar ligament and dome osteotomy of the radius reduced pain and improved the appearance of 26 wrists [35]. The Ilizarov method has also been used successfully [36]. Wrist fusion and operations such as ulnar head excision and the Sauve–Kapandji procedure are salvage options.

Multiple Hereditary Exostoses

Hereditary multiple exostosis is an autosomal dominant condition resulting from mutations in the EXT family of tumor suppressor genes [37]. It should probably be classed as a familial neoplastic trait rather than as a skeletal dysplasia.

Involvement of the forearm may cause swelling, pain, loss of motion, and unequal longitudinal growth. Exostoses that affect the radius seldom produce severe angular deformity. However, exostoses of the distal ulna are associated with restricted ulnar growth, leading to bowing of the forearm and frequently to dislocation of the radial head. The end result is a short, bowed forearm with loss of rotation. The range of forearm rotation is related to the length of the ulna and the number of exostoses [38]. The dislocated radial head is prominent and may be painful.

Excision of exostoses may be indicated to improve appearance and forearm rotation. Since exostosis size is inversely correlated with ulnar length [37], it would be logical to remove the exostoses as early as possible. However, the effect on growth is not known.

Fig. 1.22 Madelung deformity. (**a**) Anteroposterior view: inadequate growth of the ulnar half of the distal radial epiphysis allows the lunate to sink between the forearm bones. (**b**) Lateral view: the distal radius is angulated palmarward and the distal ulna is prominent dorsally

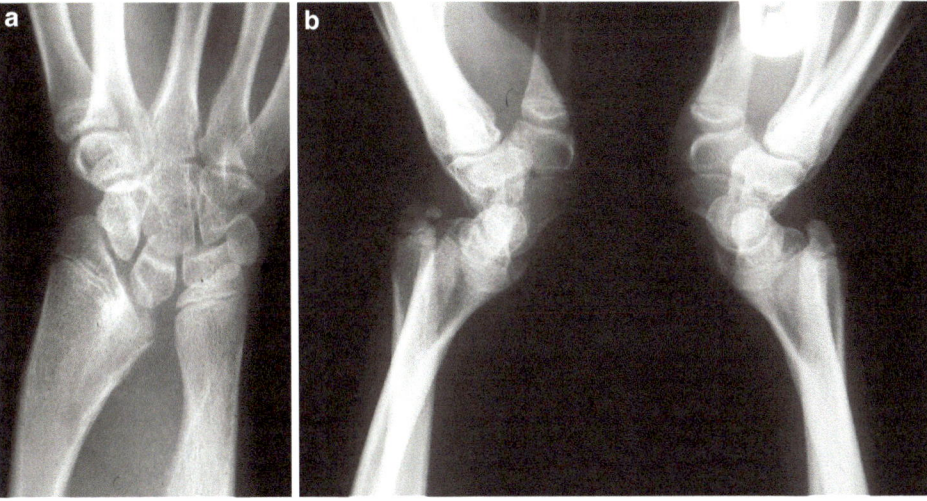

Distraction lengthening of the ulna can help to correct the length discrepancy, to improve bowing, and to maintain length. Monoaxial fixators or small circular frames can be used [39]; concomitant angular correction may also be required.

Management of established radial head dislocation associated with multiple exostoses is difficult. Relocation of the radial head requires extensive surgery and may fail to provide a congruent joint or satisfactory forearm rotation. If instability of the forearm is a problem, creation of a one-bone forearm by fusing the ulna proximally to the radial shaft distally may be appropriate.

Evidence of neurofibromatosis is present in most cases. Untreated, it produces progressive deformity, instability, and loss of rotation. Failure of ulnar growth may lead to dislocation of the radial head.

Conventional orthopaedic techniques such as nonvascularized bone grafts and internal fixation have generally failed to achieve union. Thorough excision of abnormal tissue, free vascularized fibular grafting, and stable osteosynthesis offer the best chance of healing. Creation of a one-bone forearm, providing stability at the expense of rotation, is an alternative when only the distal part of the ulna is affected.

Congenital Pseudarthrosis of the Forearm

Congenital pseudarthrosis of the forearm bones is very rare. In many respects it resembles congenital pseudarthrosis of the tibia. One or both bones may be affected (Fig. 1.23).

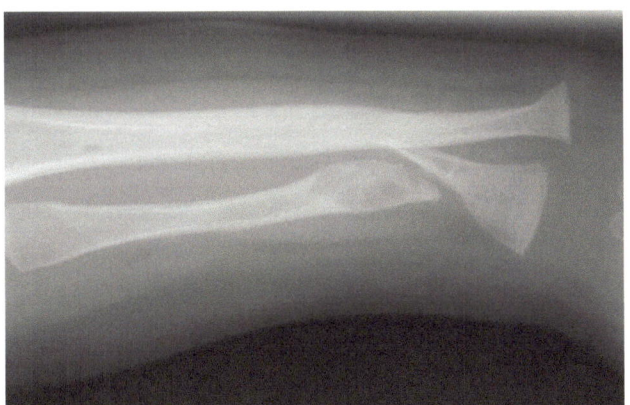

Fig. 1.23 Congenital pseudarthrosis of the radius in a 3-year-old with neurofibromatosis

Finger-Sucking Deformities

Radial deviation and supination deformities of the index finger may occur as a result of prolonged finger sucking (Fig. 1.24) [40]. Deformity is unlikely if the habit ceases by the age of 6 years. Moderate deformities may correct spontaneously once the deforming force is removed. A period of observation of 1–2 years seems appropriate, followed by osteotomy if deformity persists.

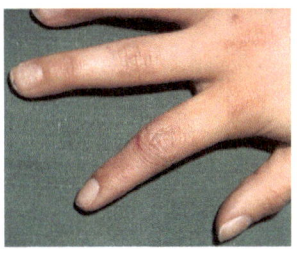

Fig. 1.24 Rotational deformity of the index finger caused by finger sucking

Arthrogryposis Multiplex Congenita

Arthrogryposis is derived from the Greek, meaning "curved joint." It is a syndrome of multiple, nonprogressive joint contractures which are present at birth. The *etiology* is unknown; in about 90% of patients, the disorder appears to be due to an underlying neuropathic process affecting the motor unit. A myopathic process has been postulated in the remaining cases.

The typical *clinical* picture comprises multiple contractures of joints in the upper and lower limbs. The limbs are atrophic, the skin is waxy, and joint creases are absent. Skin dimples may be found over contracted joints. The characteristic postures of the upper limbs are shoulder adduction, elbow extension, flexion/ulnar deviation at the wrists, and flexion deformity of the fingers with flexion/ adduction of the thumb (Fig. 1.25).

The *treatment* of arthrogryposis is difficult. As soon as possible after birth, attempts should be made to correct contractures by serial splintage and to maintain the correction by static splintage. Correction is usually incomplete. When considering operative correction, provision of independent walking should generally take priority over the upper limbs.

Loss of active and passive flexion of the elbow is a common problem in arthrogryposis. Restoration of active flexion of one hand to the mouth is desirable, but strong extension at the opposite elbow should be preserved for pushing up from the sitting position and for personal hygiene. If passive flexion of the elbow is good or can be restored by serial splintage, an elastic harness will encourage hand–mouth function until the child is old enough for tendon transfer. Posterior soft tissue release and triceps lengthening may be necessary. The pectoralis major, which is nearly always in good condition, may be transferred into the biceps tendon or into the proximal ulna, but the results tend to deteriorate with growth [41].

Flexion deformity of the wrist is managed by splintage. Soft tissue release or proximal row carpectomy may be necessary in severe cases. The aim of treatment of the flexed and adducted thumb is provision of a simple pinch, but the combined deficiency of extensors, abductors and web skin, together with contracture of adductor pollicis and flexor pollicis longus requires extensive surgery and the results may be disappointing. Function of the fingers may be impaired by flexion and ulnar deviation deformities, but their function is seldom improved by surgery.

References

1. Froster-Iskenius UG, Baird PA. Limb reduction defects in over one million consecutive livebirths. Teratology 1989; 39(2):127–135.
2. Tickle C. Making digit patterns in the vertebrate limb. Nat Rev Mol Cell Biol 2006; 7(1):45–53.
3. Daluiski A, Yi SE, Lyons KM. The molecular control of upper extremity development: implications for congenital hand anomalies. J Hand Surg Am 2001; 26(1):8–22.
4. Swanson AB, Swanson GD, Tada K. A classification for congenital limb malformation. J Hand Surg Am 1983; 8(5 Pt 2):693–702.
5. Kay SPJ. Pyschosocial aspects of the child with a congenital hand anomaly. In: Green DP, Hotchkiss RN, Pederson WC, eds. Operative Hand Surgery. 4th ed. New York: Churchill Livingstone; 1999.
6. Kallemeier PM, Manske PR, Davis B, Goldfarb CA. An assessment of the relationship between congenital transverse deficiency of the forearm and symbrachydactyly. J Hand Surg Am 2007; 32(9):1408–1412.
7. Kay SP, McCombe D. Absence of Fingers. In: Green DP, Hotchkiss RN, Pederson WC, Wolfe SW, eds. Green's Operative Hand Surgery. 5th ed. Philadelphia: Elsevier/Churchill Livingstone; 2005:1415–1430.
8. Online Mendelian Inheritance in Man. at www3.ncbi.nlm.nih.gov/omim/
9. Lamb DW, Scott H, Lam WL, et al. Operative correction of radial club hand. A long-term follow-up of centralization of the hand on the ulna. J Hand Surg Br 1997; 22(4):533–536.
10. Buck-Gramcko D. Radialization as a new treatment for radial club hand. J Hand Surg Am 1985; 10(6 Pt 2):964–968.
11. Goldfarb CA, Murtha YM, Gordon JE, Manske PR. Soft-tissue distraction with a ring external fixator before centralization for radial longitudinal deficiency. J Hand Surg Am 2006; 31(6):952–959.
12. Damore E, Kozin SH, Thoder JJ, Porter S. The recurrence of deformity after surgical centralization for radial clubhand. J Hand Surg Am 2000; 25(4):745–751.
13. Peterson BM, McCarroll HR Jr, James MA. Distraction lengthening of the ulna in children with radial longitudinal deficiency. J Hand Surg Am 2007; 32(9):1402–1407.
14. Schmidt CC, Neufeld SK. Ulnar ray deficiency. Hand Clin 1998; 14(1):65–76.
15. Cole RJ, Manske PR. Classification of ulnar deficiency according to the thumb and first web. J Hand Surg Am 1997; 22(3):479–488.

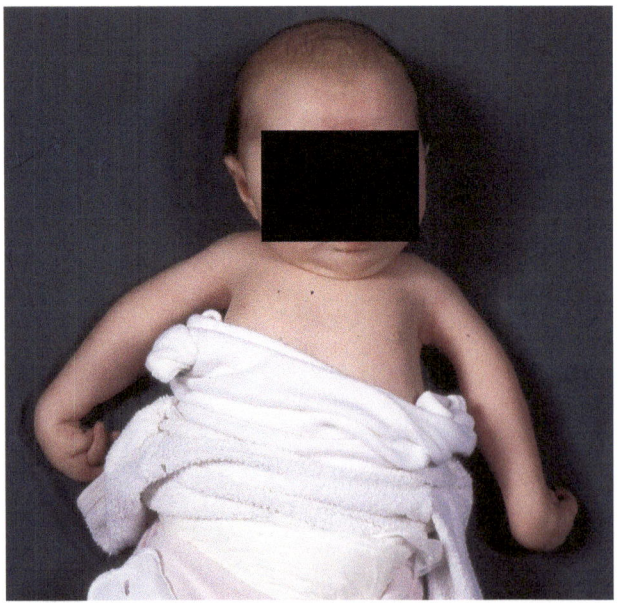

Fig. 1.25 The typical posture of arthrogryposis: elbow extension and wrist flexion

16. Kay SP, McCombe D. Central Hands Deficiencies. In: Green DP, Hotchkiss RN, Pederson WC, Wolfe SW, eds. Green's Operative Hand Surgery. 5th ed. Philadelphia: Elsevier/Churchill Livingstone; 2005:1404–1415.

17. Flatt AE. The Care of Congenital Hand Anomalies. 2nd ed. St. Louis: Quality Medical Publishing; 1994.

18. Eaton CJ, Lister GD. Syndactyly. Hand Clin 1990; 6(4):555–575.

19. McCarroll HR Jr. Congenital flexion deformities of the thumb. Hand Clin 1985; 1(3):567–575.

20. Kalliainen LK, Drake DB, Edgerton MT, et al. Surgical management of the hand in Freeman-Sheldon syndrome. Ann Plast Surg 2003; 50(5):456–462. discussion 463–470.

21. Manske PR, McCarroll HR Jr. Reconstruction of the congenitally deficient thumb. Hand Clin 1992; 8(1):177–196.

22. Buck-Gramcko D. Pollicization of the index finger. Method and results in aplasia and hypoplasia of the thumb. J Bone Joint Surg Am 1971; 53(8):1605–1617.

23. McFarlane RM, Classen DA, Porte AM, Botz JS. The anatomy and treatment of camptodactyly of the small finger. J Hand Surg Am 1992; 17(1):35–44.

24. Miura T, Nakamura R, Tamura Y. Long-standing extended dynamic splintage and release of an abnormal restraining structure in camptodactyly. J Hand Surg Br 1992; 17(6):665–672.

25. Smith PJ, Grobbelaar AO. Camptodactyly: a unifying theory and approach to surgical treatment. J Hand Surg Am 1998; 23(1): 14–19.

26. Kikuchi N, Ogino T. Incidence and development of trigger thumb in children. J Hand Surg Am 2006; 31(4):541–543.

27. Dinham JM, Meggitt BF. Trigger thumbs in children. A review of the natural history and indications for treatment in 105 patients. J Bone Joint Surg Br 1974; 56(1):153–155.

28. Lee ZL, Chang CH, Yang WY, et al. Extension splint for trigger thumb in children. J Pediatr Orthop 2006; 26(6):785–787.

29. Bae DS, Sodha S, Waters PM. Surgical treatment of the pediatric trigger finger. J Hand Surg Am 2007; 32(7):1043–1047.

30. Green WT, Mital MA. Congenital radio-ulnar synostosis: surgical treatment. J Bone Joint Surg Am 1979; 61(5):738–743.

31. Kanaya F, Ibaraki K. Mobilization of a congenital proximal radioulnar synostosis with use of a free vascularized fascio-fat graft. J Bone Joint Surg Am 1998; 80(8):1186–1192.

32. Wassel HD. The results of surgery for polydactyly of the thumb. Clin Orthop 1969; 64:175–193.

33. Tsuge K. Treatment of macrodactyly. J Hand Surg Am 1985; 10(6 Pt 2):968–969.

34. Vickers D, Nielsen G. Madelung deformity: surgical prophylaxis (physiolysis) during the late growth period by resection of the dyschondrosteosis lesion. J Hand Surg Br 1992; 17(4): 401–407.

35. Harley BJ, Brown C, Cummings K, et al. Volar ligament release and distal radius dome osteotomy for correction of Madelung's deformity. J Hand Surg Am 2006; 31(9):1499–1506.

36. Houshian S, Schroder HA, Weeth R. Correction of Madelung's deformity by the Ilizarov technique. J Bone Joint Surg Br 2004; 86(4):536–540.

37. Porter DE, Emerton ME, Villanueva-Lopez F, Simpson AH. Clinical and radiographic analysis of osteochondromas and growth disturbance in hereditary multiple exostoses. J Pediatr Orthop 2000; 20(2):246–250.

38. Watts AC, Ballantyne JA, Fraser M, et al. The association between ulnar length and forearm movement in patients with multiple osteochondromas. J Hand Surg Am 2007; 32(5): 667–673.

39. Ip D, Li YH, Chow W, Leong JC. Reconstruction of forearm deformities in multiple cartilaginous exostoses. J Pediatr Orthop Br 2003; 12(1):17–21.

40. Srinivasan J, Hutchinson JW, Burke FD. Finger sucking digital deformities. J Hand Surg Br 2001; 26(6):584–588.

41. Lahoti O, Bell MJ. Transfer of pectoralis major in arthrogryposis to restore elbow flexion: deteriorating results in the long term. J Bone Joint Surg Br 2005; 87(6):858–860.

Chapter 2

The Shoulder and Elbow

John A. Fixsen

Congenital and Acquired Dislocation of the Shoulder

Congenital dislocation of the shoulder is very rare. It is usually associated with other significant anomalies in the upper limb, such as absence of the radius and deficiency or absence of part of the humerus. On examination, the humerus is unstable in all directions and the condition is normally painless. The shoulder is small, with deficiency of the deltoid, the pectorals, and other periscapular muscles. Radiographs show a small scapula, with an underdeveloped glenoid. The proximal portion of the humerus may be deficient. There is no satisfactory surgical treatment for this condition, but function of the rudimentary shoulder and abnormal upper limb is often surprisingly good, despite the inherent instability.

Acquired dislocation of the shoulder occurring at birth in association with obstetrical brachial plexus palsy is more common, but frequently remains unrecognized for several months. The arm is flail, and only when the fixed abduction deformity persists is the diagnosis of an anterior subglenoid dislocation made, as pointed out by Babbitt and Cassidy [1]. The clinical findings were reported as fixed abduction of the shoulder with winging of the scapula. The humeral head was palpable in the subglenoid position. Closed reduction failed and open reduction was necessary to reduce the dislocation. Dunkerton [2] reported four patients who presented late with posterior dislocation and associated birth palsy. In the past, this has been considered to be the result of abnormal muscle pull after birth [3] or subscapularis contracture [4]. However, Dunkerton felt that true posterior dislocation at birth was due to the brachial plexus injury (see Chapter 23).

Recurrent dislocation, although common in adults, is rare in children, but may be seen in association with marked familial joint laxity in those younger than 2 years. The child is usually brought to the clinic by the parents who are alarmed by the shoulder apparently "slipping" or "snapping" in and out of joint when the child is being dressed or undressed. The condition is usually pain-free and the shoulder reduces spontaneously. Carter and Sweetnam [5] reported this type of joint dislocation in association with familial joint laxity. Fortunately, the shoulder usually stabilizes with time. Maneuvers that cause the shoulder to displace should be avoided. Recurrent dislocation is also seen in other conditions with excessive joint laxity, such as osteogenesis imperfecta and the Ehlers–Danlos syndrome, and should be treated conservatively if possible. More recently, Hamner and Hall [6] reported two patients with multidirectional shoulder instability in association with Sprengel's deformity, which they believed was caused by repetitive stretching of the shoulder capsule as a result of the relative immobility of the scapula in this condition. Wood et al. [7] reported progressive instability of the shoulder in Apert's syndrome, which could occur both at the shoulder and at the elbow: they suggested it was due to ligamentous laxity leading to progressive bony dysplasia.

Traumatic dislocation of the shoulder in the newborn with normal musculature is extremely rare, if it occurs at all. Bateman [8], in experimental attempts to produce traumatic dislocation, showed that epiphyseal separation occurs rather than dislocation of the joint. The capsule forms a stout protective layer over the joint which is continuous with the periosteum of the humerus. The epiphyseal plate or physis is the weakest zone and as a result traumatic epiphyseal separation, as in the hip joint, is more likely than dislocation to occur in the normal child (see Chapter 41).

Congenital Pseudarthrosis of the Clavicle

This condition is rare: approximately 100 cases have been reported [9]. It presents as a nontender lump lateral to the midpoint of the clavicle (Fig. 2.1), usually at or soon after birth. It is almost invariably on the right side and has been

J.A. Fixsen (✉)
Orthopaedic Department, Great Ormond Street Hospital for Sick Children, London, UK
e-mail: jafixsen@btinternet.com

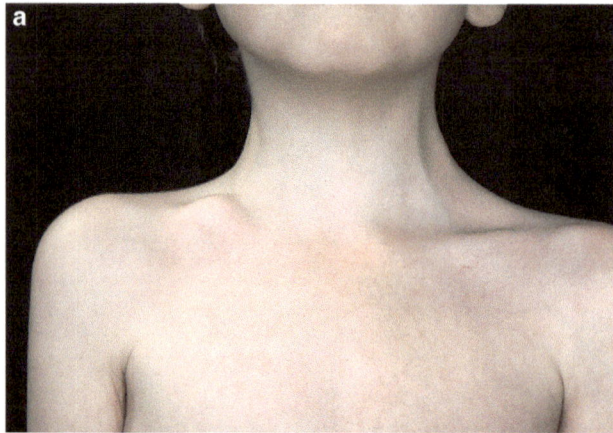

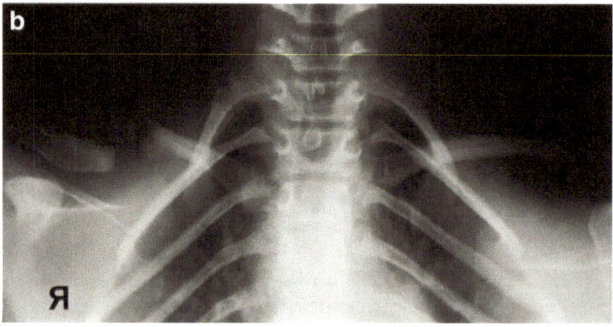

Fig. 2.1 (**a**) Clinical photograph of a child with pseudarthrosis of the right clavicle. Note the prominent lump. (**b**) Anteroposterior radiograph of the same patient showing the pseudarthrosis and the prominent lateral end of the sternal half of the clavicle

ossification. This is believed to start in membrane but, subsequently, cartilaginous growth areas develop at both acromial and sternal ends. Alldred [11] suggested that pseudarthrosis of the clavicle was the result of failure of the two centers of ossification to fuse. Lloyd-Roberts et al. [12] suggested that pressure attrition from the subclavian artery may be responsible for the pseudarthrosis. They noted that the right subclavian artery normally lies higher than the left and that this may explain the condition's right-sided predominance. They also noted that one of the very rare left-sided cases was associated with dextrocardia and an abnormally high left subclavian artery. A significant proportion of their patients also had abnormally high first ribs or cervical ribs. In the bilateral deficiencies seen in cleido-cranial dysostosis, abnormal elevation of the upper ribs is characteristic of the condition (Fig. 2.2).

Spontaneous union of the pseudarthrosis does not occur. Radiologically, there is an established pseudarthrosis, with a bulbous lateral end of the sternal half of the clavicle overlying a tapering medial end of the acromial half (Fig. 2.1). Shoulder and upper limb function is good on the affected side, but the prominent lump is unsightly. Unlike congenital pseudarthrosis of the tibia, the condition normally responds well to excision of the pseudarthrosis and bone grafting, using a block of iliac bone to bridge the gap and internal fixation with an intramedullary threaded pin to prevent migration. Alldred [11] suggested that union was easier to obtain before the child was 8 years of age and that operation was best performed around the age of 4 years. Grogan et al. [9] reported excellent results in eight children in whom the fibrous pseudarthrosis was resected early, carefully preserving the continuity of the periosteal sleeve and approximating the bone ends without grafting. All their patients healed solidly by 14 weeks after operation. They were aged from 7 months to 6 years at the time of surgery. After the age of 8 years, it appears to be more difficult to obtain fusion, and an alternative to bone grafting is excision of the prominent

described on the left side only in association with dextrocardia [10]. It may be mistaken for a clavicular fracture at birth, but it is not associated with birth injury or obstetrical palsy and, unlike a fracture, does not form callus. It should be differentiated from cleido-cranial dysostosis, in which all or part of both clavicles are deficient and associated anomalies are seen in the skull, facial bones, pelvis, and upper femora (Fig. 2.2). The clavicle is the first bone to undergo primary

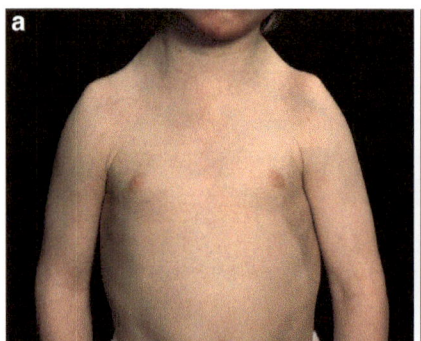
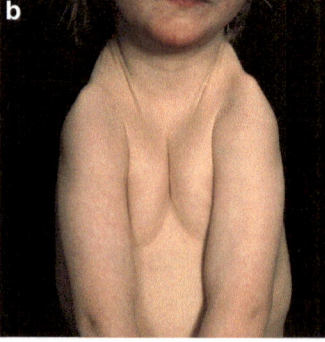
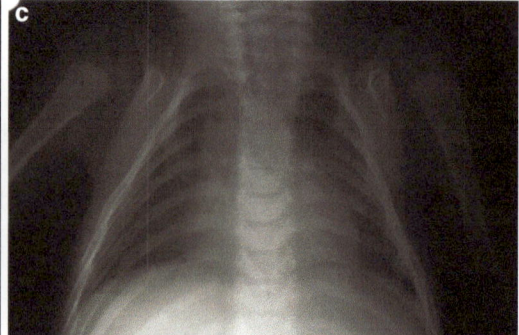

Fig. 2.2 Clinical photographs of a child with cleido-cranial dysostosis. (**a**) With the shoulders in the normal position. (**b**) With the shoulders approximated. (**c**) Anteroposterior radiograph of the chest and shoulders showing only rudimentary clavicles and abnormal elevation of the upper ribs

lateral end of the sternal half of the clavicle. This addresses the major cosmetic deformity, but ignores the pseudarthrosis, which rarely impairs function.

Congenital Elevation of the Scapula (Sprengel's Shoulder)

The limb bud for the arm appears during the fourth week of intrauterine life, between the fifth cervical and first thoracic vertebra. The scapula develops within the limb bud during the fifth week of intrauterine life and descends over the next 3 weeks to its normal position alongside the second to the seventh thoracic vertebrae. Failure to descend fully during this period gives rise to congenital elevation of the scapula, so-called Sprengel's deformity [13]. Occasionally the condition is familial, inherited as an autosomal dominant. Clinically, the scapula is elevated and rotated so that the superomedial angle is high and prominent, and the glenoid and acromion are rotated downward and forward (Fig. 2.3). In the past, the scapula was believed to be hypoplastic, but a recent 3D study by Cho et al. [14] has shown that affected scapulae have a characteristic shape, with a decrease in the height–width ratio, but were larger than the contralateral normal scapulae. The condition may be bilateral and is often associated with brevicollis and cervical abnormalities in the Klippel–Feil deformity.

The superomedial angle of the scapula may be joined to the cervical spine by a fibrous or bony omovertebral bar, first described by Willet and Walsham in 1880 [15]. The bar arises from the superomedial angle or upper one-third of the

medial border of the scapula, to which it may be fused by bone or joined by a fibrous band, cartilage, or even a true joint. The medial end is attached to the spinous process, lamina, or transverse process in the lower half of the cervical spine between C4 and C7. The muscles of the shoulder girdle are often weak and defective, particularly the trapezius, which may be absent. The rhomboids and levator scapulae are hypoplastic and often partially fibrotic. The serratus anterior, pectorals, latissimus dorsi, and sternomastoid may also be affected. Other bony anomalies are frequently seen, in particular: absent or fused ribs, cervical ribs, brevicollis with vertebral anomalies, and spina bifida occulta in the cervical and upper thoracic region. The arm itself may also be short and hypoplastic. The condition is not always noticed at birth but usually becomes obvious when the child starts to stand. In bilateral cases, the neck appears unusually short and the shoulders hunched. The sexes are equally affected. When the condition is unilateral it is more commonly left sided. Abduction and external rotation of the arm are limited on the affected side, partly because of scapular immobility on the thorax and partly because the scapular position rotates the glenoid downward and forward. An anteroposterior radiograph showing both shoulders confirms the diagnosis (Fig. 2.4). Radiographs of the cervical spine and chest should be taken because of the commonly associated spinal and rib anomalies.

Treatment

The major concern is usually the cosmetic appearance rather than the limitation of shoulder movement. This is

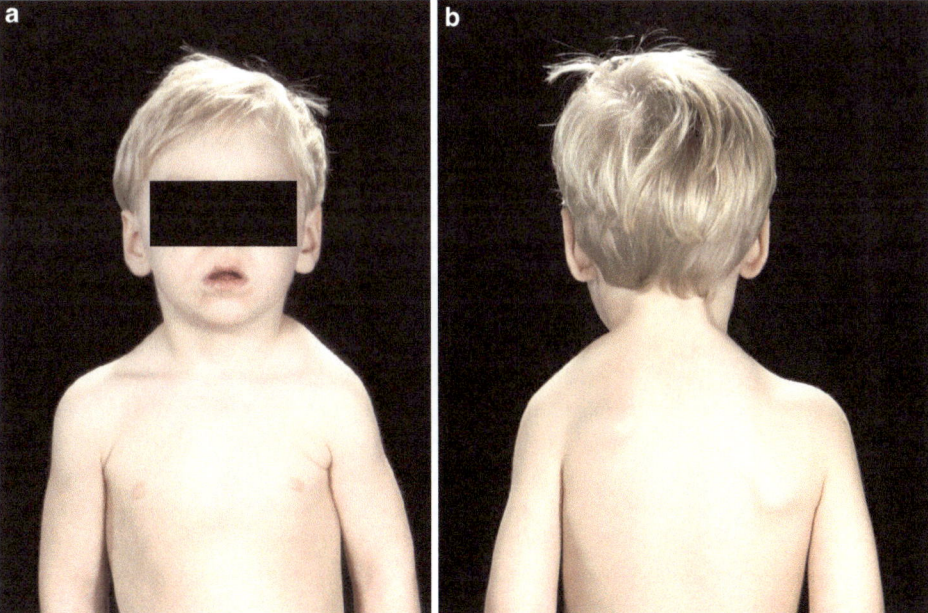

Fig. 2.3 Clinical photographs of a child with a left Sprengel's shoulder. (**a**) Anterior view. (**b**) Posterior view. Note the elevation and rotation of the left scapula

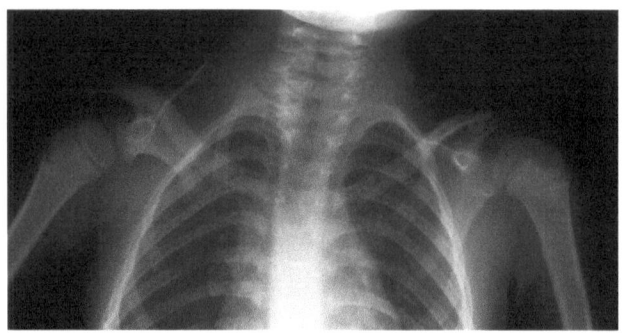

Fig. 2.4 Anteroposterior radiograph of the chest and shoulders showing congenital elevation of the right shoulder. Note anomalies in the lower cervical and upper thoracic spine and prominence of the lateral process of C7 on the right suggesting the presence of an omovertebral bar

the basis of the well-known Cavendish classification of the deformity [16], whereas the classification by Rigault et al. [17] is based on the radiographic level of the superomedial angle of the scapula at diagnosis. A program of exercises develops the maximum range of movement but does not alter the position of the scapula. From the surgical point of view, the surgeon may simply confine himself to a cosmetic procedure in which the prominent superomedial angle of the scapula is removed, together with the omovertebral bar if present. The bone should be removed extra-periosteally to avoid reformation. The patients and family must be warned that the extensive soft tissue dissection needed leaves an extensive posterior scar. The surgeon should be aware of the close proximity of the superomedial corner of the elevated scapula to the brachial plexus. This type of surgery produces an acceptable cosmetic result, but in no way alters the position of the scapula or the range of movement of the shoulder.

A more radical approach is to try to alter the position of the scapula and pull it down into its normal position. Green [18] described an extensive procedure in which the muscles connecting the scapula to the trunk are divided at their insertion along the medial border and spine of the scapula through a long posterior incision. The omovertebral bar and the superomedial angle of the scapula are removed extra-periosteally. The attachments of the latissimus dorsi muscle to the scapula are divided extra-periosteally and, by blunt dissection, a large pocket is created deep to the superior part of the latissimus dorsi. The scapula is displaced distally and secured by a traction wire, which passes from the scapula subcutaneously down to the opposite iliac crest and then out to be incorporated in an external plaster spica. Bellemans and Lamoureux [19] reported their modification of Green's procedure without dissection of the serratus anterior and with immediate post-operative mobilization; this gave satisfactory results in six of seven patients. Woodward [20] suggested that the scapular muscles be separated from the spinous processes

rather than the scapula itself, and the deformity corrected by moving the muscle origins downward. This procedure also requires a long posterior incision and may be modified by excision of the medial border of the scapula and part of its supraspinous portion [21]. Both procedures involve extensive dissection and can leave large and ugly scars. There is a well-reported incidence of damage to the brachial plexus if the scapula is displaced downward too forcefully.

Campbell and Wilkinson [22] popularized an attractive procedure, originally described by Konig in 1914 [23], in which a vertical osteotomy of the scapula 2 cm from its medial border is performed. This is combined with excision of the superomedial angle and the omovertebral bar, together with any fibrous tethering bands. The portion of the scapula lateral to the osteotomy is then rotated, correcting the abnormal downward inclination of the glenoid, improving the range of abduction at the shoulder, and the two portions are sutured together through offset drill holes, pre-drilled before the osteotomy, to maintain the corrected position.

This is a less extensive procedure than either the Green or the Woodward operations. Despite this, among the 11 patients reported, one developed mild brachial plexus palsy, but recovered, and slight winging of the scapula occurred in another patient.

Farsetti et al. [24] in a long-term study of 22 patients, 14 of whom were observed and 7 treated surgically, reported that shoulder abduction and cosmesis did not alter in the simply observed patients, but all except one were satisfied with the situation. In those treated surgically abduction was improved by an average of 38°. However, only four of the seven were satisfied, two were neither satisfied nor dissatisfied, and two were dissatisfied despite improvement in the Cavendish grade and range of abduction.

Abduction Contracture of the Shoulder

Bhattacharyya [25] reported three patients with abduction contracture of the shoulder resulting from fibrosis of the intermediate part of the deltoid. Clinically, the skin was indrawn over the contracted portion of the muscle and the arm was held in approximately 30° of abduction. In two patients this was bilateral; excision of the fibrotic muscle improved the range of movement in all three patients. There was no definite history of trauma or injection, but the condition appeared analogous to that described in the quadriceps muscle after repeated intramuscular injections. Since that time, a number of further cases have been reported in children and young adults [26–28]. The cause of the fibrosis is not usually known, but it seems likely that it follows injections into the muscle and responds satisfactorily to excision of the fibrous contracted area.

Congenital Anomalies of the Elbow

Supracondylar Humeral Spur

This is a palpable bony prominence or tubercle on the antero-medial surface of the distal humerus above the elbow. It is associated with a fibrous band extending to the medial epicondyle and was described by Struthers in 1849 [29]. Such a spur is normal in climbing mammals such as lemurs and in the cat family as a bony foramen through which the neurovascular bundle passes. It is rare but can be important as a cause of vascular and or nerve compression symptoms in the forearm and hand of a child [30]. The diagnosis can be confirmed by plain radiographs (Fig. 2.5) and, if it is clear that the symptoms are caused by it, exploration and decompression by removal of the spur and band are indicated.

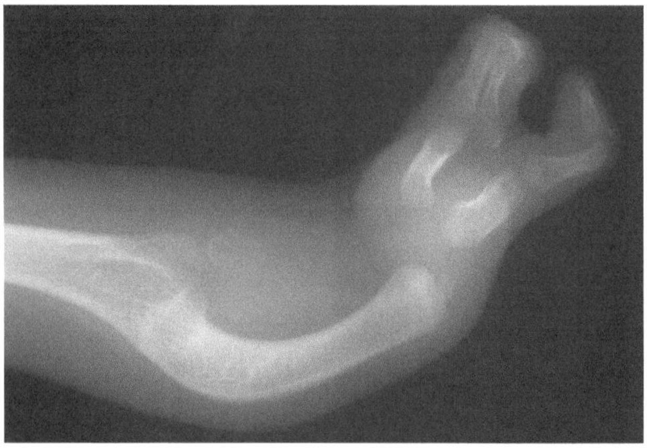

Congenital Ankylosis of the Elbow

This rare condition may involve the whole elbow joint or only the humero-ulnar or humero-radial joints in which case the uninvolved bone is commonly absent (Fig. 2.6). It may occur in isolation in which case it is usually bilateral or with other anomalies such as absent radius or ulna or cranio-facial disorders, e.g., Crouzon's syndrome (Fig. 2.7). McIntyre and Benson [31] published a useful etiological classification which highlighted the pitfalls of phenotypic variability when using a simple morphological classification and provided information on associated anomalies and syndromes. Function for activities of daily living is often surprisingly good even in bilateral cases. Attempts to construct a mobile elbow joint are unrewarding. Osteotomy to reposition the forearm and hand in a more functional position can be helpful. It should be remembered, particularly in bilateral cases,

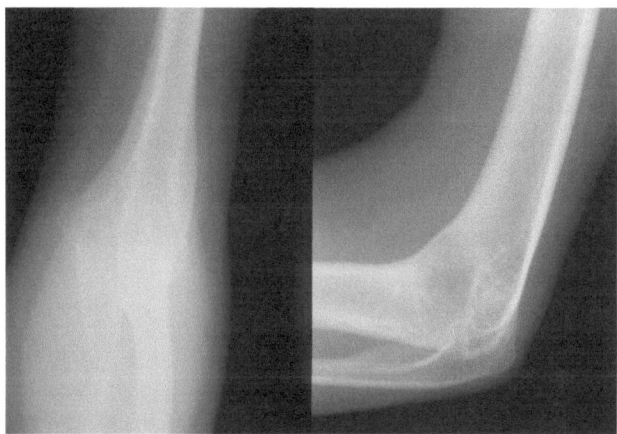

Fig. 2.6 Lateral radiograph showing congenital ankylosis of the humerus and radius with absence of the ulna and partial deficiency of the hand and fingers

Fig. 2.7 Lateral radiograph showing congenital ankylosis of the elbow in a patient with Crouzon's syndrome

that one hand should reach the mouth and the other the perineum.

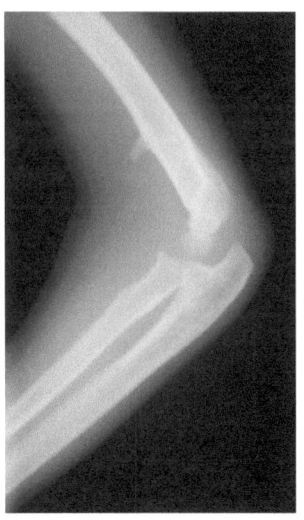

Fig. 2.5 Lateral radiograph of the elbow showing a humeral supracondylar spur. The patient presented with symptoms of vascular and median nerve compression in the forearm

Bilateral Congenital Pseudarthrosis of the Olecranon

This was first reported in the English literature in 1987 by Burge and Benson [32] who described a child born with fixed flexion of both elbows. Early radiographs showed the olecranon separated from the ulnar shaft in both arms. When this gap failed to ossify and he was suffering from weakness of extension at the age of 6 years the pseudarthroses were operated upon sequentially by excision of the fibrous and fibrocartilaginous tissue and bone grafting stabilized by tension band wiring. The results were satisfactory clinically and radiologically. This condition appears to be different from congenital pseudarthrosis of the forearm (see Chapter 21).

Osteochondritis of the Capitellum (Panner's Disease)

This condition in which changes similar to those of Legg–Calve–Perthes' disease are seen in the capitellum was first described by Panner in 1927 [33]. More rarely the radial head may be similarly affected [34]. It is commoner in boys and usually occurs between the age of 4 and 10 years [35]. The patient presents with elbow pain and stiffness. On examination there is limitation of full extension and local tenderness over the capitellum. Sometimes there is local swelling and evidence of an effusion. Radiographs show irregular areas of increased density and fragmentation in the capitellum similar to the changes seen in Legg–Calve–Perthes' disease. Treatment consists of rest in a sling or cast in the acute phase followed by gentle mobilization. Spontaneous recovery normally occurs in 1–3 years. However, there may be some permanent loss of full elbow extension, permanent deformation of the capitellum, and occasionally of the radial head [35].

The Carrying Angle of the Elbow (Cubitus Valgus/Varus)

The term carrying angle of the elbow refers to the angle between the humerus and the forearm and hand in the anteroposterior plane with the elbow fully extended and supinated. In children there is usually around 5° of cubitus valgus. The commonest cause of abnormal angulation is malunion following a humeral supracondylar fracture associated with a cubitus varus deformity (Fig. 2.8) or cubitus valgus

following nonunion of a lateral humeral condylar fracture (see Chapter 44). However, a number of inherited disorders such as the nail-patella and Turner's syndrome (45X0) are associated with an increased carrying angle (cubitus valgus). In an interesting study relating the carrying angle to sex chromosome anomalies Baughman et al. [36] showed that there appears to be a spectrum of the "carrying angle" in relation to the sex chromosome anomaly from maximal cubitus valgus X0 (Turner's syndrome) to minimal cubitus valgus or even varus in patients with supernumerary sex chromosomes as in XXY (Klinefelter's syndrome) and XXXXX (Penta X syndrome) which can also be associated with radial head dislocation and radio-ulnar synostosis. In these congenital conditions, unlike those following malunion, operative treatment is rarely indicated.

Congenital dislocation of the radial head, and congenital radio-ulnar synostosis are described in Chapter 21.

References

1. Babbitt DP, Cassidy PH. Obstetrical paralysis and dislocation of the shoulder in infancy. J Bone Joint Surg 1968; 50A:1447–1452.
2. Dunkerton MC. Posterior dislocation of the shoulder associated with obstetric brachial plexus palsy. J Bone Surg 1989; 71B: 764–766.
3. Wickstrom J, Haslam ET, Hutchinson RH. The surgical management of residual deformities of the shoulder following birth injuries with a brachial plexus injury. J Bone Joint Surg 1955; 37A:27–36.
4. Narakas AO. Obstetrical brachial plexus injuries. In: Lamb DW (ed). The paralysed hand. The hand and upper limb, vol 2. Edinburgh: Churchill Livingstone; 1987:116–135.
5. Carter C, Sweetnam R. Recurrent dislocation of the patella and shoulder: their association with familial joint laxity. J Bone Joint Surg 1960; 42B:721–727.

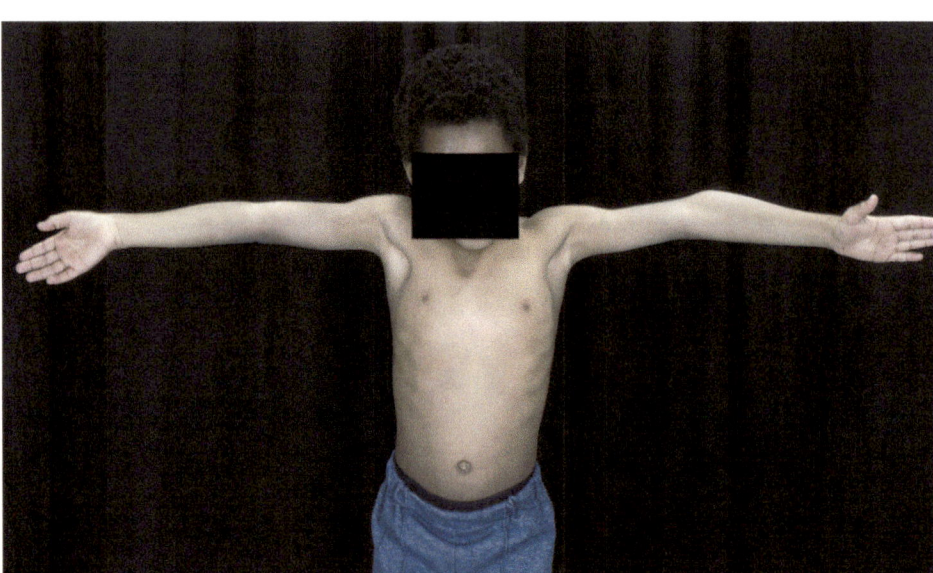

Fig. 2.8 Clinical photograph of a child with left cubitus varus following malunion of a supracondylar fracture

6. Hamner DL, Hall JE. Sprengel's deformity associated with multi directional shoulder instability. J Pediatr Orthop 1995; 15: 641–643.

7. Wood DE, Sauser DD, O'Hara RC. Shoulder and elbow in Apert's syndrome. J Pediatr Orthop 1995; 15:648–651.

8. Bateman JE. The shoulder and neck, 2nd ed. Philadelphia: WB Saunders; 1978:37.

9. Grogan DP, Love SM, Guideria KJ, Ogden JA. Operative treatment of congenital pseudarthrosis of the clavicle. J Pediatr Orthop 1991; 11:176–180.

10. Gibson DA, Carroll N. Congenital pseudarthrosis of the clavicle. J Bone Joint Surg 1970; 52B:629–643.

11. Alldred AJ. Congenital pseudarthrosis of the clavicle. J Bone Joint Surg 1963; 45B:312–319.

12. Lloyd-Roberts GC, Apley AG, Owen R. Reflections upon the aetiology of congenital pseudarthrosis of the clavicle. J Bone Joint Surg 1975. 57B:24–29.

13. Sprengel O. Die angeborene Verschiebung des Schulterblattes nach oben. Langenbeck Arch Klin Chir 1891; 42:545–549.

14. Cho T-J, Choi IH, Chung CY, Hwang JK. The Sprengel's deformity. J Bone Joint Surg 2000; 82B:711–718.

15. Willet A, Walsham WJ. An account of the dissection of the parts removed after death from the body of a woman the subject of congenital malformation of the spinal column, thorax and left scapular arch with remarks on the probable nature of the defects in development producing the deformities. Med Surg Trans London 1880; 63:256.

16. Cavendish ME. Congenital elevation of the shoulder. J Bone Joint Surg 1972; 54B:395–408.

17. Rigault P, Pouliquen JC, Guyonvarch G, Zujovic J. Congenital elevation of the scapula in childhood. Rev Chir Orthop 1976; 62:5–26.

18. Green WT. The Surgery correction of elevation of the scapula (Sprengel's deformity). J Bone Joint Surg 1957; 39A: 1439.

19. Bellemans M, Lamoureux J. Results of surgical treatment of Sprengel deformity by a modified Green's procedure. J Pediatr Orthop B 1999; 8:194–196.

20. Woodward JW. Congenital elevation of the scapula: correction by release and transplantation of the muscle origin. J Bone Joint Surg 1961; 43A:219–228.

21. Borges KLP, Shah A, Cobo Torres B, Bowen JR. Modified Woodward procedure for Sprengel's deformity of the shoulder. J Pediatr Orthop 1996; 18:508–513.

22. Campbell D, Wilkinson JA. Scapular osteotomy for the treatment of Sprengel's shoulder. J Bone Joint Surg 1979; 61B:514.

23. König F. Eine neue Operation des angeborenen Schulter blatthochstandes. Beitr Klin Chir 1914; 94:530–537.

24. Farsetti P, Weinstein SL, Caterini R, et al. Sprengel's deformity: Long term follow-up study of 22 cases. J Pediatr Orthop B 2003; 12:202–210.

25. Bhattacharyya S. Abduction contracture of the shoulder from contracture of the intermediate part of the deltoid. J Bone Joint Surg 1966; 48B:127–131.

26. Hill NA, Leibler WA, Wilson JH, Rosenthal E. Abduction contractures of both glenohumeral joints and extension contracture of one knee secondary to partial muscle fibrosis. J Bone Joint Surg 1967; 49A:961–964.

27. Goodfellow JW, Wade S. Flexion contracture of the shoulder joint from the anterior part of the deltoid muscle. J Bone Joint Surg 1969; 51B:356–358.

28. Wolbrink AJ, Hsu Z, Bianco AJ. Abduction contracture of the shoulders and hips secondary to fibrous bands. J Bone Joint Surg 1973; 55A:844–846.

29. Struthers J. On a peculiarity of the humerus and humeral artery. Monthly J Med Sci 1849; 9:264.

30. Kessel L, Rang M. Supracondylar spur of the humerus. J Bone Joint Surg 1966; 48B:765–769.

31. McIntyre JD, Benson MKD. An aetiological classification for developmental synostoses of the elbow. J Pediatr Orthop B 2002; 11:313–319.

32. Burge P, Benson M. Bilateral congenital pseudarthrosis of the olecranon. J Bone Joint Surg 1987; 69B:460–462.

33. Panner HJ. An affection of the capitulum humeri resembling Calve-Perthes disease of the hip. Acta Radiologica 1927; 8:617.

34. Trias A, Ray RD. Juvenile osteochondritis of the radial head. J Bone Joint Surg 1963; 45A:576–582.

35. Smith MGH. Osteochrondritis of the humeral capitulum. J Bone Joint Surg 1964; 46B:50.

36. Baughman FA Jr, Higgins JV, Wadsworth TG, Demaray MJ. The carrying angle in sex chromosome anomalies. J Am Med Assoc 1974; 280:718.

Chapter 3

Brachial Plexus Injuries
Peripheral Nerve Injuries

Alain L. Gilbert and Rolfe Birch

Part 1: Management of the Injury

Alain L. Gilbert

Introduction

Evolving microsurgical techniques have significantly changed our attitude to surgical reconstruction of peripheral nerve lesions, including those of the brachial plexus. However, because of the considerable distance the nerves have to regenerate after restoring anatomical continuity in the brachial plexus, the results in adults have been modest, despite the more sophisticated methods available. In contrast, similar methods in children give better results because of their superior capacity for regeneration and the shorter distances involved. The potential for regeneration diminishes gradually after birth, remaining fairly good until adolescence and then deteriorating rapidly after the cessation of growth. Obstetrical lesions occurring at birth are best considered separately, because they represent a uniform group for patient's age and type of lesion, whereas lesions occurring during childhood are more heterogeneous.

Etiology and Pathogenesis

Obstetrical birth palsy has been recognized since the late 19th century, but modern series reporting operative exploration have clarified the pathological changes.

The etiology is always a tearing force caused by traction on the head or arm. There are two basic types of lesion, which relate to presentation and birth weight:

A.L. Gilbert (✉)
Institut de la Main, Clinique Jouvenet, Paris, France

R. Birch (✉)
Peripheral Nerve Injury Unit, Royal National Orthopaedic Hospital, Stanmore, UK

1. overweight babies (over 4 kg) with vertex presentation and shoulder dystocia who require excessive force using traction, often with forceps or ventouse extraction, for delivery. This results in an upper plexus injury, most commonly of the C5 and C6, and occasionally the C7 roots. Sometimes a complete plexus injury occurs, involving rupture of the upper roots and lower root avulsions (Fig. 3.1).
2. Breech presentation, usually of small babies (under 3 kg) requiring hyperextension of the head and neck and, in many cases, manipulation of the hand and arm in a fashion that exerts traction on both the upper and the lower roots. This often causes an avulsion injury of the upper roots, or occasionally all of the roots (Fig. 3.2).

Clinical Presentation

The initial diagnosis is obvious at birth. After a difficult delivery of an obese baby by the vertex presentation or a small baby by the breech, the upper extremity is flail and dangling. A more detailed analysis of the pattern of paralysis of the various muscles of the upper extremity is now necessary, as the picture will change rapidly. Examination of the other extremities is important, to exclude neonatal quadriplegia or diplegia. Occasionally, birth palsy may be bilateral. Forty-eight hours later, a more accurate examination and muscle testing can be performed. At this stage it is usually possible to differentiate two types of paresis:

1. The *Erb-Duchenne* type paralysis of the upper roots. The arm is held in internal rotation and pronation. There is no active shoulder abduction or elbow flexion. The elbow may be slightly flexed (lesion of C5–C7) or in complete extension (lesion of C5–C6). The thumb is in flexion

Fig. 3.1 C5/C6 brachial plexus lesion: paralyzed fibers are shaded (Reproduced with permission from Narakas [34])

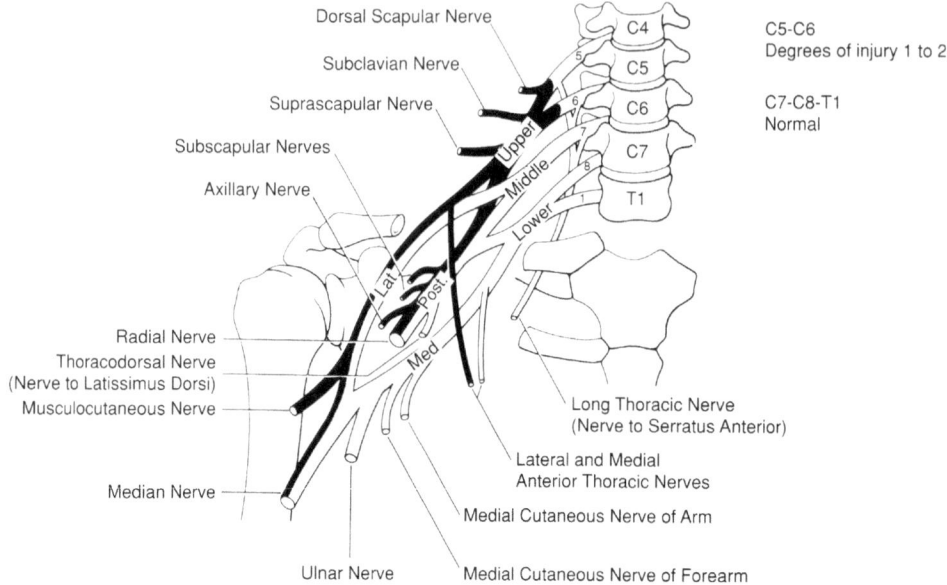

Fig. 3.2 Entire brachial plexus lesion. Rupture of the upper trunk, supraganglionic avulsion of C7 and C8, severe damage to T1 (Reproduced with permission from Narakas [34])

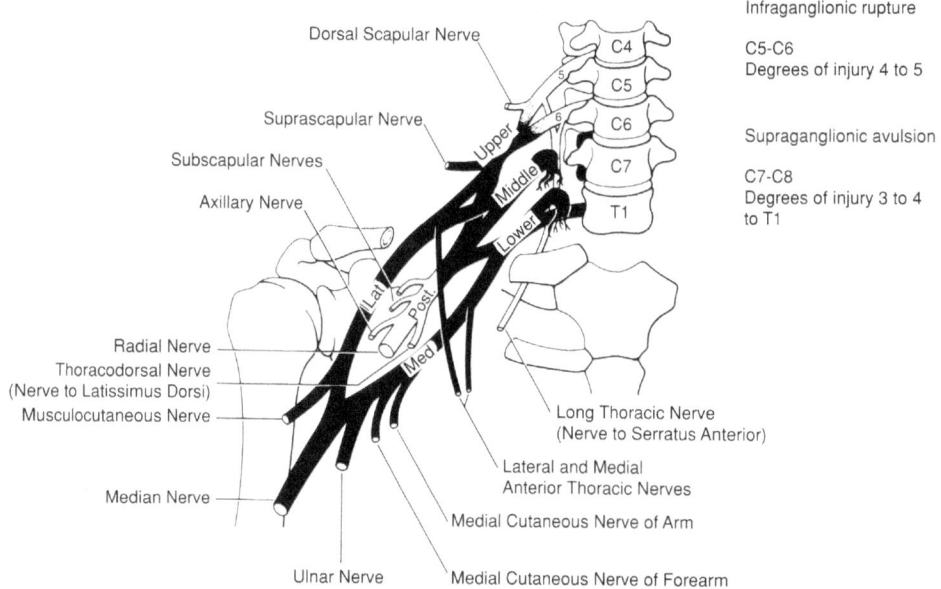

and sometimes the fingers will not extend. As a rule, the thumb and the finger flexors are functioning. The pectoralis major is usually active, giving an appearance of forward flexion of the shoulder. There are no vasomotor changes or gross alterations of distal sensation.

2. Complete paralysis (*Dejerine-Klumpke*). The entire arm is flail and the hand clenched. Sensation is diminished, and there is vasomotor impairment, giving a pale or even "marbled" appearance to the extremity. Often, Horner's sign is present on the affected side.

A shoulder radiograph should be taken to eliminate fracture of the clavicle or the upper humerus, which can occur

in association with the paresis. Occasionally, phrenic nerve palsy can be detected by diaphragmatic fluoroscopy.

The clinical development during the first month is variable, and many pareses will lessen during this stage [1]. However, Wickstrom et al. [2] reported that only 10% of total palsies recover to any useful extent. These patients should be carefully evaluated at the age of 3 months, clinically, electromyographically, and by cervical myelography. Gentle physiotherapy should be ensured during this recovery period to minimize the development of contractures while awaiting spontaneous recovery. At this stage, a complete paralysis with Horner's sign will remain unchanged so that early operation at 3 months of age should be considered for these babies.

Paralysis of the upper roots may show spontaneous recovery during the first 3 months. These babies should be treated with physiotherapy and assessed clinically and electromyographically by the age of 3 months.

Spontaneous Recovery

The literature reports varying rates of spontaneous recovery, from 7 to 80%. Useful guidelines are given in the thesis of Tassin [3] who came to the following conclusions:

Complete recovery is seen in those infants showing some contraction of the biceps and the deltoid by the end of the first month and a normal contraction by the second month.
An infant in whom neither the deltoid nor the biceps contract by the third month cannot be expected to obtain a good result. Testing the deltoid can be difficult. As a result, assessment of the biceps is the most reliable indicator for operative intervention. If there is no evidence of any recovery in the biceps by the end of the third month, operation is indicated. Clinical assessment is more reliable than electrical testing. If surgery is not undertaken, some recovery will continue to take place spontaneously, but it is likely to be less satisfactory than that after surgery.

Indications for Operation

If recovery of the biceps has not begun by 3 months, the prognosis is poor and surgical repair of the plexus is indicated [4–6]. The following clinical situations pose particular problems:

1. Complete palsy with a flail arm after 1 month, particularly with a Horner's syndrome, does not recover spontaneously and is a prime candidate for surgery. These babies are best treated by early operation at the age of 12 weeks.
2. Complete palsy of C5 and C6 occurring after breech delivery with no sign of recovery by the third month should also be considered for surgical treatment.
3. The most common C5, C6, and sometimes C7 palsies almost always show some sign of recovery, which can be misleading, and which has in the past encouraged a conservative approach. If, however, after careful examination, recovery of the biceps (and not elbow flexion) is completely absent at 3 months, surgery should be considered. Great difficulty arises when infants are seen late, by the 6–8th month, and show minimal recovery of biceps function. The parents are often encouraged by the early signs of recovery and will not accept the idea of an unsatisfactory final result. Under these circumstances, it is difficult for

the surgeon to advise an operation that cannot promise a definitive result. In order to avoid this situation, it is important to try to make decisions by the third month.

Several centers have been unable to show good correlation between electromyographic changes and the final outcome. Frequently, the pre-operative electromyogram (EMG) gives cause for over-optimism, because it takes only a few fibers to provoke an electrical response which is not associated with subsequent clinical recovery. However, a negative EMG with complete absence of signs of regeneration at the age of 3 months almost invariably signifies root avulsion.

Myelography has been used extensively in the past, but is unpredictable and associated with false-negative and false-positive results. Computed tomography with myelography has improved the quality of the results considerably.

The recent use of magnetic resonance imaging (MRI), although promising, does not always offer precise information for routine use. Both MRI and myelography need general anesthesia for the baby and should be used only if there is uncertainty about the condition of the roots (breech presentation, lower root avulsion).

Surgical Intervention

Operation is performed under general anesthesia. Usually a supraclavicular approach is sufficient, but this can de extended transclavicularly to expose the lower plexus if necessary. The neuroma usually lies between the C5 and the C6 roots and the divisions of the upper trunk at the level of the clavicle. The nerves may be ruptured totally or avulsed. The neuroma is resected back to normal tissue and one or two sural nerves are used as grafts between the sectioned nerve ends. The nerve anastomoses can be performed by fibrin glue (Tissucol). If avulsions are present, reconstruction must be tailor-made to the situation and the expertise of the surgeon. The reconstruction of the hand is a priority. Our results show that a major part of the remaining roots should be used to reconstruct C8–T1, even if the shoulder is weakened. Additional neurotizations may be used to compensate.

Neurotizations

For several years neurotizations have become increasingly popular and their usefulness confirmed. This can be used in desperate cases such as an avulsion of C5/C6 in a breech delivery where double (accessory spinal on suprascapular [7] and ulnar on musculocutaneous [8]) or triple (adding triceps branch on axillary [9]) neurotizations can give very satisfactory function at the shoulder [10]; they can also be used to complement a difficult repair if the roots are small and of doubtful quality. More classical (intercostal nerve) or more specific (phrenic nerve [11], contralateral C7 [12], and brachialis) neurotizations have been advocated by some surgeons but are not widely accepted. The outcome following end-to-side suture has not proven reliable in our hands and has not been scientifically substantiated.

Anatomical Lesions

The anatomical lesions observed at operation correspond to those described by Taylor in 1920 [13]. These include rupture at the level of the primary trunk or root, or avulsion of the roots. Unlike the reported lesions in the adult, we have never seen a double-level lesion or lesions of the secondary trunk of two branches of the plexus. Associated vascular lesions are exceptional, and we have seen only one rupture of the axillary artery, which was treated by vein graft. The upper roots are more often ruptured and the lower roots avulsed. The results in 436 surgical cases up to 1996 showed the following distribution of root lesions [14, 15]:

1. C5 and C6: 48%
2. C5–C7: 29%
3. Complete involvement: 23% (of which almost all were avulsions).

Post-Operative Care

Stretching the reconstructed region must be avoided for the first three post-operative weeks. This is best achieved by splintage. Physical therapy is then resumed by gentle passive exercises and the encouragement of voluntary movement. Every effort should be made to counteract retraction and internal rotation of the shoulder and encourage flexion of the elbow. Physiotherapy should be continued throughout the recovery period, usually for 2 years, when regular physiotherapy may be discontinued. Recovery is slow. It can be seen 4–6 months after direct suture and at 6–10 months after graft reconstruction. It can continue in upper plexus lesions for over 2 years and in complete lesions for over 3 years.

Results of Surgery

Since 1976, we have seen more than 4,330 cases. Up until April 2008, 996 have been operated upon. From this total we

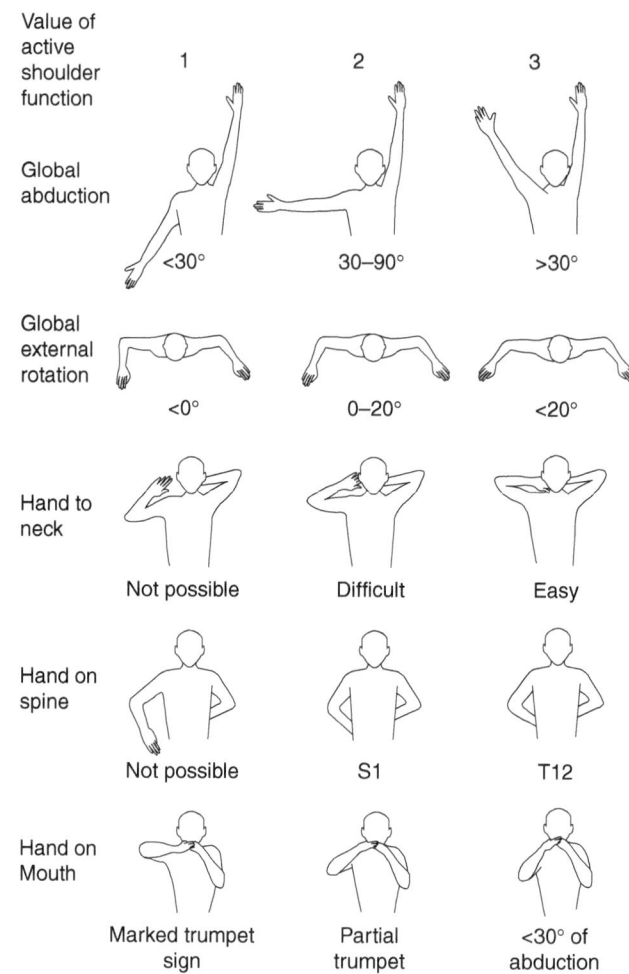

Fig. 3.3 The Mallet system of measuring function at the shoulder

have reviewed 436 patients with a minimum 4-year follow-up operated on between 1976 and 1995. The results in the shoulder, using the Mallet scale (Fig. 3.3) [16] are

C5 C6
at 2 years
>Grade IV (good–excellent)   52%
Grade III   40%
Grade II   8%

After 2 years one-third of the patients had secondary surgery:

13 subscapularis releases
33 latissimus dorsi transfers
6 trapezius transfers

and a new evaluation was completed at 4 years (after tendon transfers). The results were as follows:

Grade IV   80%
Grade III   20%
Grade II   0%
C5 C6 C7

At 2 years the results were

Grade IV   36%
Grade III   46%
Grade II   18%

After 2 years, one-quarter of the patients had secondary surgery:

7 subscapularis releases
24 latissimus dorsi transfers
1 trapezius transfer

and the results were evaluated again at 4 years.

Complete Paralysis

The results in the shoulder in complete paralysis are less satisfactory because part of the upper roots destined for the shoulder and elbow must be sacrificed in order to obtain function in the hand. The shoulder results at 4 years are as follows:

class IV: 22.5%
class III: 42%
class II: 35.5%

In the hand, however, for which the prognosis is very poor for spontaneous recovery, the results showed some function in 83% and useful function in 75% of patients, 8 years after neurotization.

Complications

In the series reviewed, there have been no operative deaths. The overall complication rate was 1%, including phrenic nerve lesions, lesions of the thoracic duct, wound infections, and vascular lesions, all of which have been managed satisfactorily, without late sequelae.

Recommendations

On the basis of the results of the author's series of patients, the following recommendations can be made:

1. Babies who do not recover biceps function by the age of 3 months should be considered for immediate operation.
2. Primary suture without tension is rarely possible. Nerve grafting is usually necessary for root or trunk ruptures.
3. In the presence of root avulsions, an internal neurotization should be attempted between different roots, particularly as children seem to have a far greater capacity to accommodate to differential neurotizations.
4. When it is not possible to perform an internal neurotization, an external neurotization can be performed, using one or more of the following donor nerves in the following order of preference: the spinal accessory nerve, the ulnar or median nerve, and the intercostal nerves.
5. The reconstruction should be protected from excessive motion for the first 3 weeks.
6. Physiotherapy should be continued up to 2 years of age, but then continued by the parents in the form of play and activities of daily living.
7. Secondary surgery can be considered when it is clear that recovery after reconstruction has failed.

Late Cases

When the patient is seen late the indications for surgery are difficult to define. It is not easy to convince a family that in order to recover some potential hand function it is necessary to scar the shoulder region and imperil natural recovery. Sometimes it is possible to use neurotizations and avoid losing existing function.

How Late Can Reconstruction Be Considered?

Children can be operated upon after several years as the muscles may stay alive much longer than in the adult, even 9 years after injury. It is necessary to record a good EMG showing fibrillations or some re-innervated fibers. Outcome is adversely affected by technical difficulties resulting from fibrosis at the sites of the lesions and by inadequate brain readjustment.

Part 2: Birth lesions of the brachial plexus Peripheral nerve injuries

Rolfe Birch

Etiology

The causes, characteristics, and consequences of this lesion were established during the latter part of the 19th century from work undertaken, for the most part, by French neurologists and surgeons (Fig. 3.4). The first reports of plexus repairs appeared in 1903, from Glasgow, Manchester, and London. Since that time the field has been plagued by controversy about causation, incidence, and natural history; about the cause and treatment of consequent deformity; and about the indications for and results of nerve repair. In 2003 Evans-Jones, Kay, and colleagues [17] published the findings of the first ever national census of the disorder. As they point out "most cases are due to trauma at delivery which is not necessarily excessive or inappropriate." The incidence, risk factors, and course to recovery during the first 6 months of life were recorded. Of 723,000 live births in the United Kingdom and the Republic of Ireland, there were 323 new cases of birth lesions of the brachial plexus (BLBP) in a period of 12 months; 143 of the 255 incomplete lesions had recovered fully by the age of 6 months. There was partial recovery in the remainder. None of the 98 complete lesions had fully recovered by 6 months. In six babies there was no recovery at all. Significant associated risk factors in comparison with the normal population included shoulder dystocia (60% vs. 0.3%), high birth weight, and instrument-assisted delivery. Evans-Jones et al. [17] point out that there was a significantly lower risk of BLBP in infants delivered by caesarean section. Breech delivery occurred in only 10 of the 323 confirmed cases which suggests that obstetricians in the United Kingdom take the matter of breech presentation rather more seriously than in some other countries. A total of 74 infants entered into the national census were followed for a minimum of 24 months after birth [18]. Recovery was full in 39 children. Operation for repair of the nerves was undertaken in nine children and for open reduction of posterior dislocation (PD) of the shoulder in 20 more.

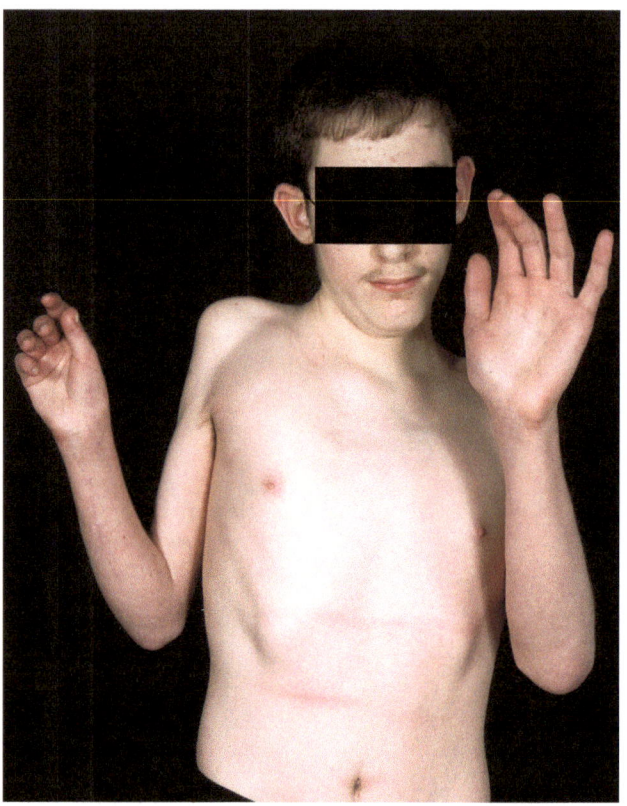

Fig. 3.4 Bilateral lesion complicating breech delivery. On the right, avulsion of C5, C6, and C7; on the left, avulsion C5, rupture of C6. The shoulders are flail; there is severe growth disturbance

The significance of risk factors has been clarified in two studies. The earlier report of 230 consecutive cases [19] found that the mean birth weight of affected babies was 4.5 kg, against the regional mean of 3.88 kg. Heavy babies had more serious nerve injuries. Shoulder dystocia was recorded in over 60% of deliveries. There was no significant correlation with social class. The later report comes from Tavakkolizadeh [20] who analyzed risk factors in over 1,000 consecutive cases. The relative risk of a baby suffering BLBP is as high as 180 when delivery is complicated by shoulder dystocia and about 10 in cases of neonatal asphyxia or maternal gestational diabetes. The relative risk of failure to perform cesarean section comes close to nine as does birth weight in excess of 3.4 kg. Tavakkolizadeh [20] confirms that increased maternal body mass index (BMI) is a significant risk factor. Anatomical variations, such as a cervical rib, may account for the 5% of cases where no obvious cause can be found [21].

Outcomes

Valuable long-term studies have been contributed by Strombeck et al. [22, 23]. Many young adults showed persisting deficits in function, exacerbated by deformity at the elbow and shoulder, and, perhaps, by continuing loss of motor neurones in the anterior horn of the spinal cord. Yang [24] found that "only 17% of children affected by right obstetric brachial plexus palsy prefer the right upper limb for overall movement." A significant correlation between defects in personal and social behavior and the extent of the lesion [25] reminds us that operations, hospitalization, and continuing dependence upon "health professionals" do the child no good.

Pathology

The nerve lesion in BLBP differs from the high-energy transfer adult injury in two important respects: traction and compression forces are expended upon the nerves for hours during a protracted and difficult delivery, and the response of the immature nervous system is very different from that seen in the adult. In the infant the spinal cord fills the cervical canal, the spinal rootlets emerging at, or close to a right angle from it. Fraher [26] states that "during development the CNS–PNS interface oscillates and continually changes its form and position as the two tissue classes establish their mutually exclusive territories." Myelination is incomplete, particularly at the junction between the roots of the spinal nerves and the spinal cord, so that conduction velocity in the neonate is only one-half that of the adult. It is even slower in premature babies. The density of nerve fibers in the neonate is higher than in the adult because of the paucity of connective tissue. Nerve blood flow is highest in the first weeks of life and thereafter declines [27]. Immature nerve fibers are more susceptible to ischemia and anoxic conduction block. Groves and Scaravilli [28] demonstrate that many neurones in the neonatal dorsal root ganglion die after axonotomy and the immature neurones of the anterior horn of the spinal cord are similarly vulnerable. Decisive evidence about defective regeneration in the immature nervous system is provided by Fullertan et al. [29, 30] who found "a selective failure of regeneration in the largest diameter fibers. . . .it seems more likely that the failure of recovery of fine movements is due to the fact that the proprioceptive pathway involving 1-α [alpha], 1-β [beta] and group 2 fibers on the afferent side and

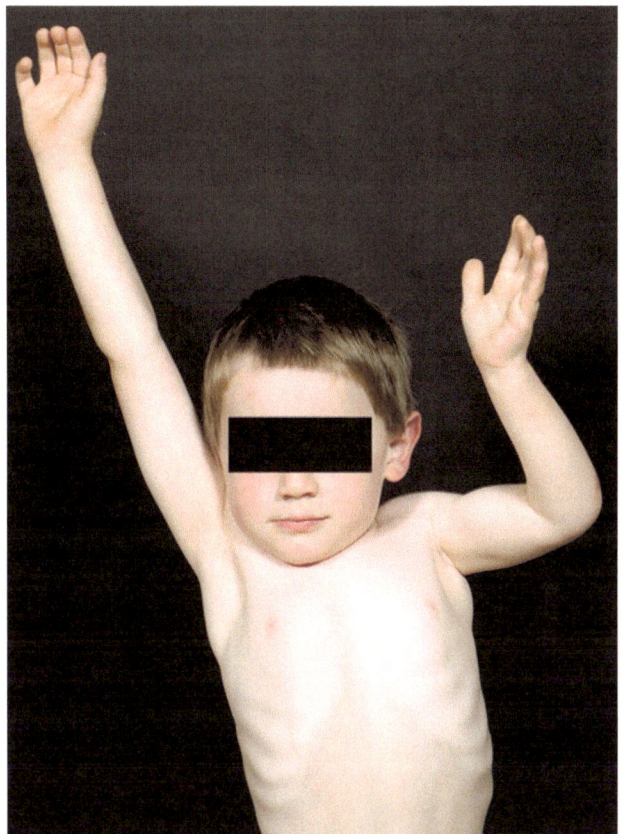

Fig. 3.5 Co-contraction of the muscles acting across the gleno-humeral joint

the process of α and γ co-activation on the efferent side, is lost." These findings may account for the simultaneous activity in antagonistic muscles seen in so many children with BLBP and explain many of the disappointing results of nerve repair (Fig. 3.5).

The injury to the spinal nerves is different from that encountered in the adult. Combined, post-ganglionic rupture and intradural lesion are common; avulsion of the roots without displacement of the dorsal root ganglion (DRG) is frequent; rupture confined to the ventral or dorsal root has been confirmed [31]. Intra-operative neurophysiological investigation (NPI) of central and of peripheral conduction is valuable in analysis of the adult case: it is essential in the infant.

Clinical Assessment

Diagnosis is usually straightforward (Fig. 3.6). Lesions complicating breech delivery are frequently bilateral and often complicated by phrenic nerve palsy requiring plication of the hemi-diaphragm as a matter of urgency [32]. Records [33] made at first attendance include the risk factor chart,

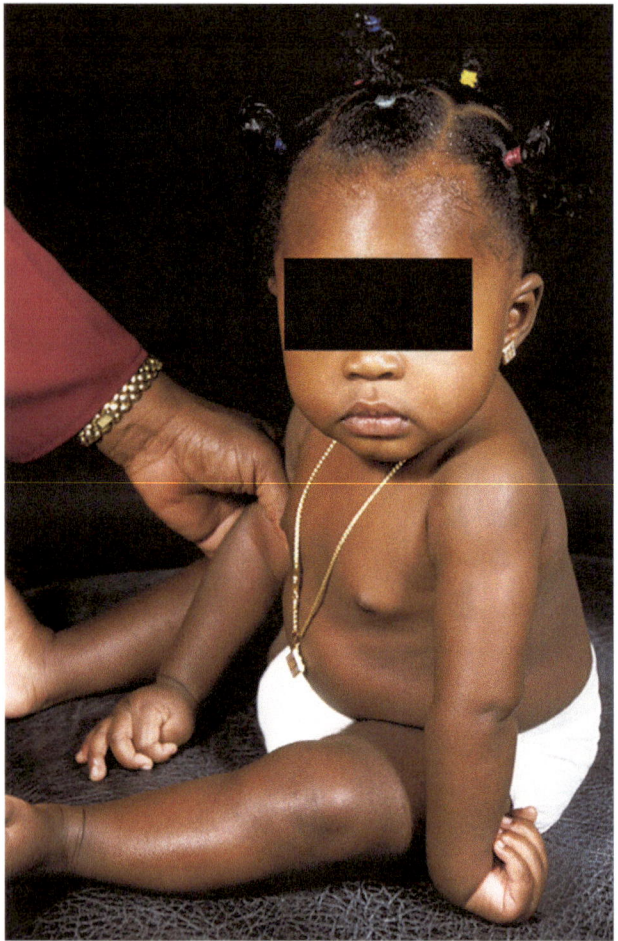

Fig. 3.6 Group 2 lesion (C5, C6, C7)

the Mallett shoulder system, and charts for operated and non-operated cases (Figs. 3.7 and 3.8). The active and passive ranges at the thoraco-scapular, the gleno-humeral, and the radio-ulnar joints are recorded. The charts are completed at every attendance in the clinic. The inferior scapulo-humeral (ISH) angle is measured between the long axis of humerus and the lateral border of the scapula. The active and the passive ISH angle is measured and recorded: the angles indicate the contributions to elevation of the thoraco-scapular and gleno-humeral joints and reveal weakness or contractures of those muscles acting across these joints. The posterior scapulo-humeral (PSH) angle subtends between the axis of the humeral shaft and the line of the spine of the scapula. The examiner holds the arm parallel to the ground and the child's hand rests on the opposite shoulder. If the PSH angle is wide, but active medial rotation is reduced, then the medial rotator muscles are defective (Fig. 3.9). Retroversion of the head of the humerus or less commonly contracture of the posterior capsule and lateral rotator muscles accounts for the narrowing of both active and passive PSH angles. Yang [24] analyzed the correlation between the different scoring

systems and function within the upper limb. The Mallett score strongly correlated with both gross and fine movements showing "the first significant correlation between actual task performance and two of the three tested obstetrical brachial plexus palsy outcome measures based on the extent of movement at different joints of the upper limb." Closer analysis of hand function requires functional assessment appropriately modified to the age of the child.

Parents should be involved in the treatment of the child from the outset. Regular and gentle exercises may prevent fixed deformity (Fig. 3.10). There is no place for vigorous manipulation. If gentle stretching movements cause pain, then there must be either a fracture or a posterior dislocation of the shoulder. The role of the therapist and the attending doctor is to teach and then to monitor progress.

The extent of nerve injury is graded using the classification of Narakas [34] in cases born by cephalic presentation. This system is not applicable to the special case of the breech lesion.

Group 1

The fifth and sixth cervical nerves are damaged. There is paralysis of supraspinatus, infraspinatus, deltoid, and biceps muscles. Good recovery is seen in 90% of cases.

Group 2

The fifth, sixth, and seventh cervical nerves are damaged. About 70% of these children make a good spontaneous recovery, but there are serious residual defects in the shoulder in the remaining 30%. Recovery of the shoulder abductors and the biceps is slower than in group 1 and these muscles often remain paralyzed or weak for the first 3 months of life.

Group 3

The paralysis is virtually complete. There is some flexion of the fingers at, or shortly after, birth. Full recovery occurs in less than one-half of these children. Defective function at the shoulder, elbow, and forearm is common. Wrist and finger extension does not recover in about one-quarter.

Group 4

The paralysis is complete. The limb is flaccid together with Bernard–Horner syndrome. Few children make a good overall recovery but we have observed useful spontaneous recovery in the hand in about one-half (Fig. 3.11).

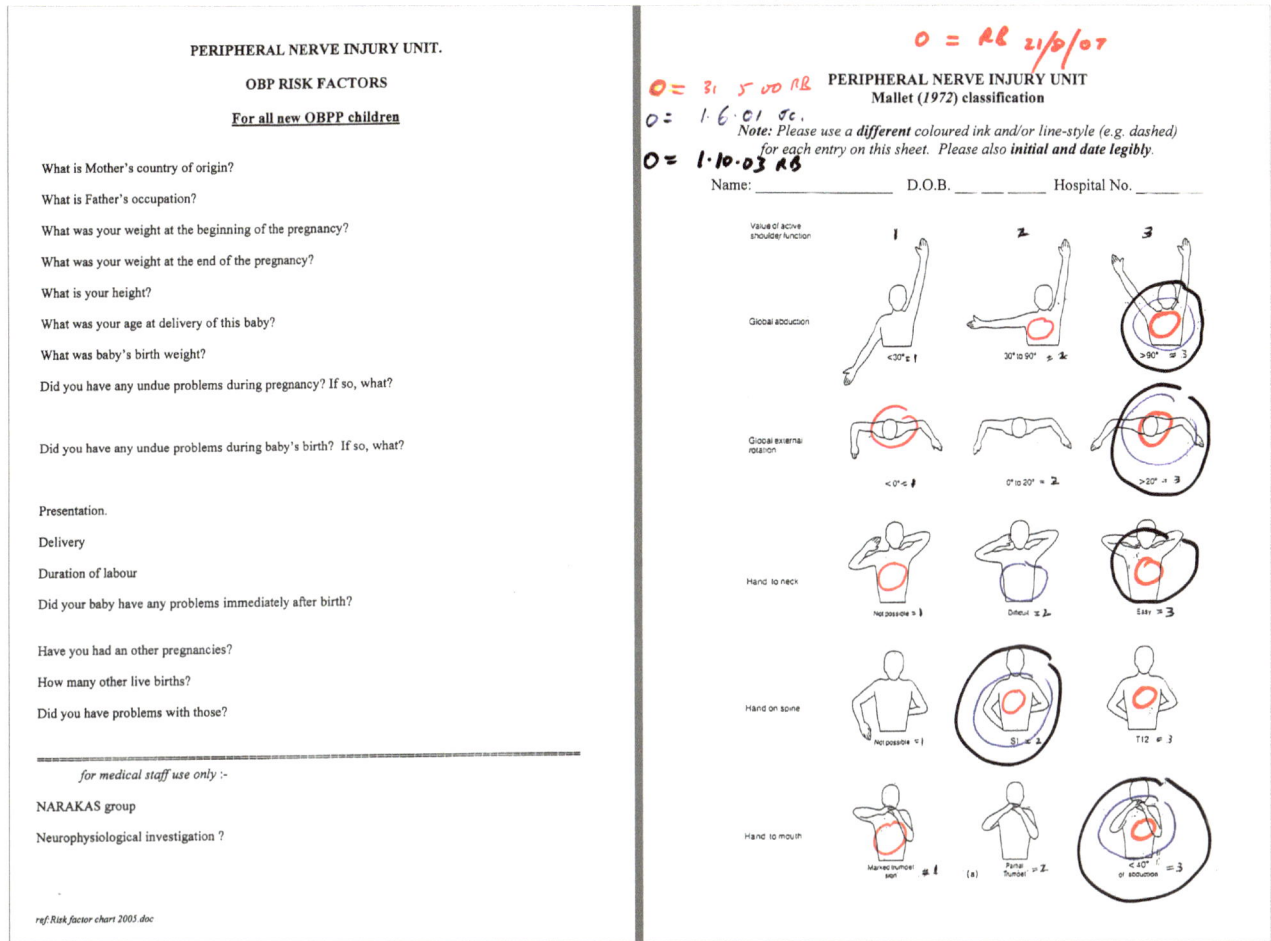

Fig. 3.7 On the left, the risk factor chart; on the right, the peripheral nerve injury Unit's modification of the Mallett system. Each entry is dated and signed by the clinician. Different colors record the dates of entry. The maximum score is 15

The Narakas classification does not recognize the rare lesion confined to C8 and T1. It may become clear that the middle nerves, C6, C7, and C8, have been severely damaged [35].

Prognosis

In favorable lesions, the parents report active grasp at 2 weeks and flexion at the shoulder and the elbow at 6–8 weeks. Return of grasp at 4 weeks virtually guarantees a useful hand. The methods of neurophysiological investigation (NPI) developed and applied by Smith [36, 37] are particularly helpful but the clinician using such information must understand the method. Nerve action potentials (NAPs) are measured from the median and ulnar nerves by stimulating at the wrist and recording at the elbow. The deltoid (C5), biceps (C6), triceps and forearm extensors (C7), forearm flexors (C8), and the first dorsal interosseous (T1) muscles are assessed by electromyography. The lesion is graded for each spinal nerve according to the degree of demyelination and axonopathy. NPI are usually pessimistic in the first weeks of life when Wallerian degeneration is at its height (Fig. 3.12). Serial NPI are reserved for cases of post-ganglionic injury of C8 and of T1 and also for some lesions of C5 where there is real doubt about progress. Bisinella [38] analyzed findings in over 350 spinal nerves in 126 children with groups 1, 2, and 3 lesions in whom elbow flexion had not recovered by the age of 3 months. Operation was undertaken in the 53 babies where poor progress was associated with unfavorable NPI grades. In these, rupture or avulsion was confirmed in at least one spinal nerve. No operation was performed in 73 children (199 nerves) with late recovery of biceps function, but with favorable NPI findings (type A or type B favorable) [38]. The predictions for recovery were matched against the clinical outcome at a mean of 4.3 years: they were confirmed in 92% of C6 and in 96% of C7 lesions. The predictions for C5 were confirmed in a smaller proportion (78%). The inability to record NAP and the high incidence of posterior dislocation (33 of 73 children) probably account for this.

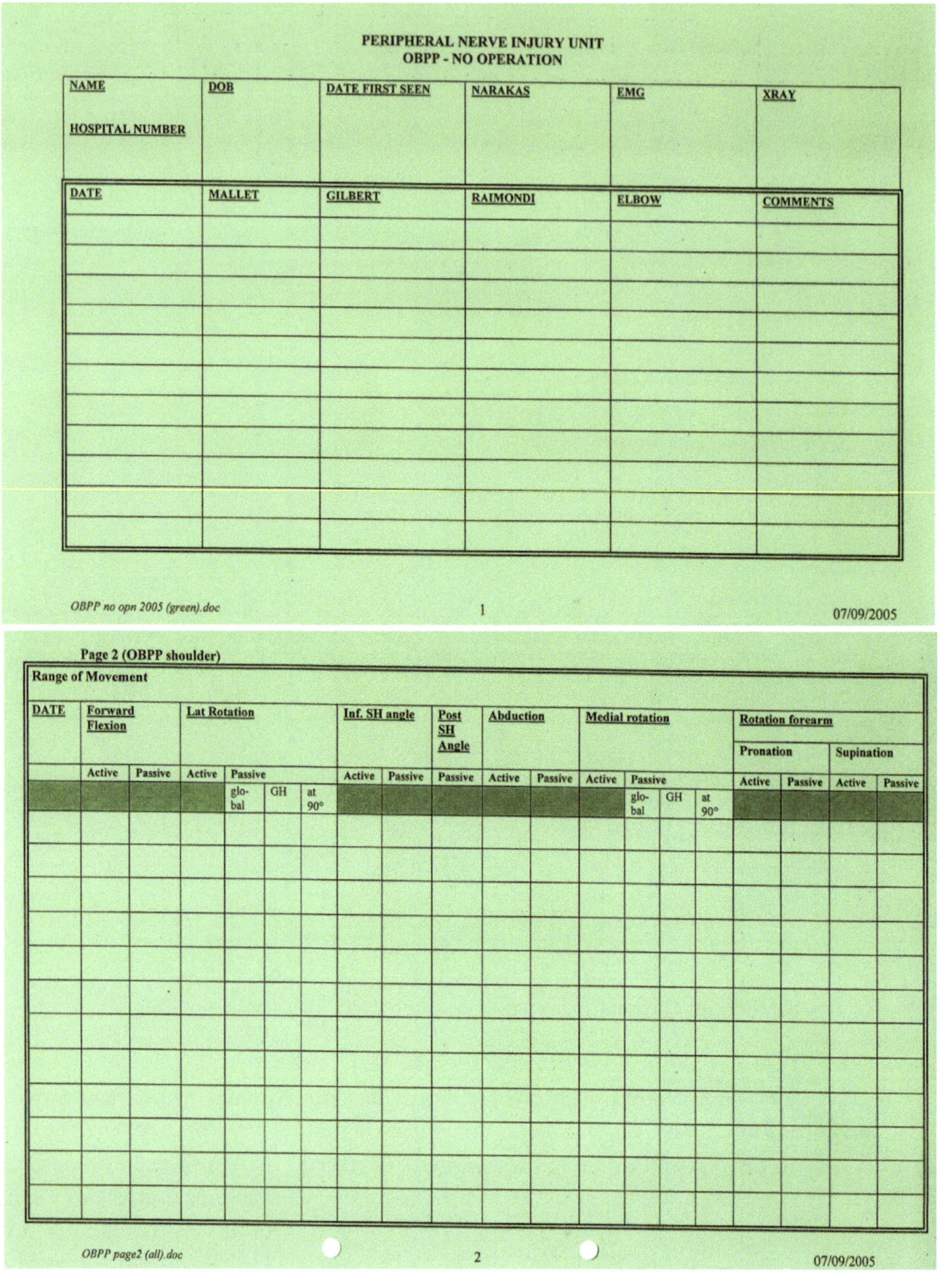

Fig. 3.8 The document used for recording progress by the Peripheral Nerve Injury Unit at the Royal National Orthopaedic Hospital

PERIPHERAL NERVE INJURY UNIT
OBPP - NO OPERATION

NAME	DOB	DATE FIRST SEEN	NARAKAS	EMG	XRAY
HOSPITAL NUMBER					

DATE	MALLET	GILBERT	RAIMONDI	ELBOW	COMMENTS

OBPP no opn 2005 (green).doc   1   07/09/2005

Page 2 (OBPP shoulder)

Range of Movement

DATE	Forward Flexion		Lat Rotation					Inf. SH angle		Post SH Angle	Abduction		Medial rotation			Rotation forearm			
																Pronation		Supination	
	Active	Passive	Active	Passive				Active	Passive	Passive	Active	Passive	Active	Passive		Active	Passive	Active	Passive
				glo-bal	GH	at 90°								glo-bal	GH	at 90°			

OBPP page2 (all).doc   2   07/09/2005

The tempo of recovery is important. Failure of biceps recovery by 3 months threatens a poor outcome [39]. Nehme et al. [40] showed that the prognosis is reliably predictable from three factors, namely birth weight, involvement of C7, and the tempo of recovery in biceps. Clark et al. [41] described a helpful scoring system which measures recovery of different segments of the limb. Combining the scores for return of elbow flexion with extension of the elbow, wrist, thumb, and fingers provides an accurate prediction of recovery. Those clinicians who rely solely on recovery of elbow flexion as a guide to prognosis for the whole limb risk serious error. Prolonged conduction block accounts for at least 15% of cases of delayed recovery of biceps function and the tearing of the muscle itself at birth explains more (Fig. 3.13) [42].

It is difficult to overstate the importance of recovery in the fifth cervical nerve. Shoulder movement is the key to function in the upper limb: far too many cases of posterior dislocation (PD) remain undetected for months or even years! The clinical appreciation of C5 recovery is greatly hindered by PD. It may be impossible to say how much lost movement is caused by the nerve injury and how much by mechanical obstruction. Operation for diagnosis and repair of the nerve lesion is justified in the following circumstances:

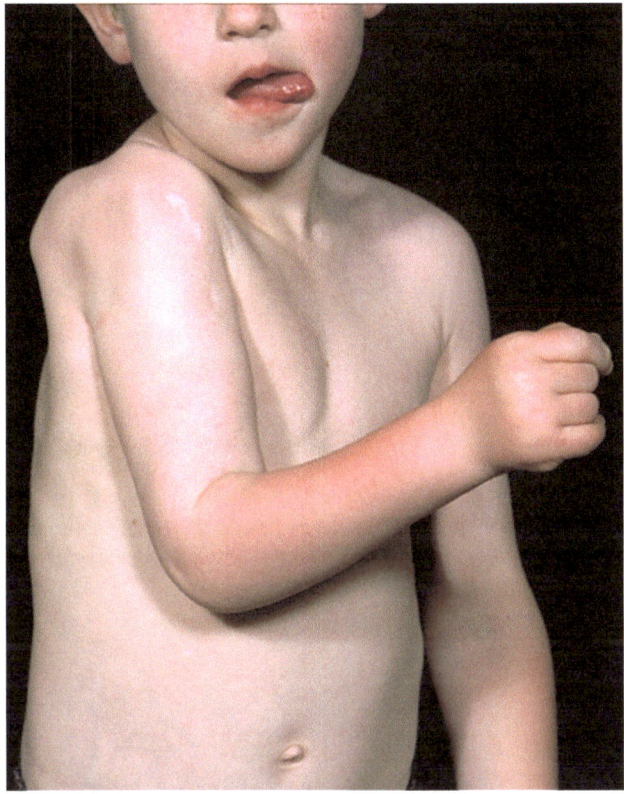

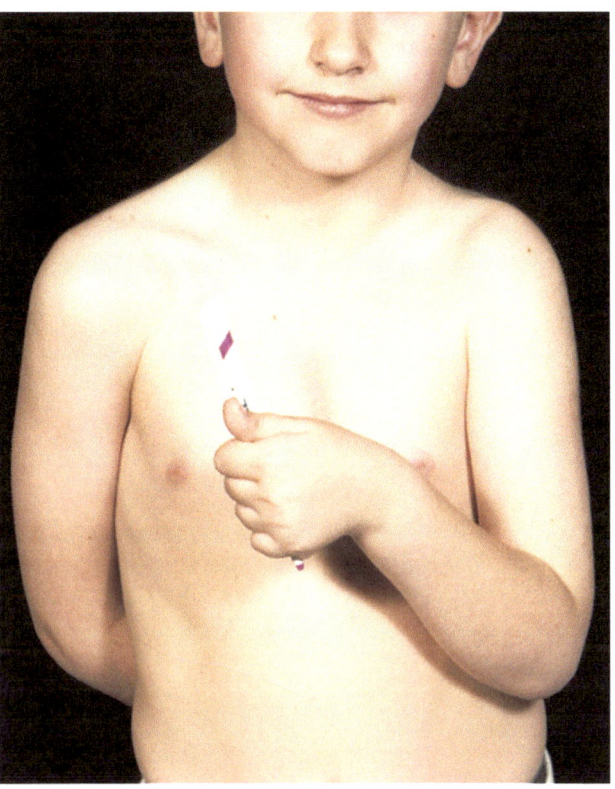

Fig. 3.9 Narrowing of the posterior scapulo-humeral angle caused by weakness of the medial rotator muscles at the shoulder

Fig. 3.11 Group 4 lesion. There was no recovery for 12 months. His parents declined operation offered at another hospital. At the age of 5 years he still has a Bernard–Horner sign. Hand function is excellent

- when failure of recovery of elevation and lateral rotation of the shoulder and of elbow flexion in groups 1, 2, and 3 by 3 months of age is accompanied by unfavorable NPI;
- group 4 lesions in which NPI and radiological evidence suggests avulsion;
- in breech lesions where there is damage to the upper cervical nerves associated with phrenic nerve palsy.

The Operation

Exposure of the brachial plexus in the infant requires a sure touch. Blunt dissection is dangerous. Scarring in the infant neck is often more severe than that seen after a closed traction lesion of the brachial plexus in the adult. After induction

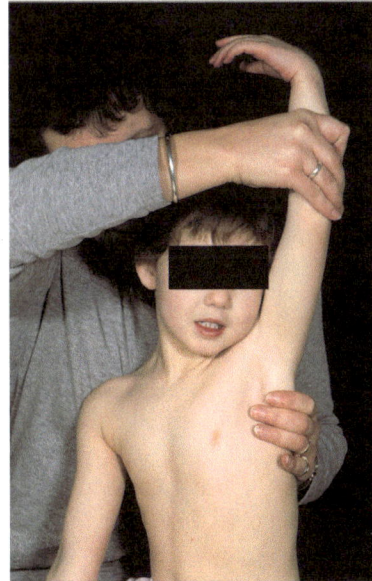

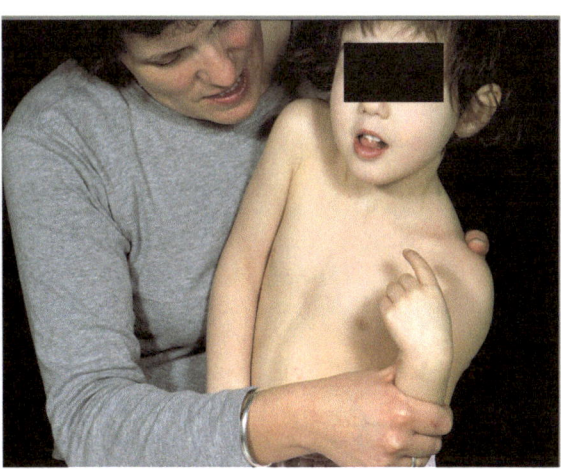

Fig. 3.10 Assiduous gentle stretching by this child's mother cured impending contractures of the shoulder and elbow. She uses one hand to block the scapula and moves the arm to open out the inferior and posterior scapulo-humeral angles

Fig. 3.12 The pre-operative analysis of lesion by Dr. Shelagh Smith was confirmed at later operation: avulsion of C5 and C6 and rupture of C7

Mixed NAP Study

	Ample (uV)	Peak Latency (ms)
Median		
Right	21	2.5
Left	24	2.4
Ulnar		
Right	5	2.6
Left	Nil seen (artefact ++)	

EMG (CNE)

Right Deltoid, Right Biceps – Small numbers of fibrillations sparse units, normal morphology, 0.2-0.5 mV.

Right Forearm extensor group – fibrillations ++. Reduced pattern, broad units firing in isolation at high rates, 1 mV.

Right Forearm flexor group, Right IDIO – No spontaneous activity. Normal units and pattern, 1-2mV.

Comments:

Median nerve action potentials are symmetrical. The right ulnar NAP is small (unfortunately, comparison with the unaffected nerve is not possible for technical reasons).

EMG findings in deltoid and biceps suggest severe axonal injury for C5 and C6, likely be pre-ganglionic in the context of the normal median NAP.
Similar EMG findings are seen in forearm extensor group, but early recover is evident.
The pattern in C8 and T1, myotomes is relatively normal.

Prediction

C5 and 6 - type C, pre-ganglionic.
C7   - unfavourable type B.
C8 and T1 - recovering.

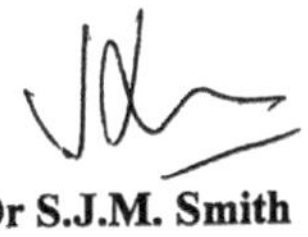

Dr S.J.M. Smith
Consultant in Clinical Neurophysiology

of anesthesia, recording electrodes are attached to the skin of the scalp and the neck. Somatosensory evoked potentials (SSEP) are recorded from the median and ulnar nerves at both wrists. The whole of the upper limb and one lower limb are prepared. A transverse supraclavicular incision is made, and the platysma is reflected with the skin flaps. The exposure is developed in the plane between the external jugular vein (medial) and the supraclavicular nerves (lateral). The omohyoid muscle and the fat pad are reflected. The external jugular, suprascapular, and transverse cervical veins are ligated with great care because of the proximity of the subclavian vein. The phrenic nerve is often deviated laterally and involved in the neuroma of the upper and middle trunks: it must be protected. The fifth and sixth cervical nerves are traced, then the middle trunk is displayed. Transection of scalenus anterior is needed to expose C8 and T1 and the subclavian artery requires careful handling. The clavicle should not be cut because of the risk of nonunion, instead the bone can be drawn up or down by a nylon tape. The findings for each spinal nerve are recorded and classified. Their

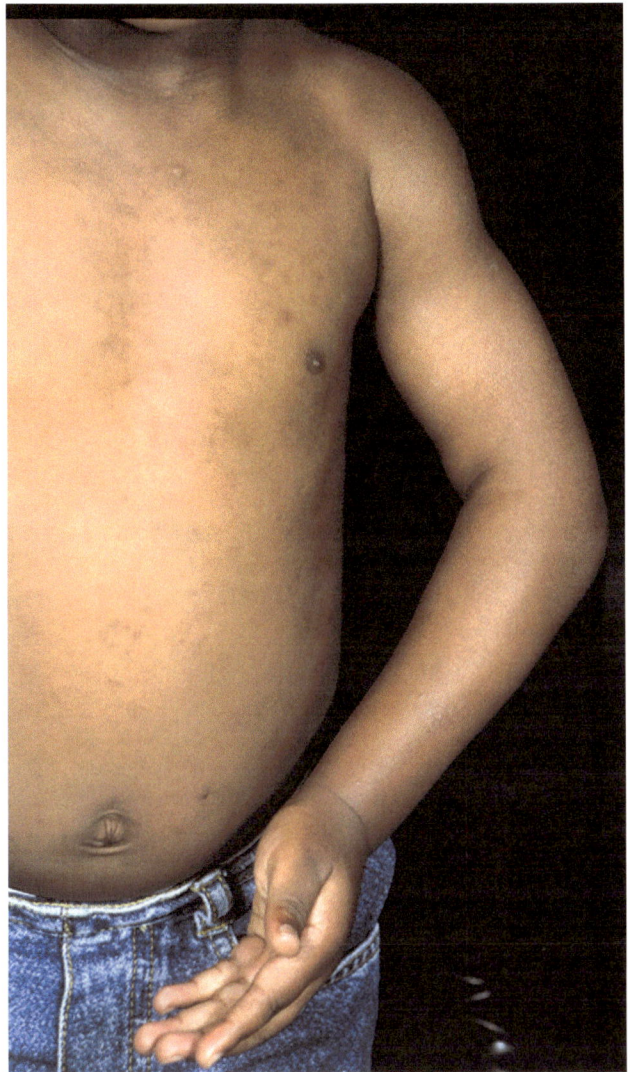

Fig. 3.13 A 9-year-old boy presenting with posterior dislocation of the shoulder and "pseudotumor" of the biceps muscle

It is worth emphasizing that the outlook for avulsed spinal nerves has been transformed by two important ideas from Gilbert [43]. In cases where rupture of the upper nerves is associated with avulsion of the lower nerves, the avulsed C8 and T1 nerves are re-innervated by one or two of the post-ganglionic stumps at C5 and C6 (intra-plexal transfer). The second concept is particularly elegant. Selective re-innervation of the ventral root of an avulsed spinal nerve is achieved by transfer of a healthy nerve, the spinal accessory, or lateral or medial pectoral nerve. I first used extraplexal transfer to an avulsed ventral root in an adult case in 1992 [33] and adopted the method in BLBP at the suggestion of Gilbert [43].

Results of Repair of the Nerves

Striking recovery of sensation and proof of central plasticity were demonstrated in a study of 24 group 4 cases [44]. The lesions to the spinal nerves included 47 avulsions, 58 ruptures, and 12 lesions in continuity. Recovery of sensibility greatly exceeded that of skeletal muscle and cholinergic sympathetic function. There was perfect localization in the dermatomes of avulsed spinal nerves which had been re-innervated by transfer of the intercostal nerves from remote spinal segments. Useful hand function was seen in just over one-half of the repaired cases. This degree of plasticity in the immature central nervous system may be a factor in the remarkable absence of neuropathic pain in BLBP, quite unlike the situation after a traction lesion in the adult. The results following grafts of ruptures are variable. In a prospective study of 100 repairs [31], a strong correlation between the pre-operative NPI and the findings at operation was found. The prediction of type C was confirmed in 177 of 191 spinal nerves. These nerves were ruptured or avulsed. Results were good in more than one-half of repair of the avulsed eighth cervical and first thoracic nerves. Extension of the wrist and fingers was regained in only one-third of the repairs of the seventh cervical nerve. A good result was seen in only one-third of repairs of the fifth cervical nerve. The outcome was worse in the 30 children who came to open reduction of PD.

It is futile to attach grafts onto poor stumps. Combined lesions of post-ganglionic rupture with an intradural component are better treated by extraplexal transfer. Every reasonable effort must be made to display avulsion, so allowing selective re-innervation of the ventral root and of the dorsal component of the spinal nerve. The undisplaced avulsion remains an enigma. Some of these recover. We leave them alone.

appearance and texture are noted. Evidence of conduction is gathered by stimulating proximal to the lesion and recording from the scalp, by proximal stimulation and noting muscle response, and by stimulation distal to the lesion and recorded from the scalp, again noting muscle response. Ruptures are repaired by nerve grafting; the small proportions of the infant make it a difficult matter to secure adequate donor nerve. The injured upper limb provides the medial and lateral cutaneous nerve of the forearm and the superficial radial nerve, which is sufficient for repairs of two ruptured spinal nerves. The sural nerve is needed for more extensive repairs and sometimes both are required. After closure of the wound the repair is protected by a plaster of Paris jacket which immobilizes the head and the affected arm.

Fig. 3.14 A 17-year-old girl who required open reduction of PD at the age of 2 years. The left clavicle is 10 cm in length and the right 13 cm. The left vertebral border of scapula is 10 cm in length, the right, 11 cm

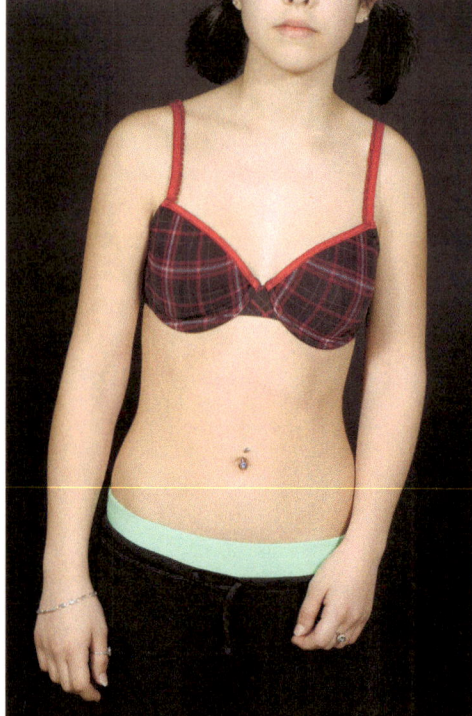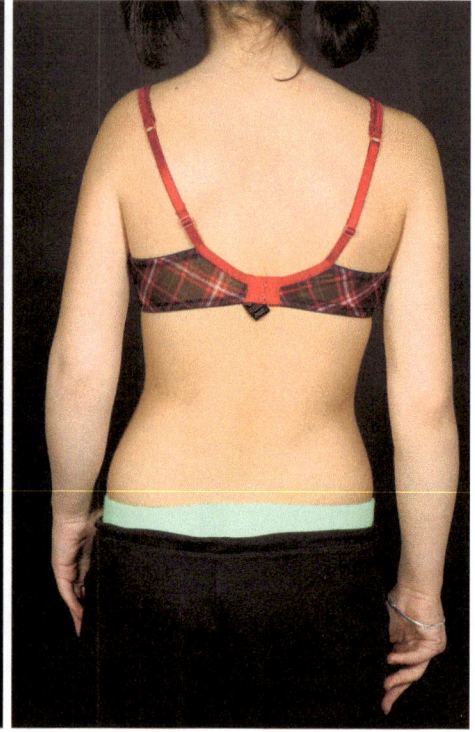

Fig. 3.15 On the left, the radiograph of the shoulder in a 10-year-old boy who had a forcible attempt at closed reduction under general anesthetic 8 years previously in another hospital. On the right, radiographs of dislocation of the elbow after over-zealous proximal advancement of the flexor origin performed in another institution

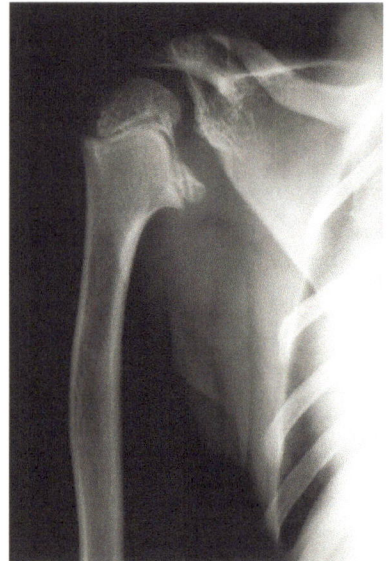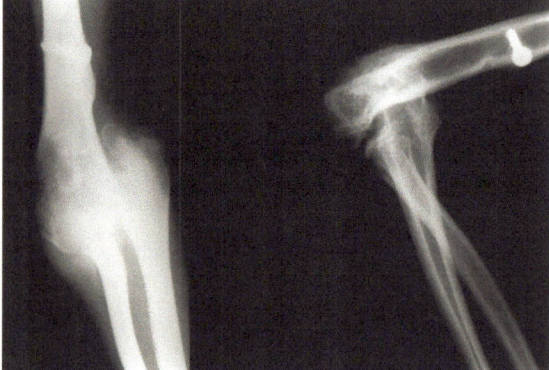

Deformity

There are four chief causes of deformity associated with BLBP:

(1) Direct damage to the skeleton and soft tissues is inflicted during a protracted and difficult delivery. Much fibrosis about the shoulder is caused during such deliveries and damage to the biceps muscle is not uncommon.

(2) There is atrophy of denervated target organs. Bone growth is impaired in all but the mildest cases of BLBP. Shortening of the clavicle, probably caused by paralysis of the clavicular head of pectoralis major may lead to serious problems at the shoulder (Fig. 3.14). The clavicle is the tie beam of the forequarter and when it is shortened it pulls the scapula forward; this pulls the acromion downward and forward and elevates its supero-medial border. The coracoid and coraco-acromial ligaments are displaced dorsally and impinge on the anterior aspect of

the head of humerus. The acromio-clavicular joint may dislocate.

(3) There is persisting muscular imbalance from incomplete neurological recovery. Imbalance between the weak lateral and the strong medial rotator muscles contributes to many shoulder dislocations. Poor medial rotation of the shoulder, a supinated forearm, ulnar deviation at wrist, and adduction of the thumb are common after a middle segment (C7, C8) lesion. Paralysis of the small muscles of the hand leads to an intractable extension deformity of the metacarpophalangeal joints.

(4) Then come the deformities provoked by treatment. Over-zealous manipulation of the incongruent shoulder damages the head of humerus and the glenoid. Incorrect muscle transfers replace one imbalance with another. Damage to the medial epicondyle during proximal advancement of the flexor muscles leads to dislocation of the elbow (Fig. 3.15). It must be restated that arthrodesis in a growing skeleton must never be performed until muscle imbalance has been corrected. The normal course of maturation of hand function and the development of limb dominance have been well described [45, 46].

Posterior Dislocation of the Shoulder

More than 500 cases have been operated upon in our unit over the last 20 years and we estimate that 100 new cases of PD occur in association with BLBP each year in the British Isles. Although the deformity may progress from a medial rotation contracture to subluxation and from there to dislocation, about one-quarter of dislocations occur at or shortly after birth. Another 50% develop during the period of neurological recovery. It is difficult to account for those cases presenting after recovery has stabilized. Fairbank [47] described the deformity and offered a logical operation which involved osteotomy of the coracoid, division of the subscapularis tendon, and anterior capsulotomy. Scaglietti [48] reported Putti's work. He considered that epiphysiolysis was common and that this contributed to retroversion of the head upon the shaft of humerus; Putti [49] also drew an analogy between the shoulder and the hip joint: "the aplasia of the glenoid corresponds exactly to that of the acetabulum in cases of congenital dislocation of the hip joint."

Valuable recent studies confirm the high incidence of incongruity at the gleno-humeral joint and the early onset of deformity of the glenoid [50–54]. Our prospective study [55] of 183 consecutive cases of PD in children with good neurological recovery, operated upon in the years 1995–2000 recorded 47 dislocations occurring at or soon after birth.

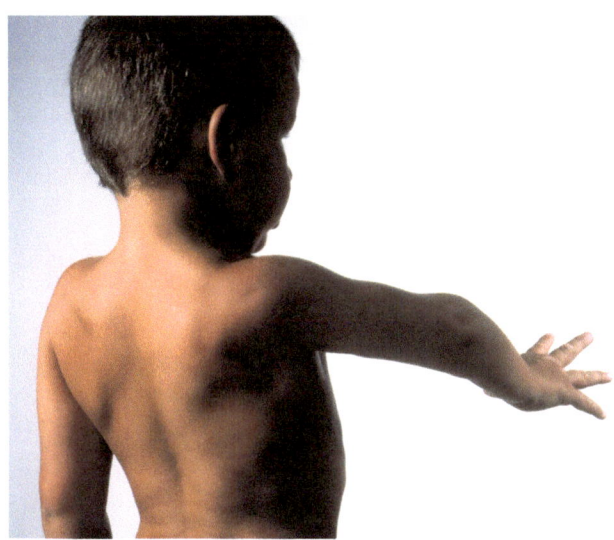

Fig. 3.16 Posterior dislocation in a 3-year-old boy

Dislocation occurred while the children were under observation in 25 shoulders and seven more children had been discharged with normal or near normal function.

Diagnosis is straightforward for the alert clinician. Palpation of the shoulder reveals dislocation in the infant. The posture of the limb, the awkward elevation of the shoulder with fixed medial rotation tells all in the older child (Fig. 3.16). Antero-posterior and axial radiographs confirm the diagnosis. Magnetic resonance imaging (MRI) is reserved for cases of unusual complexity.

It is useful to distinguish between subluxation and dislocation. In subluxation the articulation is between the head and the postero-inferior facet of the glenoid, which is lined with hyaline cartilage. In dislocation, the head lies in a distended capsular pocket adherent to the dorsal face of the scapula, and the articulation is between the hyaline cartilage of the head, the intervening capsule, and the underlying cortex of the scapula. "Telescoping" of the head of the humerus from subluxation to dislocation during forward flexion at the shoulder is a frequent finding in older children.

The Operation

The skin of the shoulder is infiltrated with local anesthetica before incisions. Interscalene block of the brachial plexus is forbidden because of the risk to the spinal cord. The shoulder is exposed through a delto-pectoral incision, which may be extended to permit exposure of the anterior shaft of humerus. Although the deltoid and pectoralis major muscles usually appear well innervated, it is common to find scarring between and deep in them. The coracoid, which is long,

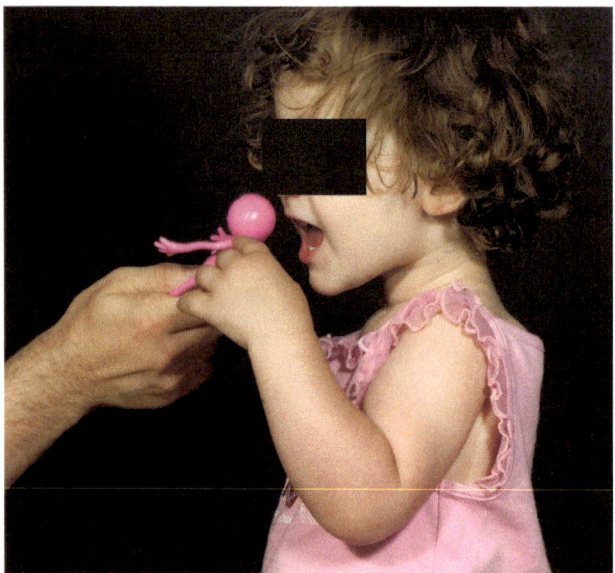

Fig. 3.17 Function 18 months after reduction of posterior dislocation with glenoplasty

rotation of the distal fragment is indicated when retroversion exceeds 40° and it is done with two objects in mind:

1. to improve stability at the shoulder after reduction
2. to ensure an adequate range of medial rotation.

The shaft of the humerus is exposed between the deltoid and the pectoralis major, preserving the upper one-quarter of the pectoralis tendon as guardian of the growth plate. A small plate is applied, the angle of rotation planned and marked by appropriate screw holes. The plate, held by one proximal screw, is rotated out of the way and the bone divided. The distal fragment is rotated medially and fixed to the plate with the planned medial rotation.

We now add glenoplasty if the head is still unstable after reduction. The posterior face of the scapula is displayed between the infraspinatus and the teres minor. The reduced head of humerus leaves behind redundant capsule which is elevated from the posterior face of the scapula. A radial incision permits identification of the posterior labrum and the edge of the hyaline cartilage of the inferior (false) facet. The posterior and the inferior rim of the glenoid is elevated by fine osteotomes and molded against the reduced humeral head. The gap is wedged open with the excised piece of the coracoid. The flap consists of the posterior inferior labrum, the inferior socket of the glenoid, and the overlying capsule. (Figs. 3.17 and 3.18) After wound closure the shoulder is protected by a plaster of Paris jacket which holds the arm in no more than 30° of abduction and no more than 45° of lateral rotation at the shoulder. The splint is retained for 6 weeks. Radiographs are taken 1 year and again 3 years after operation.

and lies vertically, is shortened to its base after releasing the coraco-acromial and coraco-humeral ligaments. A step elongation of the subscapularis muscle is done preserving as much of the anterior capsule as possible. This muscle is often fibrosed, especially in birth dislocations or after an earlier subscapularis slide. The head of humerus is now re-located. The subscapularis flaps are repaired as strongly as possible.

Retroversion of the head upon the shaft of the humerus is measured. This is the angle subtended between the coronal plane of the head and that between the lateral and medial epicondyles. Osteotomy of the shaft of the humerus with medial

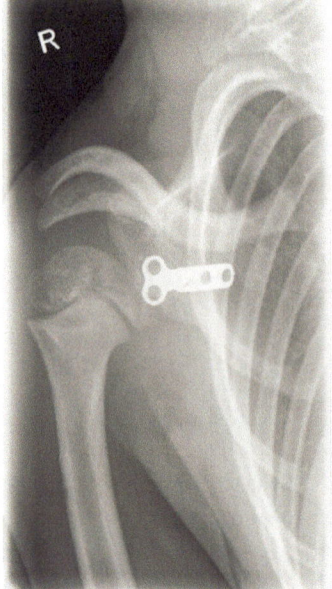
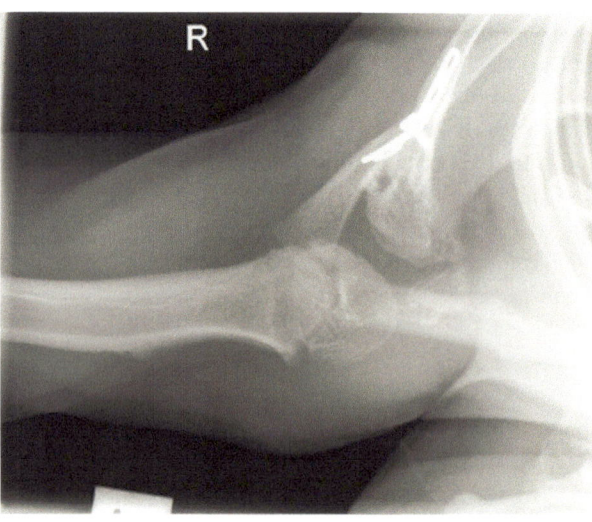

Fig. 3.18 AP and axial radiographs of the child shown in Fig. 3.17

Prolonged follow-up is essential. Dislocation recurred in 20 of the 183 children. These failures were seen in older children who showed advanced secondary deformities of the head of humerus, of the glenoid and, also of the acromio-clavicular arch. The surgeon presented with a long-standing dislocation may feel justified in advising the child, by now an adolescent, and his or her parents that it is better not to intervene. Set against this is the pain and rapid deterioration of function which led to the presentation of 24 young adults with untreated PD.

Clinicians engaged in work with these children must treat the whole child and must be alert to the significance of contractures at the shoulder, above all to restriction of lateral rotation, which usually signifies an incongruent gleno-humeral joint. These children must be observed to skeletal maturity. The early onset of a glenoid abnormality casts a shadow over the attractive idea of temporary paralysis of the medial rotators by botulinum toxin. The impressive work of Pearl et al. [56] opens the prospect of correcting medial rotation contracture and even early subluxation by arthroscopic release and muscle transfer. Nath and Paizi [57] have developed an elegant operation to deal with the deformity of the acromio-clavicular joint: the spine of the scapula and the clavicle are divided, so that the bone flap migrates upward and backward, opening out the acromio-clavicular arch. This method may contribute to the successful reduction of complex dislocations in children up to the age of about 7 years.

Lesions of the Peripheral Nerves

Most children's nerve injuries occur in the upper limb (Table 3.1). Too many are caused during treatment, usually during operation for fracture and joint injury, for "cysts" or other tumors, or during operations to correct fixed deformity. It is particularly disappointing to see cases of avoidable post-ischemic fibrosis. These iatrogenic cases account for one-third of the whole; the number of such cases continues to increase. Although the results of repair of distal nerves are generally fairly good, those following repair of the brachial plexus are rather worse than those seen in the adult. Young children ignore the insensate hand. The effect on foot posture of irreparable tibial or common peroneal nerve lesions is severe. (Fig. 3.19)

Table 3.1 Number of nerves operated in children in age from 6 months to 15 Years 1979–2007

Upper limb		Lower limb	
Cause	Number of operated cases	Nerve	Number of operated cases
Fractures and dislocations	274	Lumbosacral plexus	4
Tidy wounds	103	Femoral	3
Brachial plexus lesions	34	Sciatic	12
Cutaneous sensory nerves	39	Common peroneal	35
–	–	Tibial	9
–	–	Cutaneous sensory	26
TOTAL	450	–	89

Data assembled by Mr. Hesham Al-Khateeb, FRCS. Some of this is discussed elsewhere [69, 70]. More than 150 other children coming to operation for correction of fixed deformity or for palliation by musculo-tendinous transfer are excluded. The lesions were inflicted during treatment in one third of cases

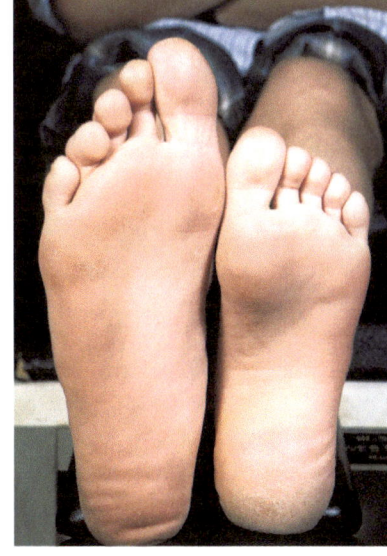
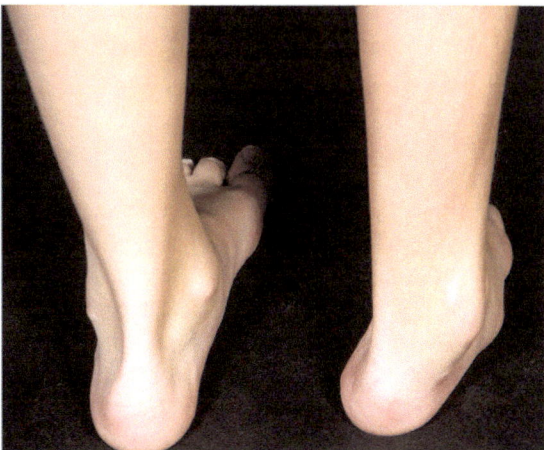

Fig. 3.19 On the *left*, the foot of a 9-year-old boy 5 years after failed repair of the tibial nerve. The painful cavus deformity was corrected by posterior transfer of tibialis anterior. On the *right*, equinovarus deformity seen 4 years after repair of sciatic nerve in a 7-year-old girl. Recovery for the common peroneal division of the sciatic nerve was poor

The surgeon must be alert to the need for muscle rebalancing operations to prevent fixed deformity in the growing skeleton and look out for progressive deformity caused by such transfers.

Diagnosis

Examination of the distressed child is not easy and is restricted if the limb is encased in plaster of Paris or other splint. It is helpful for the clinician to try to distinguish between lesions of conduction block (neurapraxia) from cases where Wallerian degeneration is occurring, the degenerative lesions of axonotmesis, or neurotmesis. The history is all important. Violent injury produces deep nerve lesions. If a nerve is not working and if there is a wound over the course of that nerve, then it is probably divided. If a nerve stops working after a surgeon has been near it with knife, scissors, or drill in hand, then that probability becomes near certainty.

A diagnosis of conduction block (neurapraxia) should be made with caution and reserved for cases where light touch sensation and the sudo- and vasomotor functions of the postganglionic sympathetic efferent fibers are preserved. One almost infallible sign is present in the first 24 h after transection of a nerve with a cutaneous sensory component: because the small as well as the large fibers are affected, the skin in the distribution of the affected nerve is warm and dry. This is particularly helpful in the diagnosis of severe lesions of the tibial, the median, and the ulnar nerves and also of the cutaneous branches of those nerves. Neuropathic pain is the most important symptom. It can be distinguished from fracture pain by irradiation into the territory of the nerve and by spontaneous abnormal or unpleasant sensory symptoms. Allodynia is a cardinal sign of serious nerve injury. It usually indicates that the noxious agent is still at work. A stimulus which is not normally painful produces pain: the child flinches when the hand or the foot is gently touched. In extreme cases, no examination of the affected part is tolerated.

Tinel's sign, when properly elicited and monitored, is an invaluable aid to the diagnosis of the depth of the injury and to the extent of regeneration. Children from the age of 4 years are very good witnesses. The examiner should explain to the child what is being done, emphasizing that it is not painful. The child is asked to say when the percussing finger, which moves from distal to proximal along the course of the nerve to be examined, induces "funny feelings" or "tingles" or "pins and needles" into the distribution of that nerve. The level of the Tinel sign is measured from a fixed bony point and recorded in the case notes. A positive Tinel sign advises

the clinician that the axons have been torn. The clinician is now in a position to ascertain the prognosis for recovery by repeating the examination at regular intervals over the next 4 weeks. If the Tinel sign remains static, recovery is unlikely. If the centrifugally progressing Tinel sign is stronger than that at the level of lesion, recovery will probably be good. If the static Tinel sign remains stronger than the advancing sign then partial transection of the nerve or the presence of an agent which is impeding regeneration is likely. In favorable degenerative lesions (axonotmesis) Tinel's sign progresses by at least 3 mm a day in the proximal part of the limb and by about 2 mm a day in the forearm and leg.

Many fracture services are poorly supported by neurophysiological investigative work, but it has to be said that timely studies of nerve conduction provide useful evidence. Electromyography is rarely necessary in the child. Conduction block (neurapraxia) is confirmed by the demonstration of persisting conduction in the nerve trunk distal to the level of the lesion at an interval of 2 weeks or more from injury. Demonstration of conduction across the lesion at any time from the day of injury proves that at least some nerve fibers are intact. I have no personal experience with ultrasound examination of the injured limb but suspect that this investigation will prove valuable to the clinician seeking confirmation of rupture or continuity of a nerve trunk or adjacent axial vessel within hours of injury.

Seddon [58] offered sound advice about the treatment of nerves injured in the arm and at the elbow. Recovery may be awaited if two conditions are met: "the first is reasonable apposition of the bony fragments and the other is *complete certainty that there is no threat of ischemia of the forearm muscles*" (original italics). The prognosis for spontaneous recovery for nerves injured in the lower limb is worse than it is in the upper limb. Of injuries to the sciatic nerve Seddon said "it is wise always to explore the nerve." Kato [59] found that spontaneous recovery was good in most cases of lesions of median and ulnar nerves caused by closed fractures or dislocations but that spontaneous recovery was very much worse for the common peroneal nerve damaged by closed injuries to the knee. The clinician will usually find it necessary to use nerve grafting in the repair of trunk nerves which have been ruptured by traction. The gaps between the stumps of the common peroneal and tibial nerves may be so reduced by flexion of the knee joint that direct suture is possible but the suture line must be protected for up to 12 weeks, gradually restoring extension at the knee by serial plaster of Paris splints.

It seems best to expose nerves damaged by fractures or by dislocations in the following circumstances: the injury requires open reduction and internal fixation; there is associated vascular injury; wound exploration of an open fracture is necessary; the nerve lesion deepens while under observation; and the nerve lesion has occurred during operation for open reduction and internal fixation. Many iatrogenic nerve lesions will be prevented or corrected urgently, if these principles are followed. Nerves and arteries become entrapped within fractures or dislocations; they are displaced by the fracture hematoma. The ulnar nerve is vulnerable to compression from hematoma in the cubital tunnel, the common peroneal nerve is similarly vulnerable at the neck of the fibula.

The Arterial Lesion

"The catastrophe of tissue necrosis after injury or surgery need never occur if complaints of undue pain in an extremity are investigated," wrote Harkess (Figs. 3.20 and 3.21) [60] Some clinicians persist in the belief that oxygenation of muscle and nerve enclosed within rigid osseo-fascial compartments can be assessed by noting return of circulation to the nail bed. Others persist with the notion that compartment syndrome is a distinct entity from the anoxia caused by interruption of flow through an axial artery. Both of these ideas are false; both were, or should have been, confined to dishonorable rest many years ago. In ischemia the final common pathway is the same: anoxia causes break down of homeostasis across the membrane of the cells of the capillaries, muscles, Schwann cells, and axons. Klenerman's [61] annotation on compartment syndrome is compulsive reading. The earliest symptom of peripheral ischemia is pain, often so intense that it does not respond to morphine. Alteration in sensibility in the extremity soon follows. The earliest fibers to suffer are the largest, those conveying proprioception and vibration sense. Deepening of sensory loss and the first signs of muscle weakness are proof positive of critical ischemia. One effect of anoxia is to increase the permeability of the capillary membrane, so that the true ischemia caused by cessation of arterial supply is added to the one caused by the rising pressure within the fascial compartments.

Perhaps it is time to replace the much misused term "critical ischemia" with the grading system for ischemia developed by The Society for Vascular Surgery and the International Society of Cardiovascular Surgery [62]. Class 2A describes a limb which is threatened, in which symptoms are limited to a mild sensory loss. Class 2B limbs are immediately at risk: there is pronounced sensory loss, mild-to-moderate motor loss and for these delay is unacceptable even with audible Doppler signals.

Those surgeons inclined to a complacent view of the loss of peripheral pulses complicating supracondylar fracture in child might care to consider Poiseuille's law which describes the volume of flow through a cylindrical tube. Among other factors volume is governed by the radius of the tube to the

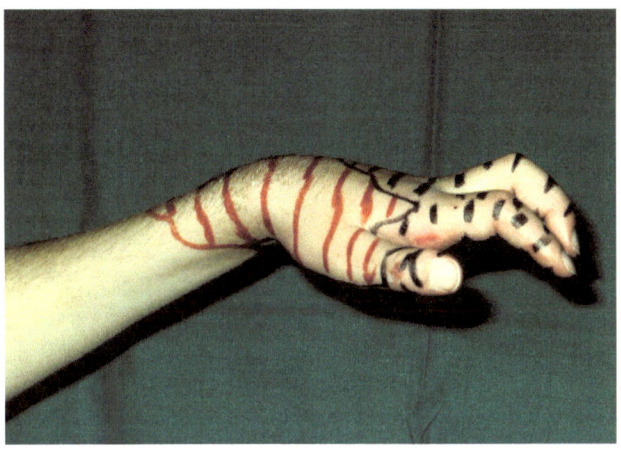

Fig. 3.20 Volkmann's ischemic contracture 10 weeks after supracondylar fracture in a 7-year-old boy. The fracture was "fixed" by Kirschner wires without exposing the brachial artery and median nerve which were entrapped within the fracture. His post-operative pain was ignored. All three nerves were involved. Black indicates complete loss of sensation; red indicates partial loss of sensation

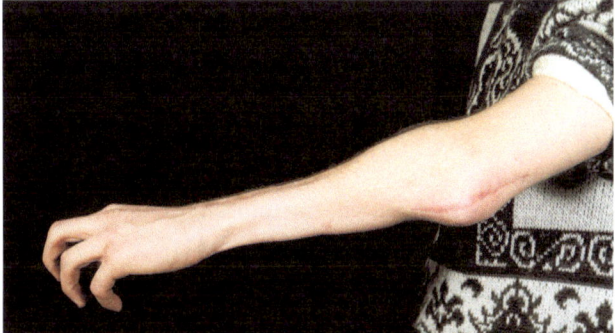

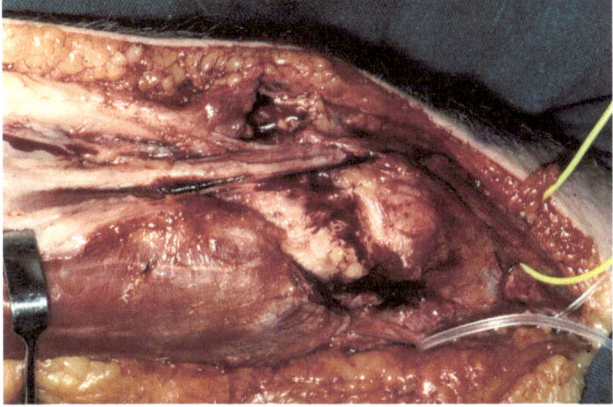

Fig. 3.21 Above: Recurrence of deformity 4 years after flexor muscle slide when the boy was aged 8 years. Below: The ulnar nerve exposed during this operation is narrowed and ischemic as it enters the infarcted muscle

power of 4 (R^4). The diameter of the brachial artery in 10-year-old children has been measured at 2.5–3 mm and resting flow is 200 ml per minute. If arterial flow is restricted to the collateral vessels running with the radial and ulnar nerves at the elbow, of a diameter of about 1 mm, then flow to forearm and hand may drop to as low as 20 ml per minute [63]. The pressure gradient is very important: Burton and Yamada [64] advise that "At a transmural pressure well above the critical closing pressure, the flow is proportional to the driving pressure but as the pressure is lowered, the flow decreases quite abruptly, to become zero at the critical closing pressure." The best advice comes from Atholl Parkes [65]: "in the absence of peripheral arterial pulses take immediate steps to relieve possible pressure on the main artery by reducing any displaced fracture or dislocation and, if still necessary, exploring the artery. With failing nerve or muscle function in a tensely swollen limb, do not be deceived by the presence of a good peripheral pulse—consider immediate decompression." Exposure of the brachial artery and of the median nerve at the elbow is, or should be, a simple enough matter. I have performed this in over 50 cases of supracondylar fracture in children. No brachial artery was ruptured, instead, they were entrapped in the fracture or compressed by hematoma. After decompression of the artery it is bathed in papaverine. It is gratifying to see the vessel dilating with the return of pulsatile flow after an interval of a few minutes. However, there have been reports of transection of the artery or of thrombosis after tearing of the intima. Repair of the brachial artery in a child is a very testing operation. Faulty technique fails. The wisest course is to involve an experienced arterial surgeon for the operation.

Pain

Neurostenalgia [66] is that pain caused by persistent compression, distortion, or ischemia and it is not uncommon in children (Fig. 3.22). The nerve is intact but is afflicted by an active, noxious agent. It is common when nerves are entrapped within fractures or joints, or when they are strangled in a swollen compartment. Causalgia is rare in children and this may account for the erroneous diagnosis of the so-called complex regional pain syndrome (CRPS) which leads to some children being subjected to protracted courses of treatment by medication or by various forms of nerve block which do not relieve the pain and which inflict physical and psychological harm (Fig. 3.23). The pathophysiological basis of CRPS is unsound. CRPS type 1 assumes no injury to a peripheral nerve. This has been discounted by Oaklander [67] who demonstrated extensive axonopathy and demyelination in cases so labeled. These findings have been confirmed by other investigators. CRPS type 2 is deeply unsatisfactory, for it is so wide-reaching as to be meaningless. The cardinal diagnostic features of causalgia include severe, intractable pain expressed throughout the limb; worsening of that pain by examination, by noise, and

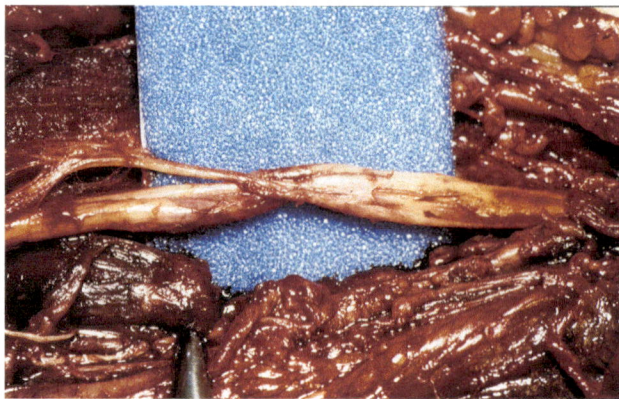

Fig. 3.22 Neurostenalgia. Mr. James MacLean (Perth) extricated this median nerve, which was entrapped in a distal fracture of humerus. The operation was done after 2 days because of pain complicating a deep median palsy. Pain was abolished; there was full recovery of the nerve

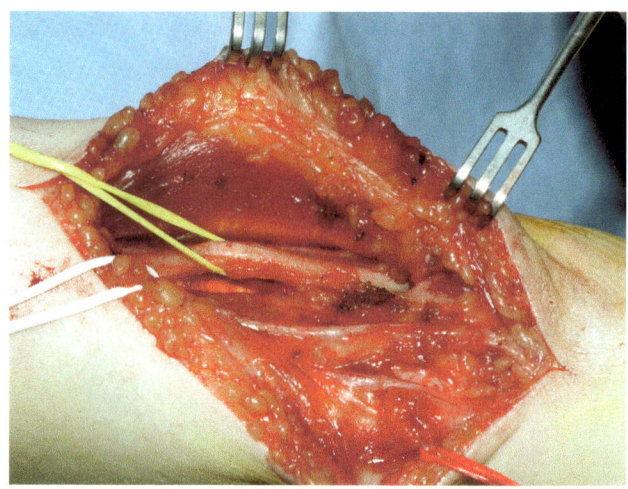

Fig. 3.23 Post-traumatic neuralgia. A branch of the dorsal cutaneous ulnar nerve was damaged during arthroscopy of the wrist in a 12-year-old girl. She developed intense pain which did not respond to a protracted course of analgesic and anti-depressant drugs. Psychological assessment revealed deterioration in cognitive skills, spatial skills, information processing accuracy, and auditory and working memories. Her reading and spelling skills declined. A request for further opinion from her educational psychologist and her mother was met with resistance but her family practitioner insisted on an urgent review. She was seen at 14 months after her first operation and the nerves were exposed 2 days later. The ulnar nerve was decompressed and a damaged branch of the dorsal cutaneous branch of the ulnar nerve was implanted into muscle. There was early relief of pain, improvement in hand function, and improvement in her psychological health

by other disturbance; vaso- and sudo-motor instability; and intense mechanical allodynia [68].

Causalgia follows incomplete transection of the lower trunk or the medial cord of the brachial plexus or the median and ulnar nerves in the upper limb, or of the tibial division of the sciatic nerve in the lower limb and is frequently associated with arterial injury or hematoma. Cure is almost always achieved by correcting the lesion of the nerve and artery. The clinician presented with a child with severe neuropathic pain must take every reasonable step to exclude a continuing provocation of that nerve before consigning that child to a pain clinic.

References

1. Bennet GC, Harrold AJ. Prognosis and early management of birth injuries to the brachial plexus. Br Med J 1976; 1:1520–1521.
2. Wickstrom J, Haslam ET, Hutchinson RH. The surgical management of residual deformities of the shoulder following birth injuries of the brachial plexus. J Bone Joint Surg 1958; 47A:27–36.
3. Tassin JL. Paralyses obstétricales du plexus brachial, evolution spontanée, resultats des interventions reparatrices precrées. Thése 1984, Université Paris VIII.
4. Gilbert A, Tassin JL. Réparation chirurgicale du plexus brachial dans la paralysie obstétricale. Chirurgie 1984; 110:76–75.
5. Gilbert A, Brockman R, Carlioz H. Surgical treatment of brachial plexus birth palsy. Clin Orth 1989; 264:39–47.
6. Gilbert A, Whitaker I. Obstetrical brachial plexus lesions. J Hand Surg 1991; 16B:489–491.
7. Dailiana ZH, Mehdian H, Gilbert A. Surgical anatomy of spinal accessory nerve: is trapezius functional deficit inevitable after division of the nerve? J Hand Surg Br 2001; 26(2):137–141.
8. Oberlin C, Beal D, Leechavengvongs S, et al. (1994). Nerve transfer to biceps muscle using a part of ulnar nerve for C5-C6 avulsion of the brachial plexus: anatomical study and report of four cases. J Hand Surg [Am] 19(2): 232–237.
9. Witoonchart K, Leechavengvongs S, Uerpairojkit C, et al. Nerve transfer to deltoid muscle using the nerve to the long head of the triceps, part I: an anatomic feasibility study. J Hand Surg Am 2003; 28(4):6.
10. Chuang DC, Lee GW, Hashem F, Wei FC. Restoration of shoulder abduction by nerve transfer in avulsed brachial plexus injury: evaluation of 99 patients with various nerve transfers. Plast Reconstr Surg 1995; 96(1):122–128.
11. Yang Y, Gu YD, Hu SN, Zhang H. Long-term impact of transfer of phrenic nerve on respiratory system of children: a clinical study of 34 cases. Zhonghua Yi Xue Za Zhi 2006; 86(17):1179–1182.
12. Gu YD, Chen DS, Zhang GM. Long term functional results of contralateral C7 transfer. Reconstr Microsurg 1998; 14:57–59.
13. Taylor AS. Brachial birth palsy and injuries of similar type in adults. Surg Gynecol Obstetr 1920; 30:434–502.
14. Gilbert A, Razaboni R, Amar-Khodja S. Indications and results of brachial plexus surgery in obstetrical palsy. Orthop Clin North Am 1988; 19:91–105.
15. Gilbert A. Long-term evaluation of brachial plexus surgery in obstetrical palsy. Rand Clin 1995; 11:583–587.
16. Mallet J. Paralysie obstetricale. Rev Chirurgie Orthaped 1972; 58(suppl 1):115.
17. Evans-Jones G, Kay SPJ, Weindling AM, et al. Congenital brachial palsy: incidence, causes and outcome in the United Kingdom and Republic of Ireland. Arch Dis Fetal Neonatal 2003; 88 F185–F189.
18. Bisinella G, Birch R. Obstetric brachial plexus lesion: A study of 74 children registered with the British Surveillance Unit. J Hand Surg Br 2002; 28B:1:40–45.
19. Giddins GEB, Birch R, Singh D, Taggart M. Risk factors for obstetric brachial plexus palsies. J Bone Joint Surg 1994; 76B:Supps. II and III 156.
20. Tavakkolizadeh A. Risk factors associated with obstetric brachial plexus palsy. Dissertation. University of Brighton for degree of M Sc. 2007.
21. Becker MHJ, Lassner F, Bahm J, et al. The cervical rib. A pre disposing factor for obstetric brachial plexus lesions. J Bone Joint Surg 2002; 84:740–743.
22. Strömbeck C, Rehmal S, Krum Linde-Sundholm L, Sejersen T. (a) Long term functional follow up of a cohort of children with obstetric brachial plexus palsy: I; Functional aspects: Dev Med Child Neurol 2007; 49:198–203.
23. Strömbeck C, Rehmal S, Krum Linde-Sundholm L, Sejersen T. (b) Long term functional follow up of a cohort of children with obstetric brachial plexus palsy: II: Neurophysiological aspects. Dev Med Child Neurol 2007; 49:204–209.
24. Yang LJ, Anand P, Birch R. Limb preference in children with obstetric brachial plexus palsy. Paediatr Neurol 2005; 33:46–49.
25. Bellew M, Kay SPJ, Webb F, Ward A. Developmental and behavioural outcome in obstetric brachial plexus palsy J Hand Surg 2000; 25B:49–51.
26. Fraher JP. The CNS PNS transitional zone. In: Dyke PJ, Thomas PK, eds. Peripheral Neuropathy, 4th ed. Philadelphia: Elsevier Saunders; 2005:67–91.
27. McManis PG, Low PA, Lagerlund TD. Nerve blood flow and microenvironment. In: Dyke PJ, Thomas PK, eds. Peripheral Neuropathy, 4th ed. Philadelphia: Elsevier Saunders; 2005:67:1.
28. Groves MJ, Scaravilli F. Pathology of peripheral neurone cell bodies. In: Dyke PJ, Thomas PK, eds. Peripheral Neuropathy, 4th ed. Philadelphia: Elsevier Saunders; 2005:683–732.
29. Fullarton AC, Lenihan DV, Myles LM, Glasby MA. Obstetric brachial plexus palsy: a large animal for traction injury and its repair. Part 1: the age of the recipient. J Hand Surg 2000; 25B:52–57.
30. Fullarton AC, Myles LM, Lenihan DV, et al. Obstetric brachial plexus palsy: a comparison of the degree of recovery after repair of 16 ventral root avulsions in newborn and adult sheep. Brit J Plas Surg 2001; 54:697–704.
31. Birch R, Ahad N, Kono H, Smith S. Repair of obstetric brachial plexus palsy. Results in 100 children. J Bone Jt Surg 2005; 87B:1089–1095.
32. Blaauw G, Slooff ACJ, Muhlig S. Results of surgery after breech delivery. In: Gilbert A, ed. Brachial Plexus Injuries. London: Martin Dunitz; 2001: 217–224.
33. Birch R, Bonney G, Wynnparry CB. Surgical Disorders of the Peripheral Nerves, 1st ed. Edinburgh: Churchill Livingstone; 1998.
34. Narakas AO. Obstetrical brachial plexus injuries. In: Lamb DW, ed. The Paralyzed Hand. Edinburgh: Churchill Livingstone; 1987:116.
35. Brunelli GA, Brunelli GR. A fourth type of brachial plexus lesion: the intermediate (C7) palsy. J Hand Surg 1991; 16B:492–494.
36. Smith SJM. The role of neurophysiological investigation in traumatic brachial plexus injuries in adults and children. J Hand Surg 1996; 21B:145–148.
37. Smith SJM. Electrodiagnosis. In: Birch R, Bonney G, Wynn Parry C. Surgical Disorders of the Peripheral Nerves. Edinburgh: Churchill Livingstone; 1998:467–490.
38. Bisinella G, Birch R, Smith SJM. Neurophysiological predictions of outcome in obstetric lesions of the brachial plexus J Hand Surg 2003; 28B:148–152.
39. Gilbert A, Tassin JL. Réparation chirurgicale de plexus brachial dans la paralysie obstétricale. Chirurgie (Paris) 1984; 110:70–75.
40. Nehme A, KANY J, Sales-De-Gauzy J, et al. Obstetrical brachial plexus palsy, predictions of outcome in upper root injuries. J Hand Surg 2001; 27B:9–12.
41. Clarke HM, Curtis C. Examination and prognosis. In: Gilbert A, ed. Brachial Plexus Injuries. London: Martin Dunitz; 2001:159–172.

42. MacNamara P, Yam A. The false tumour of the biceps—a birth injury. An analysis of 40 cases. Manuscript in preparation: data kindly released by Mr. MacNamara. 2008

43. Gilbert A. Indications et résultats de la chirurgie du plexus brachial dans la paralysie obstétricale. In: Alnot JY, Narakas A, eds. Les Paralysie du Plexus Brachiale. Monographies du groupe d'étude de la main. Paris: Expansion Scientifique Française; 1995.

44. Anand P, Birch R. Restoration of sensory function and lack of long-term chronic pain syndromes after brachial plexus injury in human neonates. Brain 2002; 125:113–122.

45. Iyer VG. Developmental maturation of the nervous system In: Gupta A, Kay SPJ, Scheker LR, eds. The Growing Hand. London: Mosby; 2000:47–52.

46. Erhard RP, Lindley SG. functional development of the hand. In: Gupta A, Kay SPJ, Scheker LR, eds. The Growing Hand. London: Mosby; 2000:71–82.

47. Fairbank HAT. Subluxation of shoulder joint in infants and young children. Lancet 1913; I:1217–1223.

48. Scaglietti O. the obstetrical shoulder trauma. Surg Gynae Obstet 1938; 66:868–877.

49. Putti V. Analisi della triada radiosintomatica degli stati di prelussazione. Chir Organi Mov 1932; XVII:453–459.

50. Waters PM, Smith GR, Jaramillo D. Gleno humeral deformity secondary to brachial plexus birth palsy. J Bone Jt Surg 1998; 80A:668–677.

51. Pearl ML, Edgerton BW. Glenoid deformity secondary to brachial plexus birth palsy. J Bone Jt Surg 1998; 80A: 659–667.

52. Sluijs JA, Van Ouwerkerk WJR, De Gast A, et al. Retroversion of the humeral head in children with obstetric brachial plexus lesion. J Bone Jt Surg 2002; 84B 583–587.

53. Sluisz JA, van Ouwerkerk WJR, de Gast A, et al. Deformities of the shoulder in infants younger than 12 months with an obstetric lesion of the brachial plexus. J Bone Jt Surg 2001; 83B: 551–555.

54. Hoeksma AF, Steeg AMT, Dijkstra P, et al. Shoulder contracture and osseous deformity in obstetrical brachial plexus injuries. J Bone Jt Surg 2003; 85A:316–322.

55. Kambhampati SLS, Birch R, Cobiella C, Chen L. Posterior subluxation and dislocation of the shoulder in obstetric brachial plexus palsy. J Bone Jt Surg 2006; 88B:213–219.

56. Pearl ML, Edgerton BW, Kazimiroff PA, et al. Arthroscopic release and latissimus dorsi transfer for shoulder internal rotation contractures and glenohumeral deformity secondary to brachial plexus birth palsy. J Bone Jt Surg 2006; 88A:564–574.

57. Nath RK, Paizi M. Improvement in abduction of the shoulder after reconstructive soft tissue procedures in obstetric brachial plexus palsy. J Bone Jt Surg 2007; 89B:620–626.

58. Seddon HJ. (a) Common causes of nerve injury. In: Seddon HJ, ed. Surgical Disorders of Peripheral Nerves, 2nd ed. Edinburgh: Churchill Livingstone; 1975:67–88.

59. Kato N, Birch R. Peripheral nerve palsies associated with closed fractures and dislocations. Injury 2006; 37:507–512.

60. Harkess JW. Acquired deformities of the upper extremity. In: Gupta A, Kay SPJ, Scheker LR, eds. The Growing Hand. London: Mosby; 2000:725–752.

61. Klenerman L. The evolution of the compartment syndrome since 1948 as recorded in the JBJS (B). J Bone Jt Surg 2007; 89B:1280–1282.

62. Barros D'Sa AAB, Harkin DW. Pathophysiology of acute vascular insufficiency. In: Barros d'Sa AAB, Chant ADB, eds. Emergency Vascular and Endovascular Surgical Practice, 2nd ed. London: Hodder, Arnold; 2005:19–27.

63. Wajcberg E, Thoppil N, Patel S, et al. Comprehensive assessment of post-ischemic vascular reactivity in Hispanic children and adults with and without diabetes mellitus. Paediatr Diabetes 2006; 7: 329–335.

64. Burton AC, Yamada S. Relation between blood pressure and flow in human forearm. J. Applied Physiol 1951; 4:329–339.

65. Parkes AR. Ischemic effects of external and internal pressure on the upper limb. Hand 1973; 5:105–112.

66. Birch R, Bonney G. Pain. In: Birch R, Bonney G, Wynn Parry CB. Surgical Disorders of the Peripheral Nerves. London: Churchill Livingstone; 1998:373–404.

67. Oaklander AL, Rismiller JG, Gelman LB, et al. Evidence of focal small-fibre axonal degeneration in complex regional pain syndrome-1 (reflex sympathetic dystrophy). Pain 2006; 120:235–243.

68. Barnes R. Causalgia: a review of 48 cases. In: Seddon, HJ, ed. Peripheral Nerve Injuries by the Nerve Injuries Committee of the Medical Research Council. Medical Research Council Special Report series 282. London: HMSO; 1954:156–185.

69. Ramachandran M, Birch R, Eastwood D. Clinical outcome of nerve injuries associated with supracondylar fractures in of the humerus in children. J Bone Jt Surg 2006; 88B:90–94.

70. Birch R, Achan P. Peripheral Nerve Repairs and their Results in Children. Hand Clin 2000; 16:579–597.

Chapter 4

Leg Deformity and Length Discrepancy

John A. Fixsen, Robert A. Hill, and Franz Grill

Part I: Classification and Management of Lower Limb Reduction Anomalies

John A. Fixsen and Robert A. Hill

Introduction

Congenital limb deficiencies or reduction anomalies in the lower limbs are the result of failure of formation of parts in the first trimester of pregnancy. They can also result from the constriction band syndrome sometimes known as Streeter's dysplasia.

Two types of abnormal development can occur, causing transverse or longitudinal deficiency. In *transverse deficiency*, the proximodistal development is normal until the level of the deficiency, although there is nearly always some attempt at the development of rudimentary digits (digital buds) on the end of the limb, which may vary from puckering of the skin to small but formed digits (Fig. 4.1). In *longitudinal deficiency,* there is a reduction or absence of a bone or bones in the long axis of the limb. However, there are often normal or near normal elements distal to the affected bone or bones. It is most important to remember that the deficiency is not simply of bone, but also of muscle and soft tissue.

Classification

In the past, many classifications have been suggested, often using Greco-Latin terms, such as fibular hemimelia,

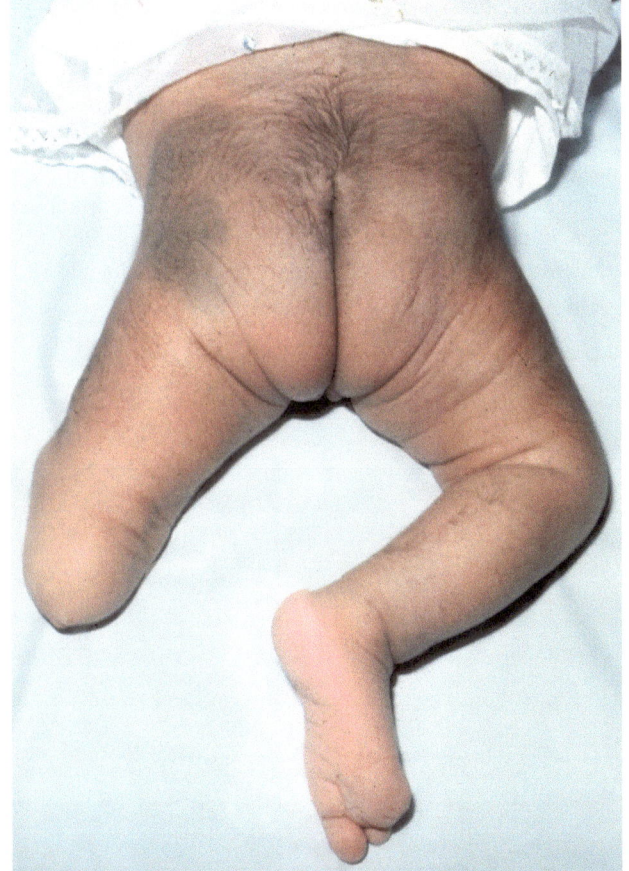

Fig. 4.1 Clinical photograph of a below-knee transverse deficiency. Transverse deficiency upper third leg (ISPO/ISO classification)

dysmelia, or amelia [1]. However, in 1989, the International Standards Organization published ISO 8548/1, "Method of Describing Limb Deficiencies Present at Birth" [2]. This has now been generally accepted by the International Society for Prosthetics and Orthotics (ISPO) and other national

J.A. Fixsen (✉)
Orthopaedic Department, Great Ormond Street Hospital for Sick Children, London, UK

R.A. Hill (✉)
Orthopaedic Department, Great Ormond Street NHS Trust, London, UK

F. Grill (✉)
Department of Pediatric orthopaedics, Orthopaedic Hospital Vienna, Vienna, Austria

organizations. It uses a simple anatomical system based on whether the deficiency is transverse or longitudinal.

Transverse deficiencies in the lower limb are described by the segment at which the limb terminates and then the level within that segment beyond which there are no skeletal elements, disregarding digital buds. The segments defined in the lower limb are the pelvis, thigh, leg, tarsal, metatarsal, and phalangeal. (Note metatarsal and phalangeal can be combined when they are termed a "ray".) Thus a transverse deficiency at upper third tibial level would be termed "transverse leg upper third" (see Fig. 4.1).

Longitudinal deficiency is described by naming the affected bones in a proximodistal sequence and whether each affected bone is partially or totally absent. If a bone is partially absent, its position and the approximate fraction missing can be described. The bones are named as ilium, ischium, pubis, femur, tibia, fibula, tarsals, metatarsals, and phalanges; the last two can be described together as a ray. Thus a case of proximal femoral focal deficiency with partial absence of the fibula and a four-ray foot (Fig. 4.2) would be described as femur, partial upper two-thirds, fibula, partial upper quarter, ray 5 total. This gives an accurate description of the whole deficiency but is clumsy to use in clinical practice. The simple terms congenital femoral deficiency, congenital fibular deficiency, and congenital tibial deficiency are simple, clear, and focus on the major site of the deficiency [3].

Etiology

The orthopaedic surgeon dealing with children should be familiar with the three main forms of congenital shortening of the lower limb:

1. Congenital femoral deficiency in all its forms, encompassing idiopathic coxa vara, congenital short femur, and proximal femoral focal deficiency (PFFD).
2. Congenital fibular deficiency associated with shortening and deformity of the tibia. Also known as congenital short tibia with absent or hypoplastic fibula or fibular hemimelia.
3. Congenital tibial deficiency. Also called congenital dysplasia or absence of the tibia with intact fibula or tibial hemimelia.

The lower limb bud appears at 28 days of intrauterine life and major development of the limb is complete in 10–14 days, after which growth and enlargement occur. A number of agents, of which the drug thalidomide is the best known, can cause abnormalities of development during this early vital period. The majority of major congenital limb deficiencies occur sporadically: a few, such as tibial dysplasia and some instances of idiopathic coxa vara, have an unequivocal genetic background. In the chick embryo, it has been possible to reproduce all the various limb deficiencies by insults

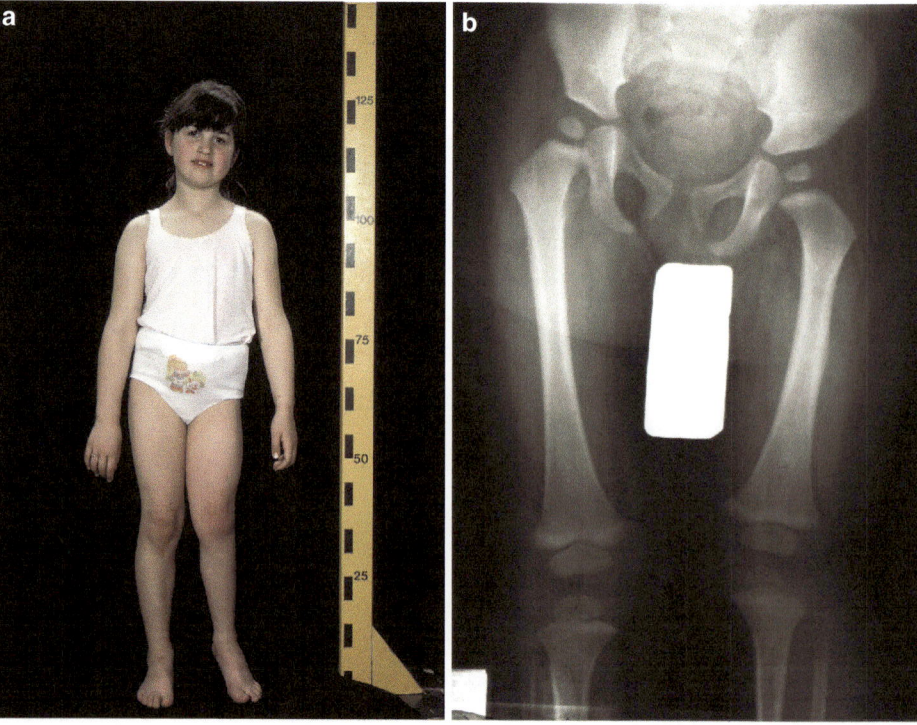

Fig. 4.2 (**a**) Eight-year-old with left congenital short femur. Note the bulky thigh, external rotation of the leg, the four-ray foot in equinus and that she can reach the floor by tilting the pelvis. (**b**) Anteroposterior radiograph of both femora and pelvis in the same patient. Note the left femur is shortened, slightly laterally bowed with some sclerosis in the diaphysis

to the limb bud: however, the cause in the great majority of children remains unknown. Abnormality in development of the normal vascular pattern in the limb has been suggested by Morgan and Somerville [4], Hootnick et al. [5] and more recently by Szeizel et al. [6], who looked at the association between smoking during pregnancy and congenital limb deficiency. Although the major deficiency is usually in one segment of the limb, a lesser degree of shortening in the other segments of the limb, which adds to the overall length discrepancy is extremely common and must be recognized. From the orthopaedic point of view particularly if limb lengthening and reconstruction are being considered it is important to remember that the bone of the major affected segment is not only short but also deformed and frequently has a sclerotic portion. A skin dimple is common over the affected bone and a degree of instability of the joints at each end of the segment must be expected

The parents of a child with a major limb deficiency are always extremely upset by the deformity and want to know the cause and the treatment as soon as possible. The advent of prenatal ultrasound screening means that parents may know before the child is born that it has a major limb anomaly and will require counseling and advice before the child is born and before the surgeon can actually examine the child. This type of counseling can be very demanding as the parents want clear and definite advice which is difficult for the surgeon to give until he has actually examined the child and apart from the few inherited forms, the cause is almost invariably unknown. Treatment should never be rushed, and it is most important to reassure parents that their children will be able to walk despite the major limb deficiency. It is usually most unwise to rush into any surgical treatment in the first year of life, although physiotherapy and splintage to stretch and mobilize deformities may be useful. Many of these children will require an extension prosthesis, extensive surgical reconstruction, and occasionally amputation. It is important to introduce the parents gently to the ideas of an extension prosthesis, extensive surgery, and possible amputation, as most will find this very hard to accept in the first instance. A visit to the prosthetic surgeon and the prosthetic unit where they can see another child with the same or similar condition is very helpful in reassuring them with regard to the child's future walking ability and function with a prosthesis. Contact with another family with a similarly affected child through a parent support group can also be very useful. An important report by the working party of the Amputee Medical Rehabilitation Society on recommended standards of care for the child with congenital limb deficiency was published in 1997 [7] and reviews the subject, recommending that there should be special limb deficiency clinics to which the child and the parents could be referred as soon as possible after birth—certainly within 3 months of birth. This would be a

major advance in the management of these children and their families.

Congenital Femoral Deficiency

Idiopathic Coxa Vara (Developmental Coxa Vara, Infantile Coxa Vara)

This condition is the most minor form of femoral deficiency. It involves the inferior portion of the capital femoral epiphysis and adjacent metaphysis. It is rarely diagnosed at birth but may cause confusion with neonatal ultrasound hip examination. It usually becomes apparent as the child grows and the leg appears short, with the development of a Trendelenburg gait, limitation of abduction, and increased external rotation of the affected side. The cause is unknown, although there are reports of families in which there appears to be a genetic influence. The child normally presents after walking age with a limp and shortening. On examination, there is limitation of abduction and usually an increased range of external rotation at the affected hip. The majority of cases are unilateral, but the condition can occur bilaterally. Its incidence is not clearly known. When first noticed clinically, idiopathic coxa vara is often mistaken for developmental dysplasia of the hip (DDH) (Chapter 26) and it is important to consider other causes of coxa vara such as trauma, infection, bone dysplasia, metabolic disease, osteogenesis imperfecta, and the common association with other forms of femoral and lower limb deficiency. The important point in idiopathic coxa vara is that the radiograph changes are confined to the femoral neck.

Radiological Changes

Radiological changes are typical once they appear. In the first year of life, they may be difficult to distinguish: until proximal femoral ossification occurs, the femur may appear relatively normal. As the femoral head and neck ossify, the classical triangular fragment (Fairbanks' triangle) on the inferior surface of the femoral neck becomes apparent, together with varus deformity of the femoral neck. The epiphyseal plate lies vertical and appears irregular. An inverted Y delineates the triangular fragment in the inferior part of the femoral neck (Fig. 4.2). If the condition is untreated the dysplasia of the femoral neck and the varus increases with proximal migration of the greater trochanter relative to the femoral head, giving rise to the so-called shepherd's crook deformity. When considering differential diagnoses it is important to remember cleidocranial dysostosis, which can give rise to bilateral coxa vara associated

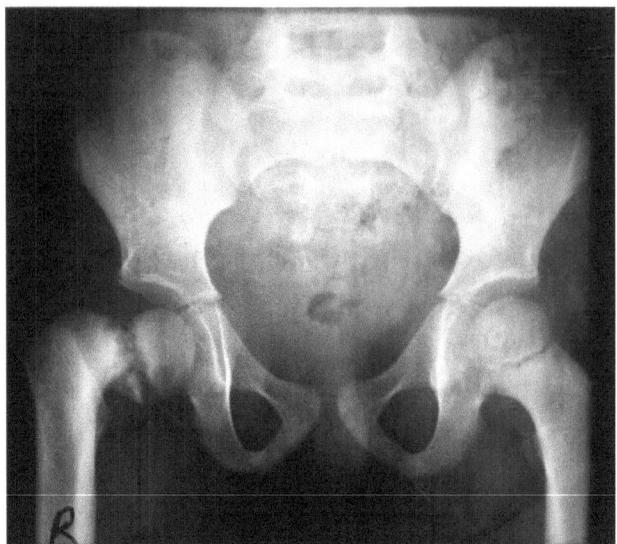

Fig. 4.3 Anteroposterior radiograph of the pelvis of a patient with idiopathic coxa vara affecting the right hip. Note the reduction in the head–neck/shaft angle, the "Fairbank's Triangle" and the inverted Y appearance of the epiphyseal plate

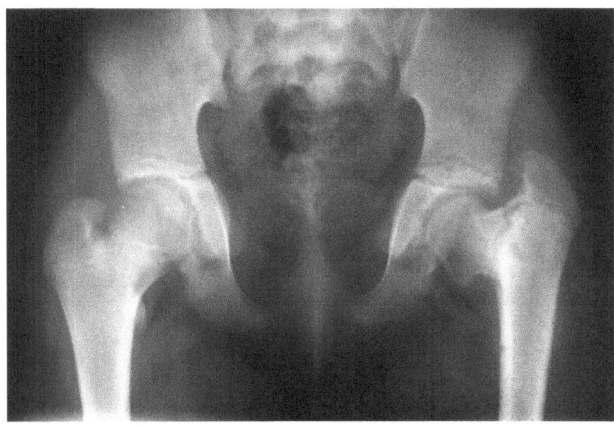

Fig. 4.4 Anteroposterior radiograph of the pelvis of a patient with cleidocranial dyostosis. Note left coxa vara with a "shepherd's crook" deformity and absence of ossification of the symphysis pubis

with absence or poor development of the clavicles, and delayed fusion of the skull suture lines and symphysis pubis (Fig. 4.4)

Management

Once the condition has been diagnosed, correction of the coxa vara should be considered. A neck–shaft angle greater than 110° should be observed as it may resolve. However, once the varus of the neck has decreased to less than 110° progression of the deformity is likely to occur. In the early

stages a simple shoe raise can be used, but if varus progresses to less than 100°, surgery should be considered to prevent inevitable deterioration. The aim of surgery is to correct the neck–shaft angle to 140° by an abduction osteotomy. Femoral retroversion can be an important part of the deformity also requiring correction [8]. Many techniques have been described including external fixation [9] but provided the operation achieves 140° of neck–shaft angle and a more horizontal position of the epiphyseal plate, the changes in the femoral neck should heal and recover. Bone grafting is not necessary. Repeat valgus osteotomy may be necessary, particularly if the initial osteotomy is performed early in childhood. Leg length discrepancy is rarely sufficient to require leg lengthening. Occasionally, in a neglected case, there is significant overgrowth of the greater trochanter and trochanteric transfer may be necessary.

Congenital Short Femur and Proximal Focal Femoral Deficiency (PFFD)

On the basis of the data from the Edinburgh birth register, Hamanishi [10] suggested that the incidence of this condition was around 1 in 50,000 live births.

The cause of this disorder is unknown. It can be associated with abnormalities not only in the lower limb but also in the upper limb and with facial anomalies as in the congenital short femur/abnormal facies syndrome.

Embryologically the hip and upper femur develop from the same anlage and so it is not surprising that the more dysplastic the upper end of the femur, the more dysplastic the hip joint. Clinically the leg appears short although minor degrees of congenital femoral deficiency (congenital short femur) may not be noticed at birth. Subsequently with growth the shortening becomes obvious. It is always associated with flexion and external rotation of the hip as a result of retroversion of the femoral neck. Early radiographs show a shortened femoral shaft or, in the most severe forms, no femoral shaft. The acetabulum may vary from virtually normal in mild cases to absent in the most severe.

It is customary to classify major congenital shortening of the femur into congenital short femur (CSF) and proximal focal femoral deficiency (PFFD). In reality, when one looks at the entire spectrum of the disorder, there is a steady progression from CSF (the femur is almost normal but short) to almost total absence of the femur with only the distal femoral condyles appearing in bone some years after birth. The first classifications by Amstutz and Wilson [11], Aitken [12], Hamanishi [10] (Fig. 4.5), and Pappas [13] were based on plain radiological appearances. Fixsen and Lloyd-Roberts in 1974 [14] pointed out the significance of the appearance

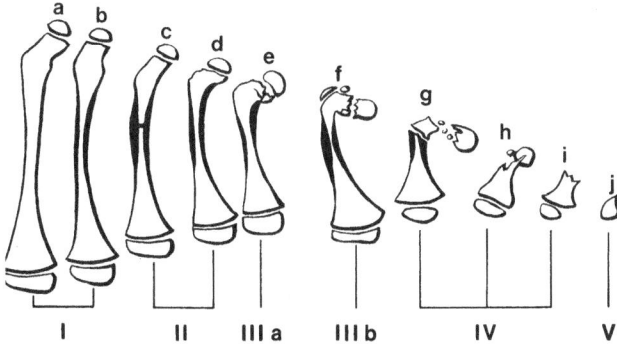

Fig. 4.5 Classification of femoral deficiency (dysplasia) as described by Hamanishi in 1980. Reproduced with permission and copyright © of the British Editorial Society of Bone and Joint Surgery. Hamanishi [10]

of the acetabulum and upper femur in early radiographs to the subsequent development of the hip and its importance in surgical treatment (Fig. 4.6). More recently, with the rapid advances in limb lengthening and reconstruction techniques, the classifications of Gillespie [15] and Paley [16] relate radiological appearance to both the hip development and the possibility for surgical reconstruction. In the Gillespie classification group A the hip is stable and if the femoral length is more than 60% of the contralateral side leg, equalization is possible. If the femoral length is less than 60%, the risks associated with lengthening increase and some surgeons would recommend a Van Nes rotationplasty [17] or fusion of the knee and amputation through the ankle joint rather than leg lengthening. In Gillespie group B the femoral length is less than 50% of the contralateral side and the hip is unstable as defined by Fixsen and Lloyd-Roberts [14]. The surgeon should aim for the best possible function with a prosthesis. In group C the femur is virtually absent or only a distal fragment is present and treatment is with a prosthesis.

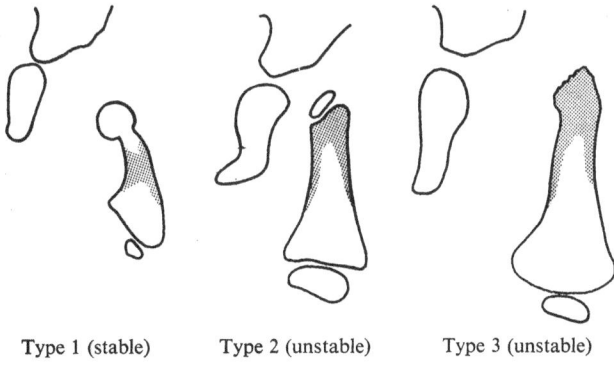

Fig. 4.6 Classification of PFFD as described by Fixsen and Lloyd-Roberts relating the appearance of the acetabulum and the upper end of the femur in the early radiograph to the future development and stability of the hip and upper end of the femur. (**a**) Type 1 (stable); (**b**) type 2 (unstable); (**c**) type 3 (unstable). Reproduced with permission and copyright © of the British Editorial Society of Bone and Joint Surgery. Fixsen and Lloyd-Roberts [14]

Paley's classification is based on what he considered necessary for reconstruction by limb lengthening with particular reference to the dysplasia and mobility of the knee as well as the hip. His type 1 is similar to Gillespie group A but with three sub-groups dependent on the state of the hip and knee. Type 2 has a mobile femoral pseudarthrosis which must be stabilized if lengthening is to be considered. Type 3 is again similar to Gillespie group C and lengthening is unlikely to be helpful. Ring [18, 19] made the important observation that the proportional shortening remains the same throughout growth, provided further displacement as a result of the coxa vara or hip subluxation does not occur. Therefore if the femur is 20% short at birth, it is likely to be 20% short in the adult, and so a reasonable estimate of the overall shortening at maturity can be made in the first year of life. In 2000, Paley et al. [20] published their multiplier method, which is very useful for predicting limb-length discrepancy at skeletal maturity in both congenital and developmental limb-length discrepancy. It is important to remember that the abnormality is not confined to the femur. The knee is nearly always to some extent unstable and there may be congenital absence of both cruciates [21, 22]. The lower leg is nearly always to some degree short, and there may be absence or hypoplasia of the fibula. The foot is often remarkably normal.

Congenital Short Femur

Congenital short femur is the milder form of congenital femoral deficiency. The femur is short with an average growth retardation of about 10%. Affected patients (see Fig. 4.2) typically have a bulky thigh with a fixed external rotation deformity at the hip and a mildly valgus and unstable knee.

Management

Congenital short femur is the most difficult of the major bone deficiencies to treat by lengthening because of the morphology of the bone, difficulty in placement of the external fixator, poor regenerate formation, and soft tissue complications particularly at the knee. Post frame removal, there is a significant risk of fracture and knee stiffness (Table 4.1). There are differing opinions as to the limits of lengthening. An individual patient's suitability may not just depend on the severity of the shortening but also on other factors including associated deformities. In general, lengthening is considered appropriate for an anticipated discrepancy at maturity of 5–20 cm. Discrepancies greater than this are probably better managed by a prosthesis although surgery may be indicated to facilitate fitting and to correct deformity.

Table 4.1 Complications of limb reconstruction for congenital limb deficiencies

Bony

1. Poor bone formation
2. Deformity and fracture after fixator removal
3. Loss of alignment during lengthening

Soft tissue

1. Joint contractures
2. Subluxation and dislocation of joints
3. Muscle weakness
4. Nerve palsy

Table 4.2 Bony abnormalities in congenital short femur

At the hip

1. Femoral neck retroversion (externally rotated leg)
2. Acetabular dysplasia
3. Coxa vara

In the femoral shaft

1. Proximal sclerosis—poor regenerate formation at this level
2. "Rib-like" shape of the bone—difficulty with fixation

At the knee

1. Hypoplasia of the lateral condyle–valgus deformity
2. Patella subluxation or dislocation

The femur is not only short but also abnormal in shape (Table 4.2). These abnormalities have to be taken into account and preferably corrected before or during lengthening. Reconstruction is a more appropriate description of management than simply lengthening as it recognizes a more comprehensive approach to the whole limb abnormality. Many patients will require more than one episode of reconstruction depending on the severity of the case. In practice, reconstruction of the congenital short femur demands the anticipation and avoidance of complications, particularly knee subluxation and stiffness, related to insufficiency of the anterior cruciate ligament and tight hamstrings. As with reconstruction for all major congenital deficiencies, management is best undertaken by an experienced surgeon working with a multidisciplinary team who can offer an expert care throughout treatment from pre-assessment and pre-admission to ongoing support for a prolonged period.

A monolateral external fixator is easier to apply and less cumbersome but may not offer sufficiently stable fixation to cope with the deforming force of the tight soft tissues which can result in bending of the regenerate bone. It is therefore a common practice to use a circular fixator but proximally to use half rings or arches for access reasons. It is also much easier to bridge the knee with a circular fixator. Correction of the associated bony abnormalities should be considered either prior to lengthening or at the time of frame application. Knee protection by extending the frame to the tibia

is almost mandatory when lengthening a congenital short femur. In order to maintain movement in a controlled manner but to avoid subluxation, the frame is provided with a hinge at the knee. There is controversy as to whether a simple or multi-axial hinge is best. Knee stiffness is a common complication following femoral lengthening despite the use of a hinge. Care must be taken with distal pin placement to try to avoid impaling the quadriceps muscle which should be on the stretch when the wires are inserted. Knee stiffness after frame removal may improve for several months with regular physiotherapy. Quadricepsplasty can be helpful in resistant cases [23].

The osteotomy should be carried out in the least damaging manner to enhance regenerate formation. A distal osteotomy has the advantage of being through more normal bone and potentially distal valgus can be corrected at the same time but the quadriceps muscle may adhere to the regenerate and become stretched and fibrotic. A proximal osteotomy above the bulk of the quadriceps does not have these disadvantages but the bone may be less normal and regenerate formation less good (Fig. 4.7).

The risk of complications after frame removal such as fracture and knee stiffness is higher after lengthenings over 5–6 cm and the surgeon should not be too ambitious when lengthening the congenital short femur.

Proximal Femoral Focal Deficiency (PFFD)

PFFD was described by Aitken [12] in 1969. He defined four types (A–D) (Fig. 4.8). He pointed out the importance of the appearance of the acetabulum with reference to the appearance of the femoral head and the increasing coxa vara that occurs with increasing severity. These patients are likely to have major shortening (Gillespie group B) and in the most severe cases the foot will be at the level of the opposite knee (Gillespie group C) (see Fig. 4.2). In those patients who develop a reasonable femoral head it seems logical to improve the range of abduction by a valgus osteotomy with internal fixation. This will also usually induce the pseudarthrosis, if present to heal thereby stabilizing the femoral head on the femoral shaft. The timing of surgery depends on the appearances and size of the bone but is not usually undertaken before the age of 3 years.

Goddard et al. [24] reviewed the natural history and treatment of instability of the hip in PFFD in 67 patients. These patients all have a degree of shortening which requires an extension prosthesis when they start to walk. Lengthening even by modern methods is very difficult and fraught with problems because of the severe shortening and abnormalities at the hip and knee (Gillespie groups B, C, and Paley types

Fig. 4.7 (**a**) Long leg standing radiograph of a patient with left congenital short femur prior to lengthening. Note blocks under the left foot. (**b**) Radiograph at the end of lengthening in the circular frame. Note lengthening over a Rush pin; the knee was controlled with a hinge and the staple across the medial growth plate of the distal femur to correct distal femoral valgus. (**c**) Postlengthening long leg standing radiograph

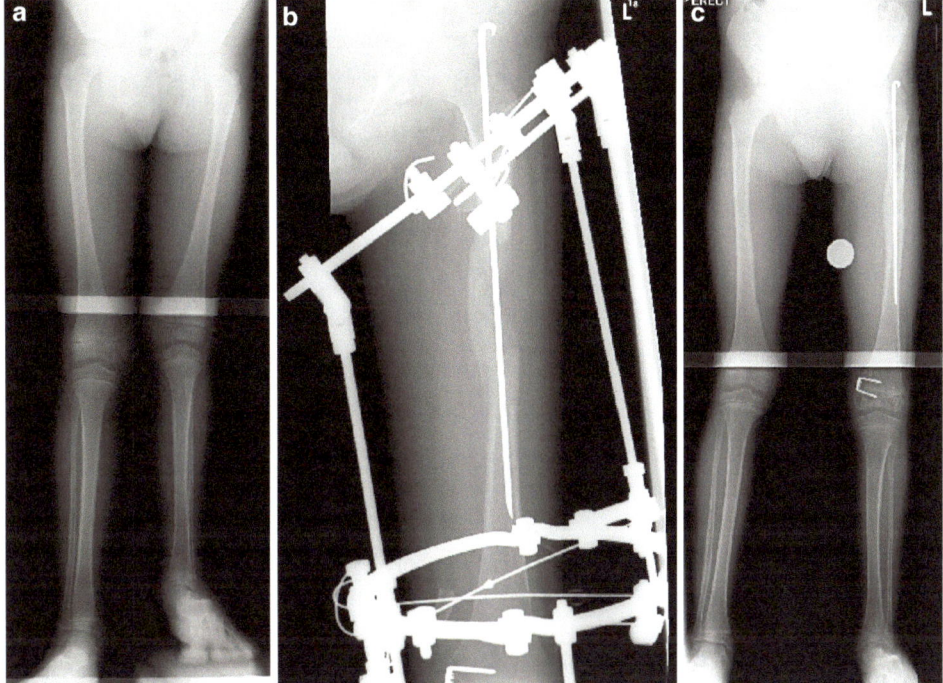

Fig. 4.8 (**a**) Child aged 1 year with severe left PFFD. Note the very short femoral segment which is flexed and externally rotated. The foot is remarkably normal and is almost at the level of the opposite knee. (**b**) Anteroposterior radiograph of a similar patient in early infancy. Note the short femoral segment, bulbous proximal end, and reasonable acetabulum suggesting this will become a stable hip despite the severe shortening

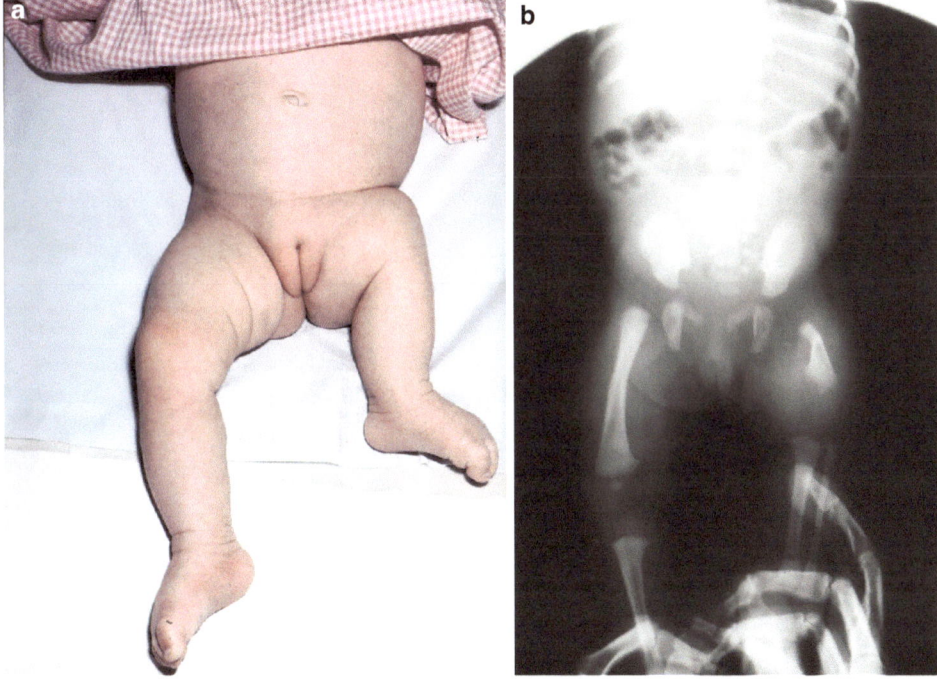

2b, 3a,b). Damsin et al. [25] published an excellent review of the problems of management of major congenital limb shortening. If the foot is at the level of the opposite knee, two possible approaches are advocated. The knee may be fused and the foot amputated to provide an adequate above-knee stump so that a good above-knee prosthesis can be fitted [26]. It is important to remember that through-joint amputations in children, unlike through-bone amputations, do not normally require revision during growth. Alternatively the Van Nes rotationplasty described by Borggreve in 1930 [27] and reviewed by Gillespie and Torode [17] may be advised. In this procedure the limb is rotated 180° and the knee fused. The foot faces backward and the ankle functions as the knee so that a below-knee prosthesis can be worn. There is considerable controversy regarding these two approaches. However, the Van Nes rotationplasty is suitable only if the foot and ankle are virtually normal and the foot will plantarflex to 180°.

In the most severe forms, where there is no satisfactory formation of the hip, it has been suggested that fusing the remnant of the femur to the ilium and using the knee as a primitive hinge hip may be useful [28]. However, in our own experience, most prosthetists find fitting and function better if the femoral remnant remains mobile.

Congenital Fibular Deficiency (or Hypoplastic Fibula)

This condition, like femoral deficiency, can vary in severity from complete absence of the fibula, with a short bowed tibia and a major reduction deformity of the foot, to simple shortening of the tibia and fibula, with no reduction deformity in the foot and a relatively minor shortening at maturity.

It is the most common form of major congenital shortening in the lower limb, occurring in approximately 1 in 25,000 live births. It does not appear to be inherited, but may be associated with other abnormalities in the same limb or the upper limb.

The clinical appearance in the classical form is typical, with marked anterior bowing of the tibia, and a dimple over the skin at the apex of the tibial kyphosis (Fig. 4.9); this dimple is also seen over the lateral side of the femur in congenital femoral deficiency. The foot is usually in valgus, with absence of one or more of the lateral radiographs. Radiographs show marked anterior bowing of the tibia with some sclerosis (Fig. 4.10). It is important not to mistake this condition for congenital pseudarthrosis of the tibia, which also shows sclerosis at the site of the bowing, but not the other features of this condition. The fibula may be totally absent or hypoplastic, being represented by a short or very small distal remnant of ossification. For many years the classification of Achterman and Kalamchi [29] (Fig. 4.11) was widely used. More recently Birch et al. [30] (Table 4.3) and Stanitski [31] have suggested classifications more closely related to modern reconstruction possibilities. The anterior bowing of the tibia often corrects spontaneously and usually does not require correction by osteotomy. If, however, the

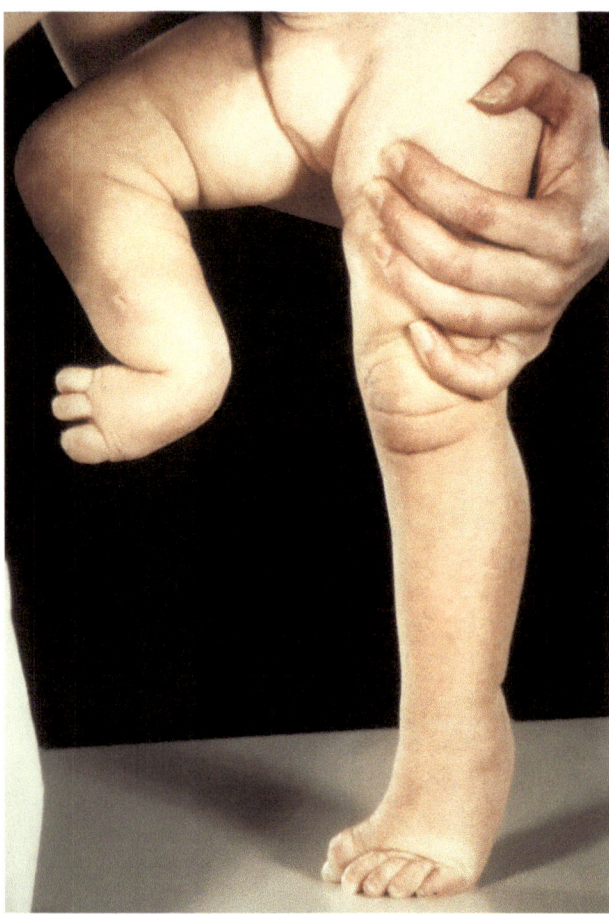

Fig. 4.9 Clinical appearance of a right congenital fibular deficiency (Achterman and Kalamchi Type II). Note the anterior bowing of the tibia with a dimple over the kyphus, severe valgus of the foot with deficient lateral two rays

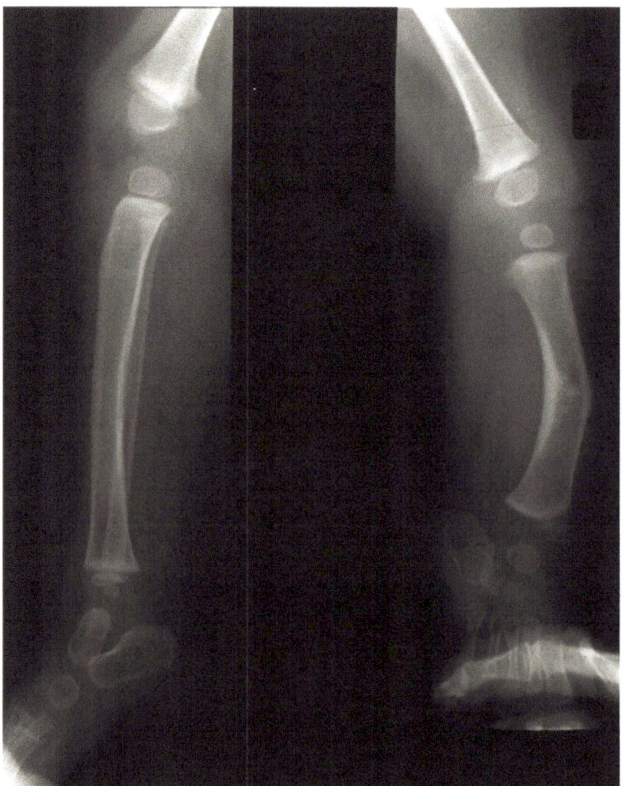

Fig. 4.10 Lateral radiographs of both lower legs showing a left congenital fibular deficiency (Achterman and Kalamchi Type II). Note the tibia is short, anteriorly bowed with complete absence of the fibula

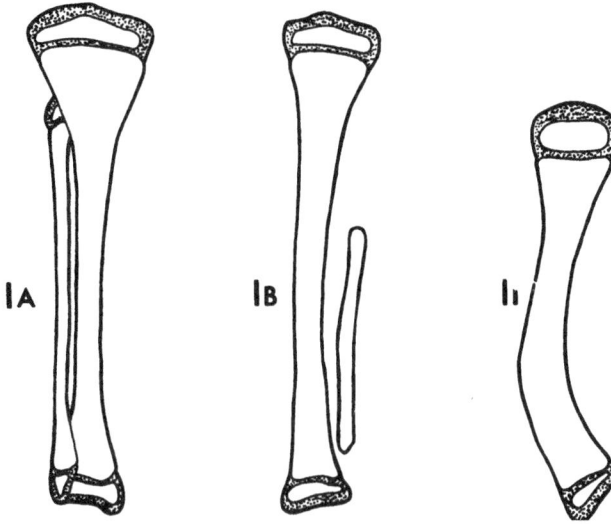

Fig. 4.11 Classification of congenital short tibia with absent or hypoplastic fibula (congenital fibula deficiency) as described by Achterman and Kalamchi. Reproduced with permission and copyright © of the British Editorial Society of Bone and Joint Surgery. Achterman and Kalamchi [29]

Table 4.3 Birch et al. classification of congenital fibular deficiency

Type based on state of foot treatment	
Type	
I	Functional foot reconstruction
IA	Leg 5% or less short orthosis/epiphysiodesis
IB	6–10% short epiphysiodesis or lengthen
IC	11–30% short 1 or 2 lengthenings or amputation
ID	>30% short >2 lengthenings or amputation
Type II Nonfunctional foot	
IIA	Functional upper limbs early amputation
IIB	Nonfunctional upper limbs retain foot

tibia is osteotomized, it will, unlike congenital pseudarthrosis, heal satisfactorily. The position of the foot in severe cases is nearly always in valgus. If the fibula is completely absent, a fibrous Thompson's band may be found. It is important to realize that, in addition to having a deficient ray or rays in the foot, there is frequently tarsal coalition, and so release of the lateral structures will not completely correct the valgus deformity of the foot. The knee often shows both cruciate deficiency and a valgus deformity associated with a hypoplastic lateral femoral condyle. Hootnick et al. [32] showed that the proportional shortening of the lower limb obeyed the same rules as that described by Ring in 1959 [18] and so it is possible in the first year of life to estimate the expected shortening at maturity. Subsequently, Hootnick et al. [5] demonstrated vascular abnormalities as a possible cause of the deformity.

Management and Limb Reconstruction

A patient's suitability for limb reconstruction is determined by the condition of the foot and the severity of the associated abnormalities especially the condition of the knee and the severity of the tibial shortening and deformity (Table 4.4). A three-ray foot is usually considered to be the minimum for reconstruction and it must be in a suitable position for weight bearing or be surgically realignable. The preliminary soft tissue realignment surgery is often carried out at around 12–18 months of age and the foot splinted until leg lengthening is commenced. If there is severe foot deformity then early treatment by amputation either through the ankle joint, a modified Syme's amputation, or retaining the calcaneum as in the Boyd amputation will facilitate prosthetic fitting and give an excellent result. It should be remembered that even patients treated by amputation may require further realignment surgery when they are older to correct, for example, progressive genu valgum due to distal femoral valgus.

The associated tibial deformities should be corrected at the time of tibial lengthening. The Taylor Spatial frame offers considerable advantages over the Ilizarov as it is easier to simultaneously correct the valgus, kyphosis, and rotation as well as lengthening (Fig. 4.12). Attention must be paid to any distal femoral valgus as this too will need correction. It is a mistake to try to correct a femoral deformity in the tibia and vice versa. Proper assessment of the whole deformity is essential prior to starting reconstruction.

Table 4.4 Abnormalities associated with congenital fibula deficiency

Foot and ankle	
1.	Lack of lateral support as fibula short or absent—tendency to valgus
2.	Tarsal coalition
3.	Ball and socket ankle joint
4.	Abnormal triangular shape of distal tibial epiphysis—tendency to valgus
5.	Absent rays
6.	Equinovalgus or equinovarus of foot and ankle
Tibia	
1.	Short
2.	Kyphotic
3.	Internally rotated
4.	Valgus
5.	Diaphyseal sclerosis
Knee	
1.	Absence or hypoplasia of anterior cruciate ligament–knee subluxation
2.	Distal femoral valgus—persistent valgus even after tibial correction.

Fig. 4.12 (a) Taylor spatial frame in use to correct both length and deformity in congenital fibular deficiency. (b) Anteroposterior radiograph after correction of length and deformity

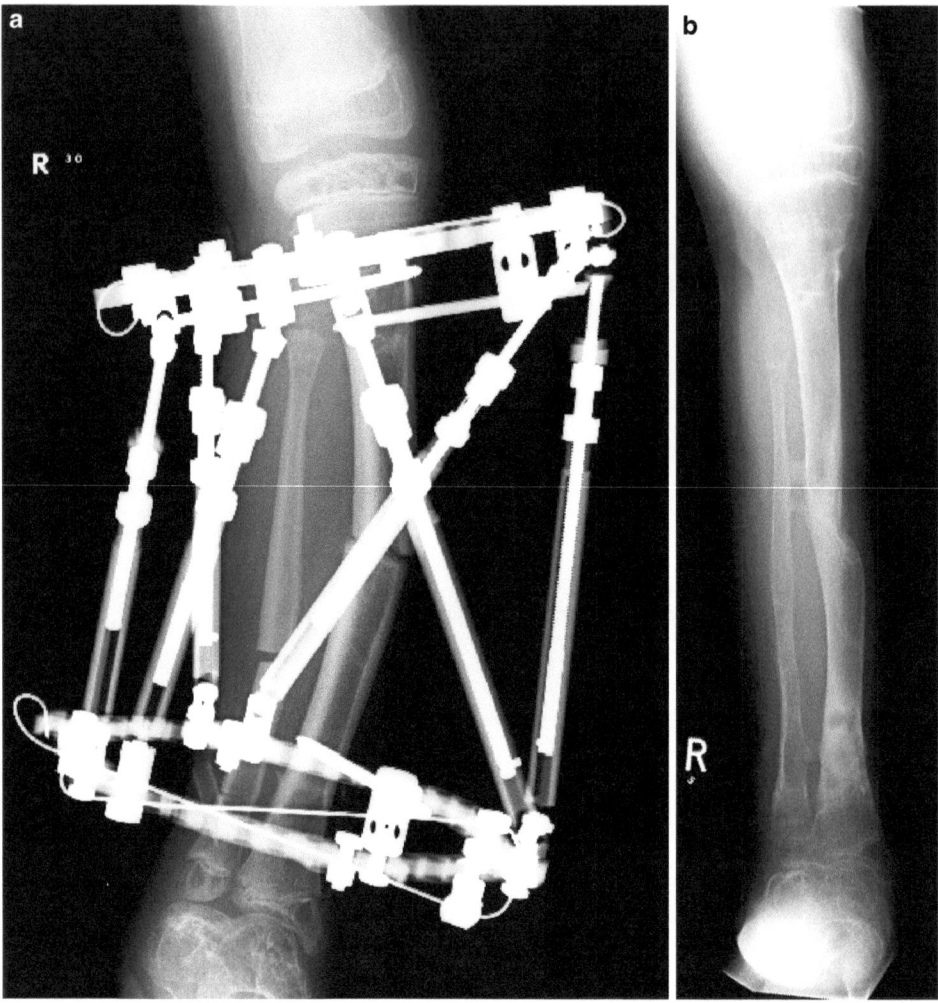

The general complications of limb reconstruction in congenital deficiencies are set out in Table 4.1 and apply to fibula deficiency. Equinovalgus of the ankle and foot are a particular problem even if the frame is extended to the foot. If the fibula appears absent on the radiograph, there may be a fibrous anlage (Thompson's band) which should be sought and resected at the time of frame application. Talocalcaneal coalition which may not be apparent on early radiographs is very common and can contribute to progressive heel and foot valgus. Late valgus of the foot and ankle may also be due to the abnormal shape of the distal tibia, lack of support from the absent or dysplastic fibula, and tightness of the tendo Achilles following lengthening. Ankle arthrodesis or an opening wedge subtalar fusion (if there is a subtalar joint) is sometimes required. Unfortunately stiffness of the foot and ankle is common and difficult to avoid.

In its more minor form, the condition may not be recognized because the fibula is present and the most obvious anomaly is the reduction deformity in the foot (Fig. 4.13). These patients are often believed to have simply a reduction deformity in the foot, and only present later with variable shortening of the lower leg. Radiographs confirm the reduction deformity in the foot, and also tarsal coalition. With the latter, there may be a ball and socket ankle joint. The fibula is present, though it may be slightly hypoplastic and, interestingly, the foot deformity is usually one of equinovarus rather than valgus. These children may present as a recalcitrant club foot. Careful scrutiny of the radiograph will show that the growth plate of the distal fibula is above the level of the ankle joint. These feet sometimes need treatment with limb reconstruction techniques as they do not always respond to conventional soft tissue surgery. Sometimes they require leg equalization, either by epiphysiodesis or by leg lengthening [33].

Congenital Tibial Deficiency or Absence of the Tibia with Intact Fibula

This is the rarest of the major congenital anomalies of the lower leg. It occurs in 1 in 1,000,000 live births. It may be inherited and associated particularly with medial duplication of both the hands and the feet (Table 4.5). Jones et al. [34] proposed a classification into four groups, based on the initial radiograph (Fig. 4.14). This was subsequently modified

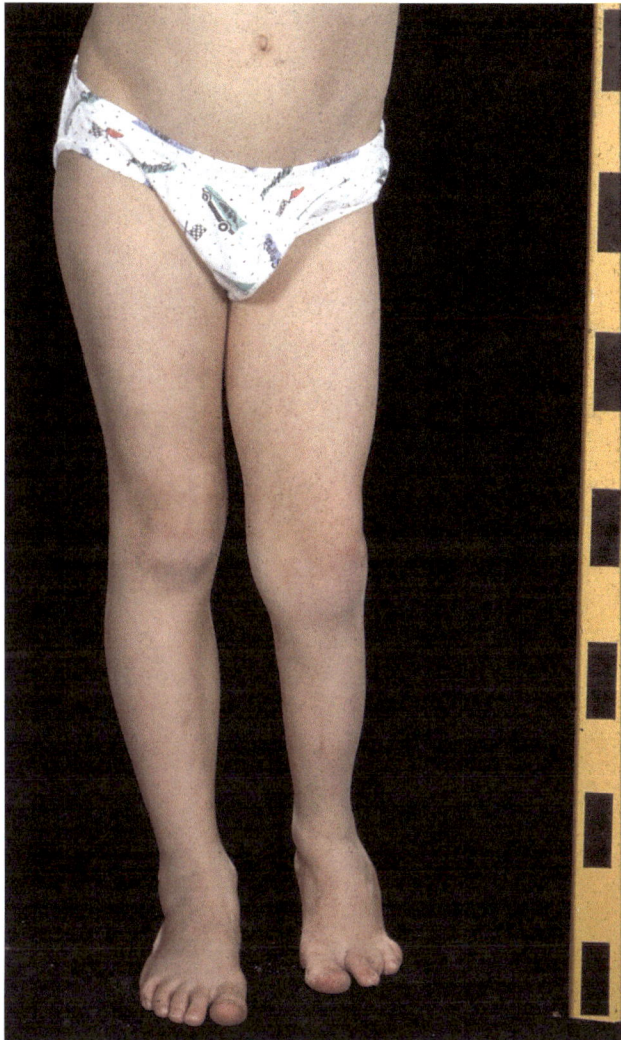

Fig. 4.13 Clinical photograph of the minor form of congenital fibula deficiency in the left leg. Note absence of the fifth ray, slight valgus at the knee, and shortening of the tibia and fibula which was present but mildly hypoplastic

Congenital Aplasia of the Tibia

Radiological Types

Type	Radiological Description	No. of limbs
1 a	• Tibia not seen • Hypoplastic lower femoral Epiphysis	6
b	• Tibia not seen • Normal lower femoral Epiphysis	12
2	• Distal Tibia not seen	5
3	• Proximal Tibia not seen	2
4	• Diastasis	4

Fig. 4.14 Classification of congenital tibial deficiency by Jones et al. Reproduced with permission and copyright © of the British Editorial Society of Bone and Joint Surgery. Jones et al. [34]

into three types by Kalamchi and Dawe [35] (Fig. 4.15). However, Schoenecker et al. [36], in a major review of 71 limbs in 57 patients, felt that the Jones classification into four groups was preferable.

Table 4.5 Abnormalities associated with congenital tibial deficiency

1. Polydactyly—sometimes also in the hands
2. Severe equinovarus
3. Tarsal abnormalities
4. Talus articulates with enlarged distal fibula

Tibia

1. Variable degree of absence (Jones' classification)
2. Deformity of shaft when present

Fibula

Overlong relative to tibia and prominent proximally

Knee

Instability

The clinical appearance is typical, with gross equinovarus deformity of the foot, which may show medial duplication (Fig. 4.16). The fibula is intact and there may be severe varus at the knee. As in femoral deficiency the radiograph at 1 year gives a clearer picture of the dysplasia than the radiograph at birth.

Management and Limb Reconstruction

Reconstruction for Jones Type 1a Tibial Dysplasia

In type 1a deformity, with complete absence of the tibia and no quadriceps apparatus, the best treatment is through knee amputation and a prosthesis. If this is not acceptable to the parents the alternative is the procedure described by Brown [37] in which the intact fibula is moved under the femoral condyles to replace the absent tibia. The results are usually poor because of inherent knee instability and lack of the quadriceps, requiring an orthosis, and a tendency to

Fig. 4.15 Classification of congenital tibial deficiency as modified by Kalamchi and Dawe. Reproduced with permission and copyright © of the British Editorial Society of Bone and Joint Surgery. Kalamchi and Dawe [35]

KALAMCHI AND DAWE CLASSIFICATION

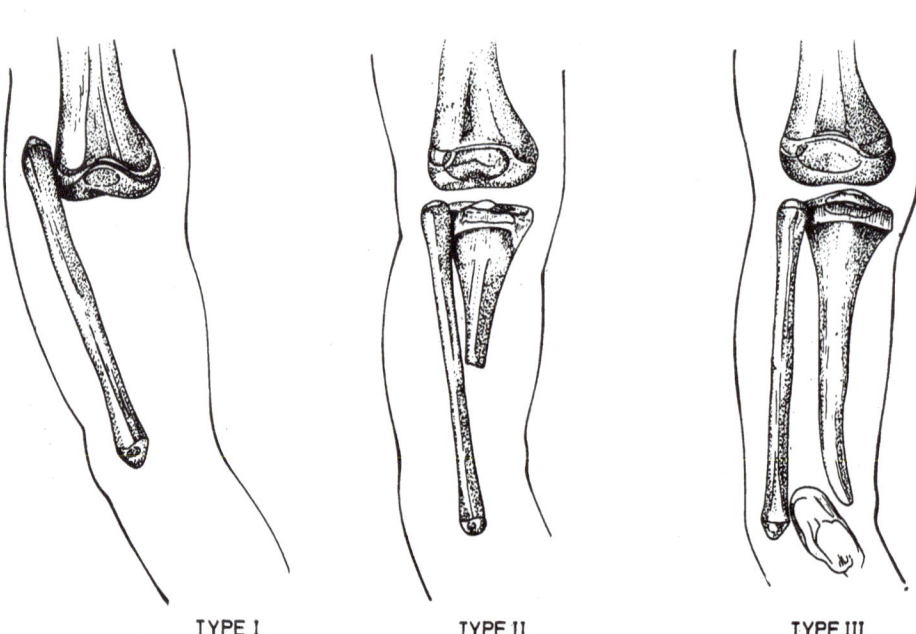

TYPE I   TYPE II   TYPE III

Fig. 4.16 (a) Child with Jones' type 2 congenital deficiency of the right leg. Note the severe equinovarus foot and duplication of the hallux. (b) Anteroposterior radiograph of the right showing the proximal end of the tibia is present in bone, the fibular is in marked varus with severe equinovarus of the foot and duplication of the hallux

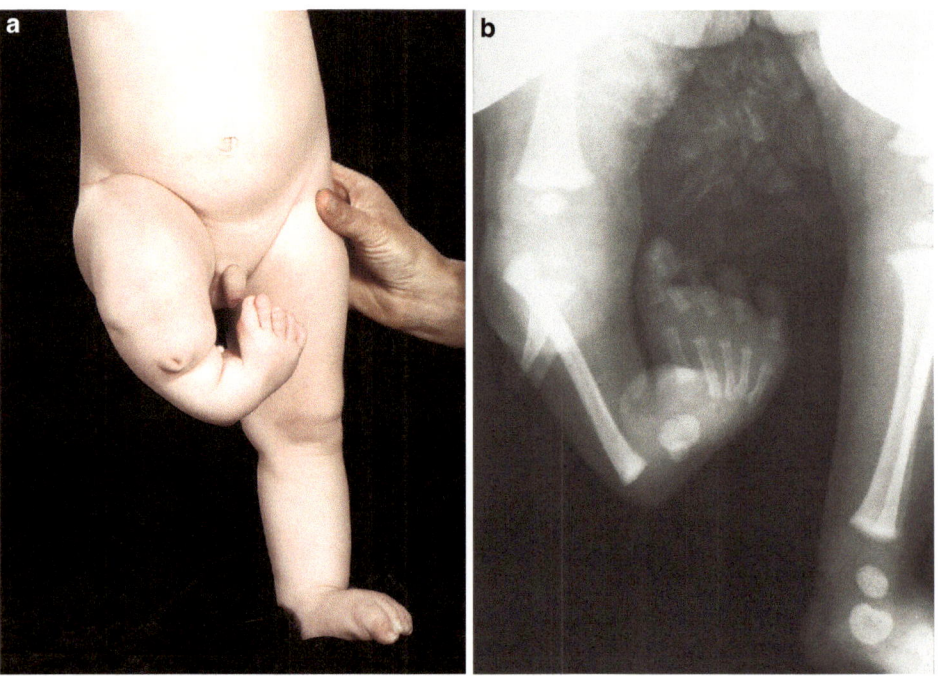

develop a knee flexion deformity. There are anecdotal reports of subsequent lengthening of the hypertrophied fibula.

Reconstruction for Type 1b Tibial Dysplasia

In type 1b the proximal tibia is present in cartilage and not visible on the early radiograph but can be seen on ultrasound and magnetic resonance imaging (MRI). The quadriceps

apparatus is also present and these patients can be treated as type 2 patients.

Reconstruction for Type 2 Tibial Dysplasia

In type 2 patients the upper end of the tibia and the quadriceps apparatus are present. Reconstruction is possible depending on the condition of the foot and ankle. If there is severe deformity then a below-knee amputation at

Fig. 4.17 (a) Anteroposterior radiograph of a patient with congenital tibial deficiency Jones type 2. (b) Anteroposterior and lateral radiographs following reconstruction by fusion of the fibula to the tibia using a screw. Note how the fibula is bowed and has hypertrophied. The foot has been stabilized on the distal end of the fibula. Further lengthening and deformity correction will be necessary later

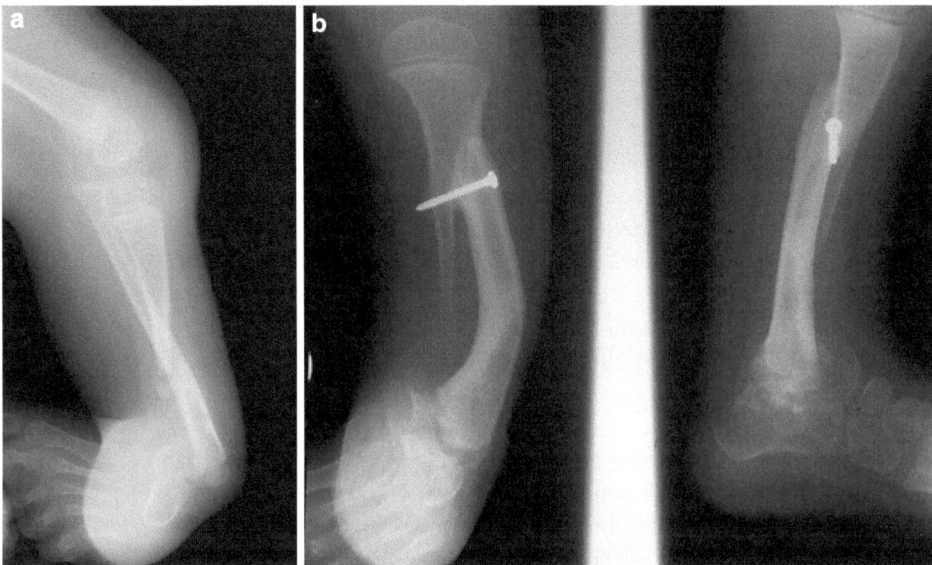

the level of the distal end of the tibia is probably the best option. As this is a through-bone amputation, stump revision, particularly for overgrowth of the fibula, is usually necessary. If the foot deformity is not too severe and the foot can be positioned by surgery for weight bearing then satisfactory reconstruction may be possible. As the distal tibia is absent the talus articulates with the fibula. It is usually necessary to explore the ankle and foot to correct an equinovarus deformity and position the talus under the fibula. Accessory toes may need excision. Later a one bone leg has to be created fusing the distal fibula to the tibial remnant usually with resection of the proximal fibula as this can be prominent and cause problems at the knee (Fig. 4.17a, b). Bone lengthening of the one bone leg can be carried out when the child is older together with adjustment of alignment either using an Ilizarov or using a spatial frame. These patients often have significant shortening and several lengthenings including femoral lengthening may be necessary. Knee and foot deformities can be troublesome [38].

Reconstruction for Type 3 Tibial Dysplasia

This is the rarest type of tibial dysplasia in which the tibia is represented by an amorphous segment of bone more distal than proximal. An MRI scan can be very helpful to assess the extent of the dysplasia as occasionally the proximal tibia is present in cartilage particularly if the femoral condyles appear normal. True type 3 cases are best treated by amputation which gives a good result and there is insufficient experience to recommend reconstruction.

Reconstruction for Type 4 Tibial Dysplasia

The tibia is present but short and there is a diastasis between the lower end of the tibia and fibula. The fibula is long relative to the tibia and is prominent proximally. The foot is usually in equinovarus. The talus may articulate with the tibia, fibula, or both bones. Although type 4 dysplasia is of variable severity, it is overall the mildest form of tibial dysplasia and reconstruction is often feasible. The foot position needs early correction at about 1 year of age. A decision has to be made at the time of surgery whether the talus is best positioned under the tibia or the fibula. The foot is then splinted until the patient is old enough for lengthening. It is important to control the foot in the frame and to consider differential lengthening of the fibula and the tibia to restore their normal relationship proximally. It is often necessary to include the foot in the frame to protect the ankle and most patients will have a stiff foot.

Congenital Pseudarthrosis of the Tibia

Congenital pseudarthrosis of the tibia is rare with an estimated incidence of 1 in 140,000 live births. Its etiology is unknown and its management difficult. The name is confusing, in that fracture at birth is rare; the condition is better called infantile pseudarthrosis of the tibia. Fracture commonly occurs in the first 2 years after birth, but may be delayed until very much later.

Clinical and Radiological Appearances

The tibia is bowed anteriorly, and commonly laterally, often with shortening (Fig. 4.18). The most common site of the deformity is at the junction of the proximal two-thirds with the distal one-third of the tibia. A number of classifications based on the clinical and radiological appearances have been described, of which the best known is that of Boyd [39], who describes six different types. Radiologically, however, there are two main types of deformity. The more common shows narrowing, and often obliteration, of the marrow cavity, with surrounding sclerosis related to the apex of the anterior bowing, usually at the junction of the middle and lower thirds of the tibia (Fig. 4.19). The less common type shows a cystic lesion at the site of the deformity in the tibia; it is important not to confuse this with fibrous dysplasia, which can cause a similar deformity and fracture, but responds much better to treatment in the form of curettage, grafting, and intramedullary rodding. The fibula is often involved in the disease process (Fig. 4.19). Isolated congenital pseudarthrosis of the fibula (CPF) is very rare and has a generally more benign prognosis [40]. Between 40 and 80% of patients will show neurofibromatosis, and it is important to look for the

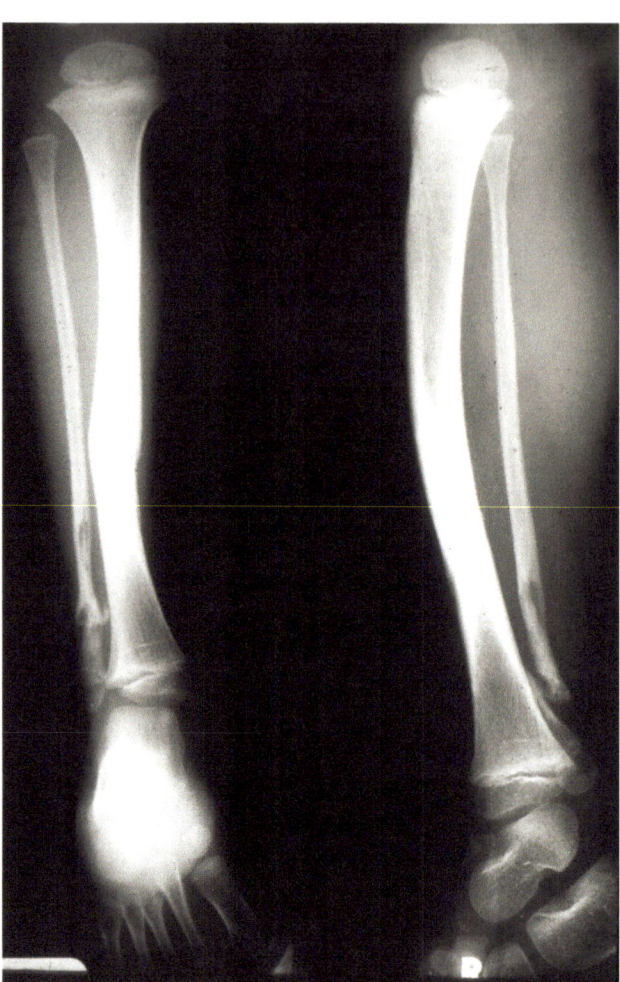

Fig. 4.19 Anteroposterior and lateral radiographs of a patient with congenital pseudarthrosis of the tibia which has not yet fractured. Note the anterior bowing, sclerosis and loss of the marrow cavity; the fibula is also affected and has already fractured in its distal third

stigmata of this condition, which may be present when the pseudarthrosis is diagnosed, or may develop later. The characteristic "cafe au lait" spots of pigmentation in the skin often do not appear until the age of 2 years. Other members of the family should be examined, because relatives very reasonably do not relate their child's bowed tibia to the occurrence of skin nodules, pigmentation, or nerve tumors in other members of the family.

Management

Management is complex. Once fracture has occurred union is very difficult to achieve. It is most important to recognize the condition in the pre-pseudarthrosis stage and not to osteotomize the bowed tibia and precipitate nonunion. Prophylactic bracing from the time the child is first diagnosed seems to be very worthwhile if compliance can be maintained. Murray and Lovell in 1982 [41] reported

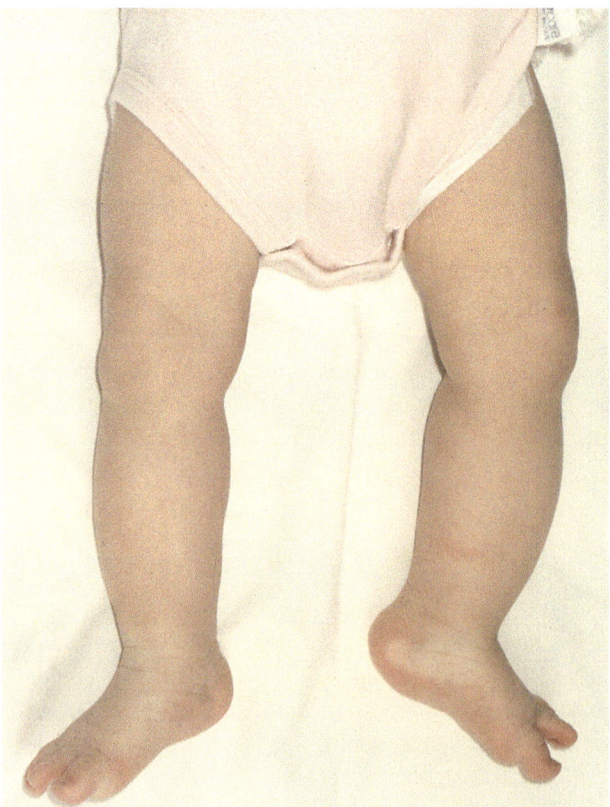

Fig. 4.18 Child aged 9 months with congenital pseudarthrosis of the left tibia. Note the anterior bowing and slight shortening. The tibia has not yet fractured and he was treated with a protective orthosis

good long-term results in a small group of patients treated by bracing alone. Fibular bypass grafting was described by McFarland in 1951 [42] and subsequently prophylactically by Lloyd-Roberts and Shaw [43] and Strong and Wong-Chung [44]. Once a pseudarthrosis becomes established it is extremely difficult to heal. Many methods of grafting have been advocated in a condition that is so rare that most experience is of small numbers and therefore anecdotal. In two large reviews by Hardinge [45] and Baker et al. [46] amputation rates of 29 and 22% were reported.

Three methods have emerged as useful in obtaining union in this difficult condition:

1. Intramedullary rodding and grafting as described by Charnley in 1956 [47] (Fig. 4.20). Anderson et al. [48] reported union in 10 out of 10 patients, but subsequent

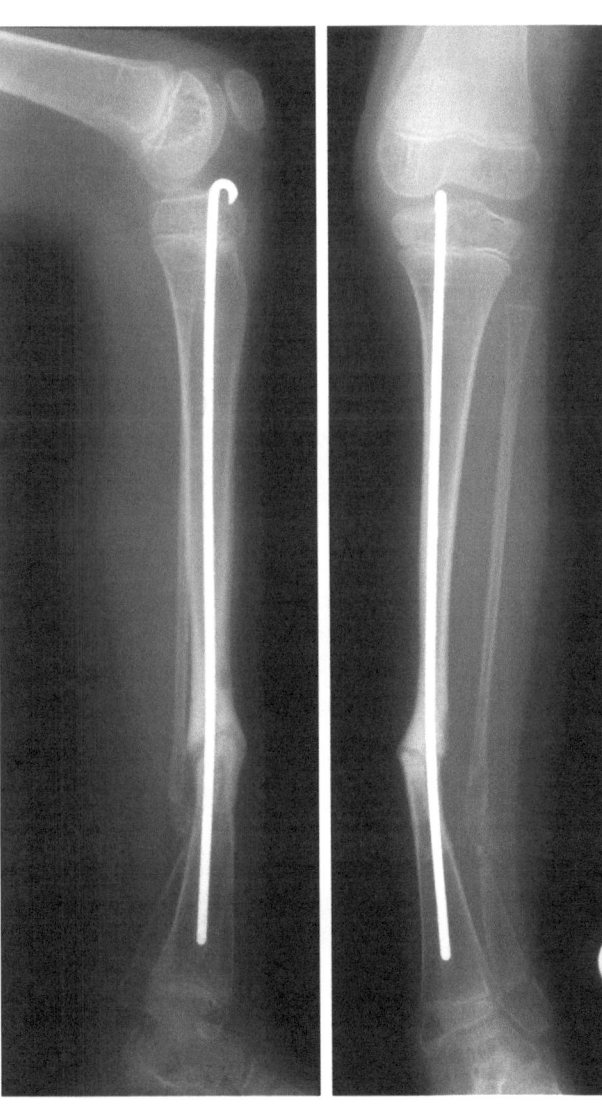

Fig. 4.20 Anteroposterior and lateral radiographs showing intramedullary rodding with a Rush pin for congenital pseudarthrosis of the tibia. Note a valgus deformity of the distal fragment has already developed

re-fracture required further grafting or re-rodding in 5. Paterson and Simonis [49] used electrical stimulation from an implanted stimulator (Osteostim) in addition to intramedullary rodding and obtained union in 20 of 27 tibiae. They emphasized the importance of retaining the intramedullary rod until maturity to avoid re-fracture.

2. Free vascularized fibula graft. Gilbert [50], Pho et al. [51], and Simonis et al. [52] have reported satisfactory results using a free vascularized fibula graft from the contralateral leg.

3. Bone transport. Grill [53] reported good results with a modification of the Ilizarov technique [54] in nine patients, seven of whom had failed several previous operations.

In view of its rarity it is important that in any one geographical area a particular surgeon or group of surgeons undertakes the management of this rare disorder to gain sufficient numbers and experience in its treatment. To try to overcome the problem of small anecdotal series the European Paediatric Orthopaedic Society (EPOS) set up a European multicenter study of treatment and published the results in 2000 [55]. They obtained detailed validated data from 172 patients and drew the following conclusions regarding management:

1. Prophylactic splintage in the pre-pseudarthrosis stage was very useful.
2. There was a clear correlation between the age of surgery and the final outcome with better results being achieved with increasing age.
3. Intramedullary rodding could be used to manage early fracture together with an orthosis.
4. The two most successful surgical treatments in the survey were the Ilizarov technique and the free vascularized fibula graft with union rates of up to 75%. Both methods gave better results if delayed until at least 4–6 years of age. An important observation, which has been supported by a more recent publication in 2006 [56], was that despite union of the tibia, function was often severely limited by residual problems such as valgus deformity and degenerative change in the ankle joint.

Reconstruction Techniques with a Circular Fixator

Treatment with the Ilizarov technique is more likely to be successful after the age of 6 years [55]. In the infant and young child the question of management before definitive treatment at the age of 6 years arises. It is undoubtedly easier to attempt limb reconstruction in a relatively straight tibia with well-aligned foot. If the foot and ankle have been neglected in this condition a troublesome valgus deformity may develop. If the tibia has fractured or there is a significant deformity it is worthwhile correcting the deformity and stabilizing the tibia by a simple osteotomy (without attempting to resect the pseudarthrosis) and rodding the tibia. The lower leg and foot should then be splinted. Unfortunately, particularly with a very distal pseudarthrosis, replacement of the rod will be required at regular intervals. Some surgeons have tried telescopic or extending rods to obviate the need for frequent exchange. Occasionally the pseudarthrosis will heal with rodding alone.

Once the child reaches 6 or 7 years (although the older the child the better), definitive treatment can be attempted with a circular external fixator. The options are resection of the pseudarthrosis and bone transport or resection of the pseudarthrosis, acute compression, and lengthening above in as normal bone as possible. If an intramedullary rod (Rush pin) is still in situ it is useful to leave it in place to protect against fracture when the frame is removed. The principles of fixator

treatment include correction of the mechanical axis, a very stable frame, and apposition of viable bone. With a distal pseudarthrosis it is frequently necessary to extend the frame to the foot to gain adequate stability.

Tibia Recurvatum (Posteromedial Angulation of the Tibia)

This is a very rare deformity. The tibia is bowed posteriorly and, commonly, medially at the junction of the middle and lower thirds. It occurs in association with marked calcaneus of the foot (Fig. 4.21). The appearance is alarming, but the prognosis benign. The majority of cases respond readily to stretching and splintage of the foot into equinus. If the surgeon is prepared to wait long enough, probably all cases will correct with time. Pappas [57] reviewed a large group of 33 patients with this rare condition. He pointed out

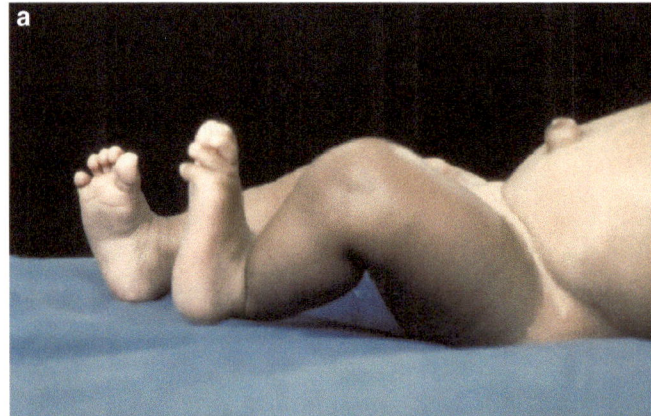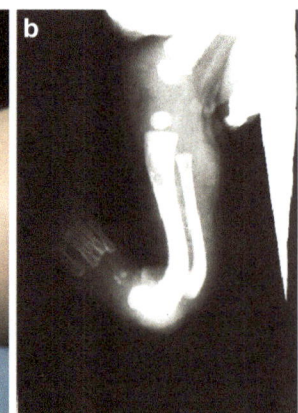

Fig. 4.21 (**a**) Child aged 5 months with left tibia recurvata. Note the calcaneus foot and posterior bowing of the tibia. (**b**) Lateral radiograph of the same patient showing the marked posterior bowing of both the tibia and the fibula

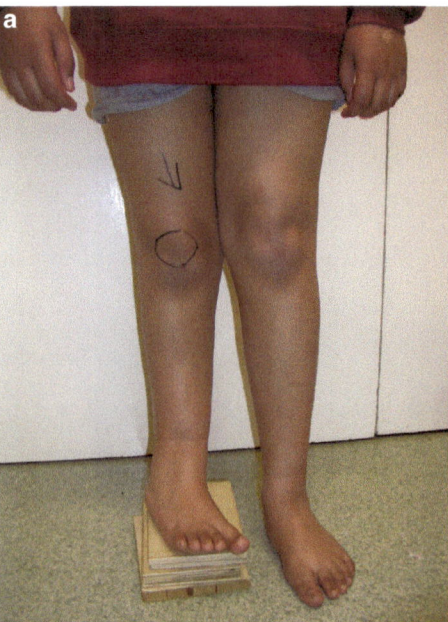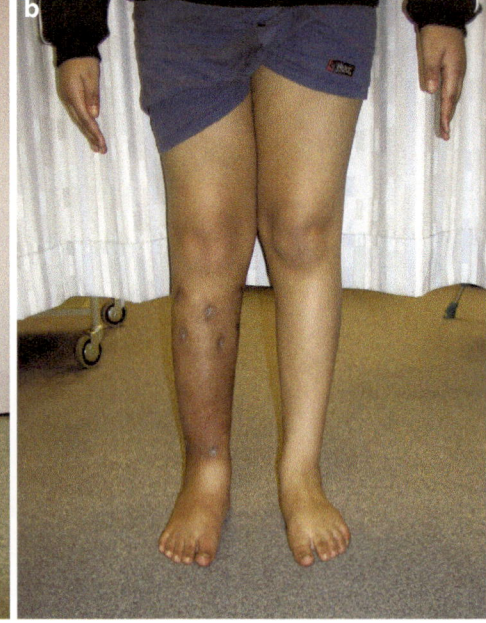

Fig. 4.22 (**a**) Patient with right tibia recurvata showing shortening and inward rotation of the foot. (**b**) Clinical photograph after correction using a Taylor spatial frame

that, in general, the greater the initial bowing the greater the ultimate leg length discrepancy and that the proportionate length differences between the normal and the bowed tibiae remain stable after the child had reached 12 months of age. The maximum leg length discrepancy seen in this series of patients was 6.9 cm. However, if there is persistent deformity when the child starts to walk, corrective osteotomy can be undertaken. Unlike congenital pseudarthrosis of the tibia, the osteotomy will heal, despite the sclerosis at the site of the angulation. However, union may take some time and an intramedullary rod is a useful way of splinting the tibia while awaiting union. Once the deformity has corrected, the child normally manages extremely well, but should be followed up as he or she is liable to be left with some residual shortening, which may require leg equalization procedures near maturity [58]. Any persistent deformity may be corrected at the time of lengthening near maturity using a spatial frame (Fig. 4.22).

Part II: Leg Length Inequality

Franz Grill

Introduction

Leg length discrepancy (LLD) is defined as a condition in which the lower extremities are noticeably unequal.

LLDs are relatively common. Knutson reports a prevalence of 90% in normal adults, with a mean inequality of 5.2 mm. LLD exceeding 20 mm affects at least one in every 1000 individuals [59].

The etiology of LLD may be subdivided into two categories: *anatomical leg length discrepancies* are caused either by shortening of bone structures, angular deformities, or by functional disorders. *Functional length discrepancies* usually result from joint contracture. At hip level, a contracture of the adductor muscles leads to functional shortening, while abduction contracture causes functional lengthening in the standing position. A fixed pelvic obliquity may also be due to a deformity of the lumbar spine. Additionally, flexion contracture of the hip and the knee joint may cause functional shortening, leading to foot deformities such as the equinus [60].

The question as to how much limb-length inequality creates a significant impact on the locomotor system is controversial [59].

According to gait studies in the laboratory, the crucial magnitude is between 2 and 3 cm [61–64]. The authors state that the body is well able to compensate for minor LLD below 2 cm.

Any greater difference in leg length will cause postural imbalance in standing and uneven gait. A common effect of anatomic LLD is rotation of the pelvis. Walsh found that pelvic obliquity was the most common method of compensation for LLD below 22 mm [65]. This compensation mechanism is not without consequences. When LLD exceeds 15 mm the prevalence of chronic back pain is 5.3 times that in the normal population [66].

In addition, an association was found between the LLD and the development of osteoarthritis in the knee and hip joint. Osteoarthritis was found to occur more commonly in the hip of the longer (84%) than the shorter (16%) leg [67, 68]. This conclusion was supported by Golightly, who also reported a higher rate of osteoarthritis in the knee joint of the longer leg [69].

Patellar apicitis in athletes is much more common in the longer leg because of the significantly increased quadriceps activity [70].

Children usually compensate for discrepancies by pelvic obliquity, flexion of the knee on the longer side, or equinus on the shorter side, resulting in significantly greater plantar flexion in the shorter limb.

Etiology of Limb-Length Inequality and Malalignment

Structural causes of limb-length discrepancy and malalignment are numerous. The etiology may be congenital or acquired. The natural course depends upon the degree of inhibition or acceleration of growth and varies according to etiology. In cases of congenital defects, LLD can be calculated and predicted more easily because growth remains proportional. The growth rate in vascular, infectious, traumatic, or neoplastic disorders, however, is variable (Table 4.6) [71].

Deformity

Deformities of part or all of the lower extremity are frequently associated with LLDs. Deformities may be present in the frontal, sagittal, or coronal planes. They may be single level, multilevel, uniplanar, or multiplanar. The biomechanical effect of malalignment exerts a negative impact on the function as well as the longevity of a joint.

Genu varum occurring at the age of 2–3 years is physiological and has an excellent prognosis. Mild bow-leg is common in many adult athletes. Genu valgum is physiological up to the age of 8 or 10 years and persists in mild degree in many adults, particularly women (Table 4.7).

Table 4.6 Etiologies of limb-length discrepancies

	Inhibition of growth	Acceleration of growth
Congenital	Proximal femoral focal deficiency	Klippel Trenaunay syndrome
	Tibial/fibular deficiencies	Proteus syndrome
	Coxa vara congenita	Hemihypertrophy
	Congenital hip dislocation	Hemophilia
	Silver–Russel syndrome	Arteriovenous malformation
	Hemiatrophy	–
	Ollier's disease	–
	Clubfoot	–
Infection/ inflammation	Osteomyelitis (metaphyseal), septic arthritis with growth plate damage	Osteomyelitis (diahyseal)
	–	Juvenile rheumatoid arthritis
Neurological Diseases	Poliomyelitis	–
	Myelomeningocele	–
	Cerebral palsy	–
Posttraumatic	Traumatic growth plate lesson	Metaphyseal fracture, diaphyseal fracture
	Slipped capital femoral epiphysis	Postoperative (osteotomy)
Tumor	Osteochondroma	Neurofibromatosis, malalignment
	Neurofibromatosis	Bone tumors
Other	Legg–Calvé–Perthes disease	Fibrous dysplasia
	Irradiation	–

Table 4.7 Different etiologies of malalignment

Cause	Genu valgum	Genu varum
Congenital	Fibular hemimelia	Tibial hemimelia
	Skeletal dysplasia	Skeletal dysplasias
Trauma	Partial physeal arrest	Partial physeal arrest
Arthritis	Juvenile rheumatoid arthritis	–
Infection	Partial growth arrest	Partial growth arrest
Metabolic	Rickets	Rickets
Others	Burns	Blount's disease

Assessment of the Patient

History

Eliciting a careful past medical history is essential when dealing with acquired discrepancy. A positive family history may indicate a syndrome.

Clinical Assessment

It is fundamental to distinguish between true and apparent shortening and to bear in mind the fact that some patients may have both.

As the causes of LLD are numerous, a meticulous, standardized clinical assessment must be performed to determine all associated abnormalities.

Discrepancies are commonly compensated for by altered function. Limping, circumduction, varus and valgus deformity, equinus on the shorter side, and knee flexion or hyperextension on the longer side may be present, depending upon the magnitude of the LLD.

Height, the relationship between the trunk and the extremities, thigh and lower leg proportions, as well as alignment and posture must be evaluated in the standing position. Pelvic obliquity is present in any LLD and the physician must determine by clinical examination whether this is due to a fixed deformity of one or more of the three lever arms attached to the pelvic ring, or secondary to structural spinal deformity.

In the supine position, joints have to be clinically tested in respect of instability or restriction of motion.

Measurement of Discrepancy

In the absence of fixed joint deformities, two methods for measurement of LLD provide reliable results:

- Assessment in the standing position by placing blocks of known height under the short leg to level the pelvis: each segment should be assessed visually by this method. Forward flexion of the spine allows the pelvic alignment to be reviewed from behind, along with rotation and tilting of the back.
- Tape measurement in the supine position of the distance between the anterior superior iliac spine and the medial or lateral malleolus: this method may be misleading in cases of pelvic asymmetry or hind foot deformity or if the legs are not positioned parallel to the pelvis and spine.

Clinical assessment of minor length inequalities may be difficult and imprecise when performed before the child begins to walk. Standing with blocks under the foot of the shorter leg is the best measurement in the older child.

Imaging

Radiography has long been considered the gold standard for LLD measurement and will determine any associated bone or joint deformities.

Radiographs in standardized reference planes are necessary to analyze deformity and obtain reproducible measurements. Angular deformities are better analyzed by the use of radiographs in the standing position. For the antero-posterior (AP) radiograph in the frontal plane, the knee is positioned with the patella exactly centered and pointing forward, regardless of the foot position [72]. In cases of fixed dislocation or subluxation of the patella, the tibial tuberosity is used to align the limb. A further option is to assess the knee flexion–extension axis and position the knee perpendicular to this axis. For a more accurate assessment of the impact of ligament laxity or joint laxity, a radiograph in single-leg stance may be obtained.

The knee must be exactly positioned in order to obtain a projection in the same plane as that used for the initial analysis. A long focal distance is necessary in order to visualize the hip, knee, and ankle joint on a single film. The advantage of the long distance is that magnification is minimized so that measurements and planning of the hardware can be performed more accurately. The majority of the digital radiograph systems currently in use permit digital synthesis of two or more separate images, enabling reconstruction of a full standing radiograph. Sagittal view films are particularly important to evaluate abnormal or diminished range of motion in the joint (flexion contracture or hyperextension). For the full standing lateral radiograph, the patient is positioned with the pelvis of the contralateral side rotated posteriorly by about 35° and the knee in full extension. However, in most instances a lateral radiograph of the femur and a lateral view of the tibia are sufficient to evaluate the respective joint alignment in the sagittal view. Full standing radiographs cause significantly greater radiation exposure than do ordinary ones because of the long film focus. They should be performed only if additional information about the femur and the tibia is needed to decide appropriate treatment, such as preoperative planning or fine-tuning of the final alignment when performing gradual correction of a deformity using an external fixator.

Assessment of LLD can be performed by the use of long, standing films or orthoradiography (Fig. 4.23). Orthoradiography is performed with the patient lying supine with a full scale between the legs on the table [73, 74]. Three separate sequential exposures with the central ray directed successively over the hip, knee, and ankle joints are necessary. As the scale is magnified by approximately the same factor as the bones, the true length of the femur and tibia can be calculated. However, this method does not provide any information about functional LLD or pelvic obliquity, or the role of foot height as a contribution to total LLD. A second imaging technique to assess LLD is the long, standing radiograph with extra-long film cassettes. Extra-long films of 51 in. in length (more than 1 m) are widely available in the United States, while smaller long films of 90 cm are available in most European countries. These provide images of the entire lower extremity including the foot and pelvis in adolescents as well as adults.

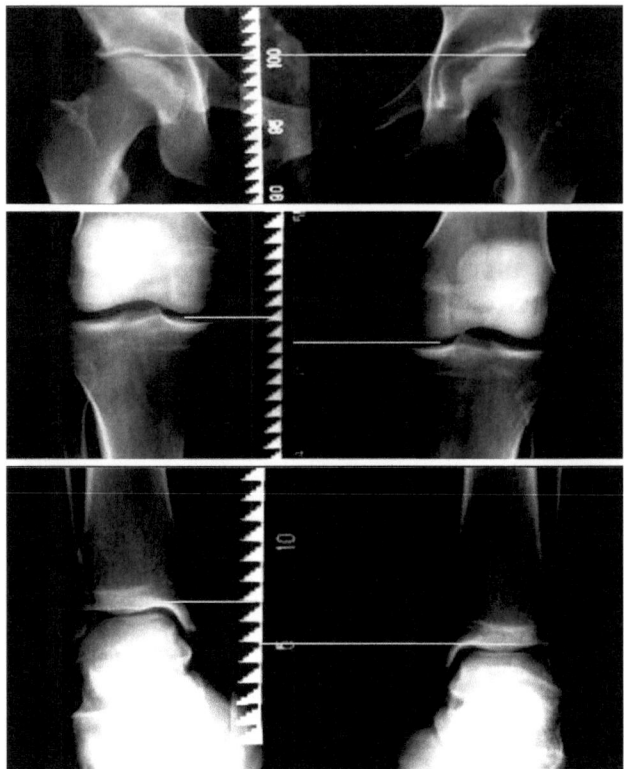

Fig. 4.23 Orthoradiography for measurement of LLD

Digital radiography imaging systems are increasingly used and usually offer a software solution to paste together two or more exposures, combining them into a single, continuous image. The advantage of such films is the ability to calculate precisely leg length, foot height, and the magnitude of a potential functional shortening.

Deformity Analysis

Deformity analysis and preoperative planning should be performed to compare the anatomy of the patient with the mean values of a normal population, to assess the exact location and magnitude of the deformity, and to predict the outcome in respect to the osteotomy and correction. In the past, the femorotibial angle was used to describe varus or valgus alignment of the knee and the Mikulicz line was used to assess the position of the mechanical axis. While the Mikulicz line is still used to describe the mechanical axis deviation (MAD), the center of rotation of angulation (CORA) planning method permits exact analysis of angular deformities of the lower limbs (Fig. 4.24) [75–77].

CORA can be analyzed for every angular deformity. A basic understanding of the nomenclature is necessary to plan the treatment. Alignment refers to the colinearity of the hip,

Fig. 4.24 Normal values for joint orientation according to Paley and Tetsworth

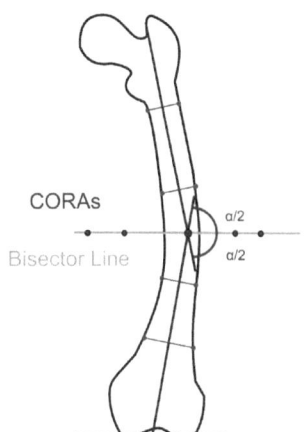

CORAs

Bisector Line

α/2

α/2

- if the osteotomy line and the ACA pass through the same CORA, the bones will angulate relative to each other without translation.
- when the ACA passes through a CORA but the osteotomy is at a different level, the ends of bone at the osteotomy level will angulate and translate to each other. The proximal and distal axis lines will realign fully when the correction is complete.
- if the ACA does not pass through the CORA, the proximal and distal axes of the bone will be parallel but will translate to each other. The same principles are applicable for multi-apical deformities or deformities of the upper extremity or the foot (Fig. 4.25).

Prediction of growth is a prerequisite prior to epiphysiodesis or distraction lengthening of a shortened extremity

knee, and ankle joints. Joint orientation refers to the position of an articular surface in relation to the axis of the limb segment. In mid-diaphyseal deformities it is relatively intuitive to draw a line along the axes of the respective segments. However, in deformities close to the joint or in juxta-articular deformities, the line for the short segment has to be constructed using predefined angles. The angles can be determined by drawing the axis of the long segment and the joint orientation line. Average figures based upon values for the normal population have been provided for all joint lines of the lower extremity.

Two modes of planning have been proposed for the frontal plane. For anatomical planning one uses the anatomical axis of the femur, the mid-shaft axis, and the anatomical axis of the tibia; the respective joint lines define the CORA. Mechanical planning is based upon the mechanical axis of the femur which is inclined 7° to the anatomical axis and usually connects the center of the femoral head with the center of the knee joint. In the tibia the mechanical axis is nearly identical to the anatomical axis; there is no difference here between the two planning modes. However, the two modes should never be mixed.

The CORA is the most important assessment for the correction of an angular deformity. The line that runs through the CORA and bisects the lateral and medial angle formed by the proximal and distal axes at the bone is named the transverse bisector line.

The other two important factors are the angulation correction axis (ACA) and the osteotomy level. ACA is the axis line around which the deformity is corrected. While the CORA is determined by deformity analysis and cannot be selected by the surgeon, the ACA and the osteotomy level can be freely selected. However, if ACA is not on the bisector line of CORA, a secondary translational deformity will occur. Paley and coworkers formulated three osteotomy rules to describe the relationship between the CORA, the ACA, the osteotomy level, and the result of correction:

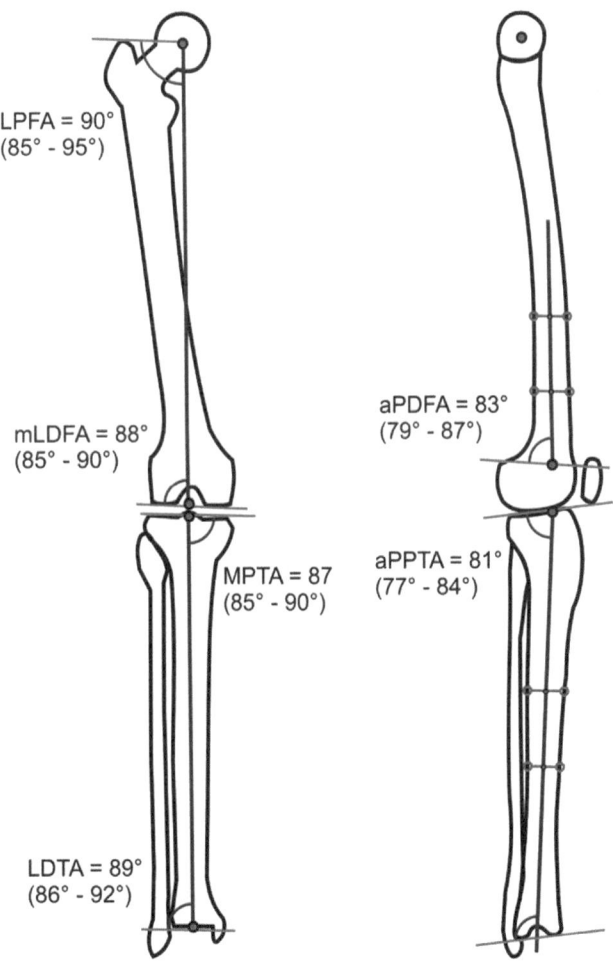

LPFA = 90°
(85° - 95°)

mLDFA = 88°
(85° - 90°)

MPTA = 87
(85° - 90°)

LDTA = 89°
(86° - 92°)

aPDFA = 83°
(79° - 87°)

aPPTA = 81°
(77° - 84°)

Fig. 4.25 Analysis of malalignment; determination of CORA. CORAs along the bisector line. Correcting around CORA on the convex side will result in shortening of the bone; the magnitude of lengthening increases in direct proportion to the distance of CORA from the bone and the concave side. This is particularly important in correction using unilateral fixators in the immature patient. Various methods have been proposed to calculate the magnitude of the remaining growth. The majority of these methods are not based upon chronologic age but on bone age, which can be estimated using specific indicators.

Calculation and Determination of Bone Age

Several disorders are associated with a delay in bone age, such as Perthes' disease, cerebral palsy, or Ollier's disease. The atlas of Greulich and Pyle uses gender-specific details of anteroposterior radiographs of the left hand to determine bone age [78]. However, the radiographs used for this atlas were obtained from children born between 1917 and 1942. An atlas produced by the French authors Sempé and Pavia provides similar data [79]. However, changes on radiographs may not be obvious during puberty, thus raising the likelihood of inaccurate interpretations.

The Sauvegrain method employs a scoring system to evaluate the AP and lateral views of the elbow. This method has been evaluated by Diméglio and coworkers [80] and was found to provide more details than the atlas of Greulich and Pyle [78, 81]. However, the method is restricted to the growth spurt during puberty, which occurs between the age of about 10 and 13 years in girls and between 12 and 15 years in boys.

The Tanner and Whitehouse system uses 20 indicators on the AP hand radiograph [82]. It is very time-consuming and cumbersome despite being available in computerized form on the Internet.

Prediction of the Progression of Deformity

In cases of posttraumatic hemiepiphysiodesis secondary to a bone bridge, the margin of the growth plate can be calculated. The width of the physis, the percentage of growth in relation to the growth of the entire bone, bone length, and age-specific multipliers must be determined. However, the proportion of growth from the distal femur and the proximal tibia is not the same at all ages [71]. As a temporary hemiepiphysiodesis by staples or a plate is recommended to correct angular deformities in the growing child, the prediction may only be necessary at the end of growth in order to ensure that the remaining growth is adequate to bring about full correction of the deformity.

Remaining Growth

The Green and Anderson method is based upon growth data [73, 74]. These longitudinal data include the length of the femur and the tibia for females and males from the age of 1 year to maturity. A total of 700 children, 87% of whom had residual paralysis in one lower extremity and a normal extremity on the other side, and 158 normal children were included in this study.

The patients were Irish children from South Boston; the majority of them had poliomyelitis. It should be noted that the study did not account for differences in ethnicity, height, or socioeconomic status.

Straight Line Graph

The straight line graph was introduced by Moseley [83] and is based upon data provided by Green and Anderson. Moseley transformed the normal growth curve of Anderson data into a straight line by adapting the data points on the x- and y-axis of the chart. The result is a 45° line that represents normal growth and can be used to predict geometric growth and the effects of an epiphysiodesis. However, the straight line graph should ideally be used by performing three separate measurements at different ages, not always possible if the patient reports to the surgeon in later childhood or adolescence.

Minimum requirements for the calculation are the length of the long leg and the short leg, and skeletal age. The greatest difficulty associated with this method is to determine the percentile of the patient within the skeletal age range. This determination is improved by taking skeletal rather than chronological age into account.

Arithmetic Method

The arithmetic method was introduced by Westh and Menelaus and is used for the purpose of timing epiphysiodesis [84]. The method employs chronologic age and the difference in leg length by blocks. It should not be used when chronologic age and bone age differ by more than 1 year. As a rule of thumb, distal femur growth is 0.95 cm and proximal tibial growth 0.64 cm per year. However, this assumption does not account for growth spurts or the fact that the growth plates at the knee joint increase their percentage of total bone growth when approaching the end of growth.

Paley's Multiplier Method

Paley and coworkers introduced the multiplier method to predict bone length, adult height timing of epiphysiodesis, and even prenatal prediction of LLD at maturity

[20]. The multiplier method is a simple arithmetic formula. The data for this formula have been derived from the Anderson and Green growth data [73, 74] and compared with multipliers calculated from 19 other databases, including radiographic, clinical, and anthropological information from a variety of different populations. In all of these calculations, the same multipliers were established for the different data sets and populations. The method appears to be independent of percentile groups and is the same for the prediction of femoral, tibial, and total limb lengths.

The multiplier method can also be employed to calculate adult height. It is simpler to use than the percentiles of Bailey and Pinneau [85].

Error in Using Growth Charts

Little et al. [86] compared eight methods of predicting limb-length discrepancy, including those of Anderson [87] and Moseley [83]. They found that the methods using skeletal age were no more accurate than those based on chronological age. They evaluated the techniques for timing epiphysiodesis as described by Green and Anderson [73, 74], Moseley [83], and Westh and Menelaus [84] and registered similar accuracies for all, independent of whether chronologic or skeletal age was used.

All of these methods are valid only when there is constant growth inhibition of the short limb. Thus, they cannot be used in patients with conditions involving accelerations and decelerations of growth, such as rheumatoid arthritis.

Management of LLD

The goals of any treatment of LLD are to level the pelvis and avoid secondary problems such as low back pain or early osteoarthritis.

Treatment guidelines for limb-length equalization are well established. There is general consensus that no treatment is required in adults with discrepancies less than 2 cm unless these are symptomatic. Only about 10% of adults with a length discrepancy of up to 2 cm use a shoe lift.

In discrepancies of more than 2 cm, a shoe raise is indicated. The shoe raise should be about 1 cm less than the actual discrepancy. Adjustments can be applied inside or outside the shoe or as a combination of both. A shoe raise is generally not well accepted. Children as well as adults feel awkward when asked to use one and usually opt for surgical correction.

Surgical management of LLD depends upon age, basic pathology, severity, projected height at the end of growth, and associated deformities. Equalization can be achieved surgically either by shortening the longer limb or by lengthening the shorter limb, or both.

In a growing child, a prerequisite for any intervention is exact preoperative planning based upon the estimation of skeletal age, calculation of discrepancy, and body height at maturation. Ideally, relevant growth data should be collected over a number of years prior to surgery, permitting precise calculation.

In principle, correction of LLD should remain at the same level as the deformity. The two knees should be at the same level and the pelvis should be balanced after correction.

Surgical Limb Equalization

Shortening the Long Leg in Children

The pros and cons of shortening as a means of leg length equalization have to be discussed with the patient and the parents. In a child of normal height at maturation and an anticipated discrepancy of 2–5 cm, shortening should be the method of choice. It is safe and effective if there is sufficient growth left to effect a correction. The preferred method is epiphysiodesis, which is defined as surgical interruption of the growth of the physis of the longer leg. Epiphysiodesis of the distal femoral epiphysis is used to shorten the femur, while shortening of the tibia is best achieved by epiphysiodesis of the proximal tibia, including the fibula if there are more than 2 cm of expected skeletal growth. Using different techniques, epiphysiodesis can be either temporary or permanent. In case of valgus or varus deformity, the surgeon may perform a gradual correction by means of hemiepiphysiodesis (unilateral medial or lateral). When remaining growth is inadequate to achieve full correction by epiphysiodesis, surgical shortening by bone reSection may be indicated.

Epiphysiodesis

This is a simple method for equalizing leg lengths but is frequently neglected or not undertaken at the appropriate time. As it is a biological method, the final outcome is not entirely predictable. Nevertheless, the method is important not only for LLDs of 2–5 cm predicted at skeletal maturity but also in cases of severe LLD in congenital limb deficiencies as an adjunct to lengthening procedures. Parents tend to feel anxious when the healthy leg of their child is suggested as the site for operation. The surgeon must explain the method accurately so that the parents comprehend its benefits for their child. They should be made aware that procedures that lengthen the leg, or a shortening operation after skeletal maturation, are more complex and carry greater risk. An epiphysiodesis or hemiepiphysiodesis can be performed relatively simply by different techniques that bring about a permanent or temporary arrest of the physis [88]. The impact on final height is moderate, nevertheless the method should be avoided in patients of short stature

Permanent Growth Plate Arrest by Mini-invasive Techniques [92]

Under image intensifier guidance, a K-wire or small Steinmann pin is inserted through the middle of the physis from the medial aspect of the distal femur or proximal tibia using the Canale technique [89] or the lateral side using the Macnicol technique [90, 91]. The latter approach allows the proximal fibular physis to be ablated if appropriate. After performing a 10 mm skin incision directly over the epiphyseal guide wire, the epiphysis is entered using a cannulated drill [89]. The size of the drill bit is gradually increased from 6 to 12 mm (Fig. 4.26). The growth plate is drilled out along the K-wire to the opposite side. After withdrawing the K-wire, the drill bit is used to destroy the growth cartilage. The tubesaw method allows access from the lateral side [91], with removal of a 1 cm diameter core of the growth plate and neighboring bone followed by thorough removal of the physis which can be accessed by small curettes. The bone plug is reinserted transversely at the end of the operation, thus controlling postoperative hemorrhage. A plaster cast is unnecessary but crutches

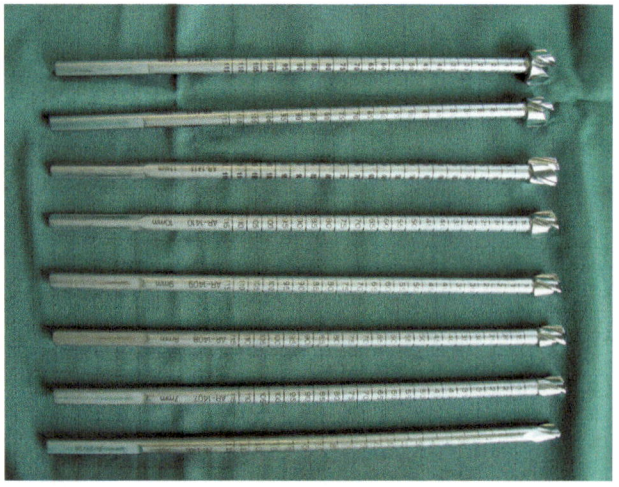

Fig. 4.26 Special design for drill bits used for Canale mini-invasive technique of epiphysiodesis. Diameters from 6 to 12 mm

are provided initially, with full activity permitted after 6 weeks.

Permanent Growth Plate Arrest—Phemister's Open Surgery Technique

A longitudinal 3-cm incision is made both medially and laterally over the physis. Using an osteotome, a cortical bone block (2 cm × 2.5 cm), centered over the physis, is removed on each side. A curette is used to excise part of the growth plate, especially in the central area of the physis. The bone blocks are then rotated 90° or 180° and impacted into the respective defects medially and laterally.

Postoperative immobilization with a knee immobilizer and partial weight bearing is advised for 4 weeks. Full activity is permitted after 6 weeks. However, postoperative morbidity is greater after the Phemister method than following the less invasive methods described [90]. Complications include postoperative hemorrhage or hematoma, under- and overcorrection of the discrepancy and angulatory deformity.

Permanent Hemiepiphysiodesis

These techniques can be used for permanent hemiepiphysiodesis although the rate of correction of angulation is unpredictable.

Temporary Arrest of the Growth Plate: Stapling

Physeal stapling consists of placing 2–3 staples medially and laterally across the physis (distal femur, proximal tibia) extraperiosteally. As long as the staples are in place, growth is inhibited. The staples should be left in position until the scheduled correction has been performed. They should not remain for more than 18–24 months because of the potential risk of permanent damage to the physis.

Several complications may be associated with this procedure, such as extrusion and breakage of staples, permanent arrest, overcorrection, growth abnormality (axial deviation), or rebound of longitudinal growth after removal of staples.

Temporary Arrest of the Growth Plate—Epiphysiodeses and Hemiepiphysiodeses—The 8-Plate Technique

Under C-arm control, the growth plate is identified. A small skin incision is made. Either from the lateral (varus deformity) or from the medial (valgus deformity) aspect, an

8-plate is fixed strictly extraperiosteally using two self-tapping cannulated screws, one fixed distally and one proximally to the growth plate. The plate should be perfectly positioned on the AP as well as lateral views. Inserted medial and lateral to the physis, the 8-plate can also be used to achieve a temporary growth arrest (Fig. 4.27).

The postoperative course is usually uneventful. The patients are able to walk the same day and clinical follow-up investigations must be performed every 3 months. The 8-plate (or staples) must be removed on time in order to avoid overcorrection.

The 3-month follow-up investigation is mandatory to identify overcorrection or any other disturbance of growth. In general, the staples or the 8-plate should not remain for longer than 18–24 months since exceeding this may lead to definitive damage of the physis.

The 8-plate is superior to conventional staples in several respects. A longer skin incision is required for stapling.

Usually the surgeon has to insert two or three staples. Postoperative rehabilitation takes longer and the technique is associated with greater risk.

Shortening Osteotomies

Acute shortening is indicated in patients with a discrepancy of 2–5 cm in adolescence with an absence of sufficient residual growth, or in young adults. The magnitude of shortening should not exceed 4 cm.

Femoral Shortening Techniques

From the lateral aspect, a segment of bone is resected at the proximal femoral level either at the subtrochanteric level or by a z-shaped interochanteric approach. After resection of the bone segment the osteotomy is coapted, compressed, and fixed by the use of a blade plate (Fig. 4.28) or a dynamic hip screw. Shortening should not exceed 10–15% of the total femoral length. Acute shortening is mainly indicated in patients with a discrepancy of 2–4 cm. Postoperatively the patient has to use crutches for at least 3 months until bony consolidation of the osteotomy has occurred.

A further technique is closed femoral shortening. By placing a saw in the intramedullary canal from proximally, a segment of the femur is excised and displaced by splitting the separated fragment. The femur is fixed with an intramedullary nail.

Tibial Shortening

The magnitude of the shortening should not exceed 3 cm. Resection is performed proximally, and fixation is achieved by the use of a plate or an interlocking nail.

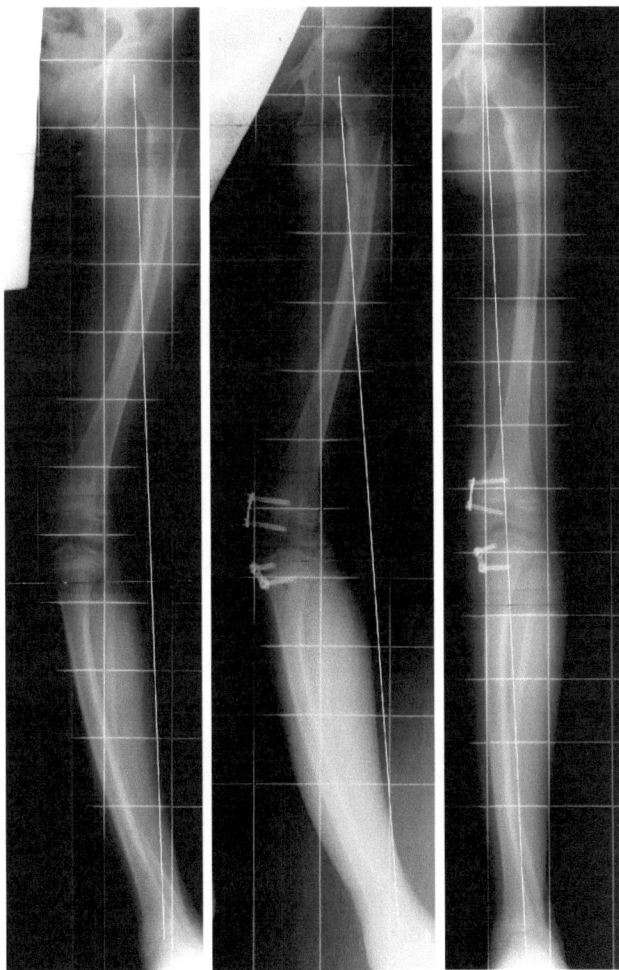

Fig. 4.27 Temporary arrest of growth plate in a 9-year-old female with valgus knee deformity treated by hemiepiphysiodesis at the distal femoral and proximal tibial level using 8-plates

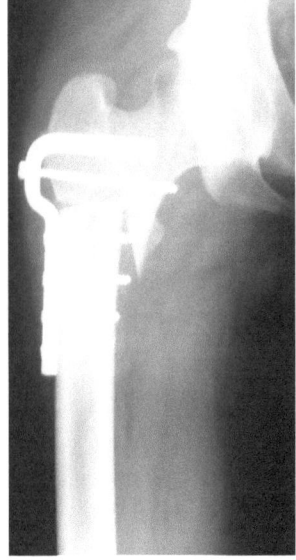

Fig. 4.28 Shortening osteotomy in a case of LLD secondary to poliomyelitis. The Wagner technique was used to preserve the lesser trochanter. Fixation used an AO-blade plate

In general, shortening of the femur is preferred to shortening of the tibia because the latter is associated with a greater risk of compartment syndrome, persistent muscular weakness, and delayed bone union.

Leg Lengthening

History

Long bone lengthening has been undertaken for more than 100 years, dating back to Codivilla who performed femoral lengthening in several steps using traction after femoral osteotomy, with a Steinmann pin placed in the calcaneus [93]. Codivilla reported on 26 patients whose femora had been lengthened by 3–8 cm.

Modern lengthening techniques have evolved and been refined gradually [72, 94–99]. The Wagner technique is now historical. It consisted of fixing a monolateral external fixator with a distraction unit on the bone, then performing a diaphyseal osteotomy followed by distraction. After having achieved the desired lengthening, the gap was filled with cancellous bone grafts and stabilization was achieved by inserting an AO plate.

The principle of distraction osteogenesis for bone healing during lengthening was described by Abbott, Anderson, and by Ilizarov [96, 100, 101].

Biology of Lengthening—Distraction Osteogenesis—Bone Regenerate

As in any fracture, after osteotomy bone healing starts by callus formation. Gradual distraction of living tissues creates stresses which stimulate and maintain active regeneration. This early reparative tissue is distracted by lengthening and followed by intramembranous ossification with the formation of a bone regenerate. Ossification occurs on both sides of this structure and columns or osteoid appear, a process known to occur in membrane bone formation as well. On radiographs these columns look striated in the line of the distraction force.

Callus formation is enhanced by performing a low-energy osteotomy (corticotomy). This minimally invasive procedure preserves blood supply and causes less damage to soft tissues and bone marrow. Under ideal conditions, distraction should start 5–7 days after corticotomy. Delays of 2–3 weeks are associated with a high risk of premature bone consolidation. On the other hand, unstable mechanical fixation and a distraction rate of more than 2 mm daily lead to poor bone formation and eventual nonunion.

The rate of lengthening for optimal bone formation is 1 mm per day. Lengthening is best achieved in increments of 0.25 mm.

The mechanical lengthening device must ensure stability in order to produce the distraction stress phenomenon. Undesirable angular or shearing movements will result in the formation of fibrous tissue and not fibrocartilage. Smoking delays bone healing, so patients should refrain from smoking at least during the period of their treatment, failing which they should be regarded as unsuitable candidates for lengthening [102].

There is good reason to believe that axial micromovements are beneficial or even essential for producing the correct tissue response. Axial micro motion signifies that the bone is dynamized throughout the lengthening process.

After the desired lengthening has been achieved, the external fixator is kept in place until full bone consolidation is evident. The fixator may be removed as soon as cortical bone has appeared.

Usually the index healing period for full consolidation per centimeter of lengthening biologically normal bone is around 25–35 days, depending upon the patient's age.

Up to 20% of any given bone can be safely lengthened. Larger magnitudes can be achieved at the expense of a higher complication rate.

The Gigli saw or the De Bastiani corticotomy method permit a more controlled bone cut [95]. When using the De Bastiani technique the cortical bone is predrilled using several circumferentially applied drill holes and the bony bridges between the drill holes are cut using a chisel or osteotome.

Chondrodiatasis lengthens by growth plate distraction. It can be achieved without rupture of the growth plate by increasing growth through the hypertrophic zone, between the proliferating cells and the zone of provisional calcification. Currently this procedure is only indicated in exceptional cases confined to individuals approaching skeletal maturity.

The results of Ilizarov's research and clinical work provide a clear understanding of the basic principles of bone lengthening, deformity correction, and treatment of bone defects [96, 97, 100, 101]. Such knowledge is mandatory for the surgeon performing limb lengthening.

Mechanical Devices for Leg Lengthening

Mechanical methods of lengthening include external fixation, external fixation in combination with an intramedullary nail (lengthening over nail), and intramedullary distraction devices.

A perfect device should allow for lengthening, permit simultaneous accurate correction of deformities in all planes and dimensions, provide stability of the bone regenerate, be user-friendly, painless for the patient, devoid of complications, and acceptable to the patient. The ideal device has not yet been developed. However, a large number of systems are available, depending upon the pathology and the respective anatomical conditions.

The Ilizarov Ring Fixator

The fixator consists of rings connected by threaded rods. Tensioned Kirschner wires are fixed to the ring and cross within the bone. The K-wires are made of either titanium or stainless steel. The wire tip is shaped like a bayonet and measures 1.5 or 1.8 mm. Smooth and olive types of wires are available. They have to be tensioned in the full ring to 130 kg and in the half ring to 70 kg. Fixation is not secure unless the rings are positioned in pairs. Two wires are used at each level. For maximum stability the two wires should cross at right angles. Anatomical limitations must be taken into account. It is mandatory for the surgeon to always remain in an anatomical safe zone. The advantages of wires are that they can be placed in tight spots, permit micro motion in axial loading, and stable fixation in porotic bone. A combination of wires and half pins increases stability and avoids the risks of limb transfixion.

The Ilizarov system consists of numerous items that permit the surgeon to construct a tailored device for any deformity, including those of the foot and the knee. The rings are connected by threaded rods. If angular deformities have to be corrected, the surgeon may include hinges in the construct. Hinge placement is performed according to the rules of deformity correction [72]. Angular, rotational, and translational deformities can be corrected by this procedure.

Extending the frame across a joint will protect it and permit progressive correction to occur either before or during lengthening. An equinus deformity can be corrected by placing hinges at the level of the ankle joint.

Lengthening can be combined with multilevel correction using proper ring and hinge placement. In bifocal lengthening both metaphyses within the segment may be lengthened simultaneously.

Other conditions that can be treated with the Ilizarov ring fixator are bone defects and pseudarthrosis. In these conditions a segmental bone transport is an effective technique for achieving bone consolidation and healing.

Lengthening Over a Nail

Lengthening over a nail is an option to shorten the duration of external fixator support. When using this technique in conjunction with an Ilizarov device or a monolateral fixator, an intramedullary locking nail is inserted. As soon as the desired lengthening has been achieved the nail is locked and the fixator can be removed.

Taylor Spatial Frame

The Taylor spatial frame is a hexapod system consisting of two rings connected with six telescope struts at universal joints. By adjusting only strut length, one ring can be repositioned in relation to the other. Simple or complex deformities are treated using the same frame. The multiple angles and translations of a given deformity are addressed by adjusting the length of struts only. The Taylor spatial frame fixator is capable of correcting 6-axis deformity, guided by a web-based software program. Six deformity parameters, three frame parameters, and four mounting parameters are required to achieve correction using the program. In the event of failure the program can be restarted by entering new and more accurate parameters [98]. The system permits correction of complex foot deformities using special foot applications and a foot correction computer program and can also be combined with Ilizarov items (Fig. 4.29). Joints can be bridged with the Ilizarov system. Multiple-plane correction can be achieved at three levels in the same limb segment. The Taylor spatial frame is much easier to handle than the conventional Ilizarov system, especially for correction of rotational and translational deformities. The Taylor spatial frame produces more accurate corrections of deformity than those achieved with the Ilizarov device. Patients find the system easy to use because a daily adjustment schedule is provided. The strut exchanges are listed and explained in chronological sequence (Fig. 4.30).

Monolateral Devices

The first widely used monolateral fixator was the Wagner device, which was designed for diaphyseal lengthening followed by cancellous grafting and plating. Unlike the Wagner technique, the earlier Abbott/Anderson method recognized the biological importance of gradual distraction, thus avoiding the use of bone grafting, but these early, double frames were torsionally weak and therefore did not allow walking. The Wagner device was replaced by the Orthofix fixator, a much more sophisticated monolateral system allowing bone lengthening, axial correction, segmental transport, and multilevel correction.

A new device (Multi-Axial Correction MAC Biomet) now makes it possible to obtain optimized multiplanar deformity correction by the use of a unilateral system. The latter is highly modular, can be integrated into a rail system and

Fig. 4.29 A Taylor spatial frame for lengthening in an 8-year-old boy at the proximal tibial metaphysis. Hybrid mounting with conventional Ilizarov items to avoid knee dislocation by bridging the knee and ankle joint to avoid equinus. (**a**) AP view. (**b**) Lateral view

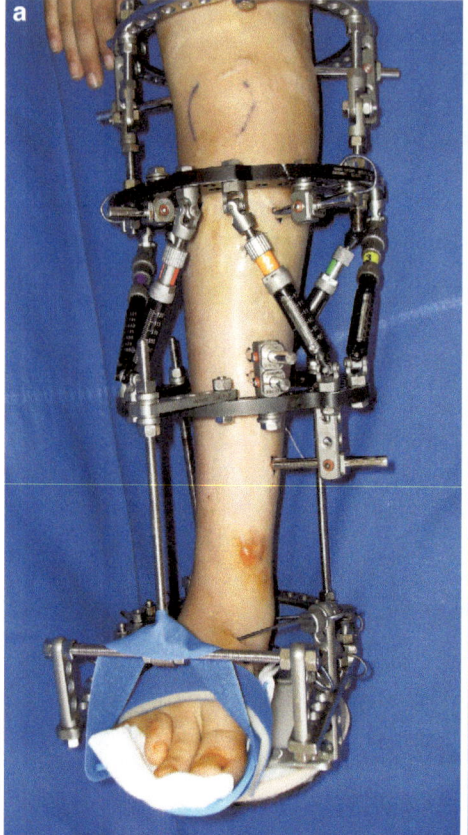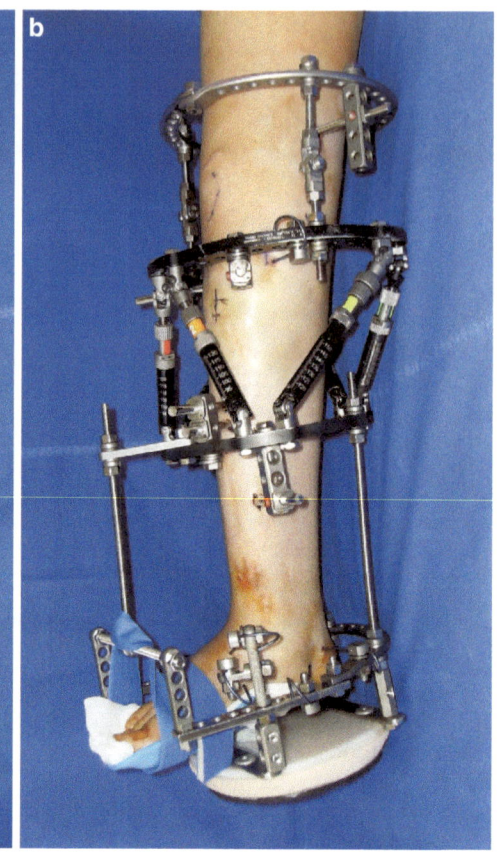

Fig. 4.30 (**a**) Twelve-year-old boy with posttraumatic shortening and valgus deformity of the left knee, treated using a TSF shortening of 5 cm with valgus knee deformity. (**b**) TSF in situ after deformity correction. (**c**) Radiograph showing perfect alignment, correction of valgus deformity, and shortening. (**d**) Final outcome after removal of the external fixator

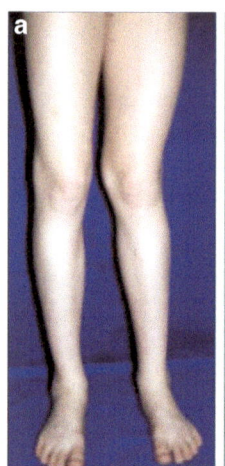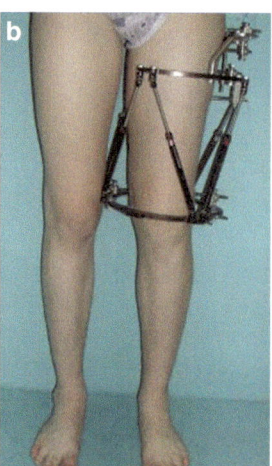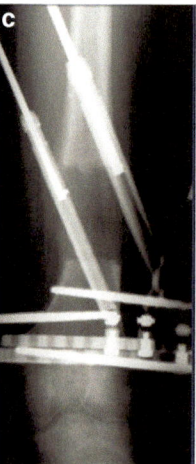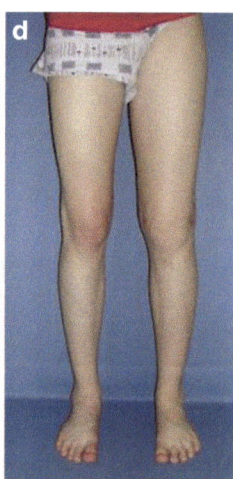

a hybrid ring construct, and also offers the possibility of articulated joint distraction.

The advantage of monolateral fixators is that they are less bulky. Their main indications in paediatric orthopaedics are trauma, lengthening of small bones such as metatarsals or metacarpals, as well as lengthening of the humerus. A further common indication is articulated distraction of the hip and elbow joint using dynamic monolateral fixators (Fig. 4.31).

Intramedullary Bone Lengthening

Patients with a discrepancy in limb length as well as short stature generally prefer to undergo a lengthening procedure that does not involve the use of external fixators. The disadvantage of external fixators is that the activities of daily life are severely limited. Painful pin site infection occurs in

Fig. 4.31 Monolateral fixator for hip joint distraction

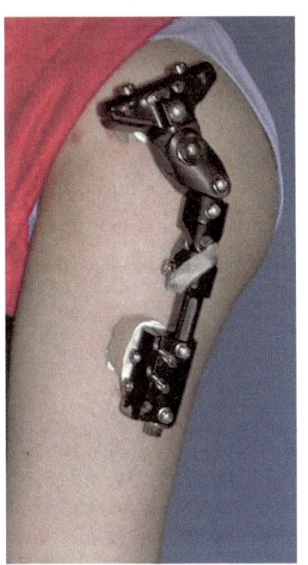

Fitbone

Fitbone is a further innovative concept that recognizes the biological importance of callus distraction. It consists of a fully implantable computer-controlled motor-driven distraction device. The internal drive system is provided with an electromechanical segment and an integrated electronic module that receives electric power through high-frequency transmission from outside the limb. There is no connection between the implant and the surface of the human body. The nail is very well accepted by patients because elongation occurs continuously and very slowly without rotational movements. It is also painless and does not limit joint movement. The metal is removed approximately 2 years after lengthening has been concluded and tibial or femoral bone union is assured (Fig. 4.32).

nearly all cases if skin is allowed to tent and is not regularly cleansed. Furthermore, the risk of fracture after removal of the fixator remains a concern. The development of an intramedullary bone lengthening implant was achieved in Germany by Götz and Schellmann in 1975 [103], Baumann and Harms [104], and Witt and Jäger [105]. Bliskunov in Russia has also developed a system [106–108]. The most recent innovations in this regard are the Albizzia nail developed by Guichet [109], the intramedullary skeletal kinetic distractor (ISKD) nail by Cole [110], and the Fitbone by de Baumgart et al. [111].

The implants can only be used if the medullary cavity is wide enough and the growth plates are about to close.

Albizzia Nail

Gradual lengthening is achieved by efforts of the patient who is required to produce rotational movements of 20° to lengthen the nail together with the bone. Manual rotation of this sort is painful and poorly tolerated by a large number of patients.

ISKD Nail

The ISKD was developed by Orthofix. Small rotational movements of 3–9°, effected by the patient, cause the telescopic nail to be lengthened. Analogous to Ilizarov's method, the ISKD nail is associated with gradual lengthening of callus. The rate of distraction depends on how frequently the patient rotates the limb. A monitor enables the patient to follow the progress of distraction.

Up to 8 cm of lengthening can be achieved but patients may overlengthen the limb and produce problems in bone regeneration.

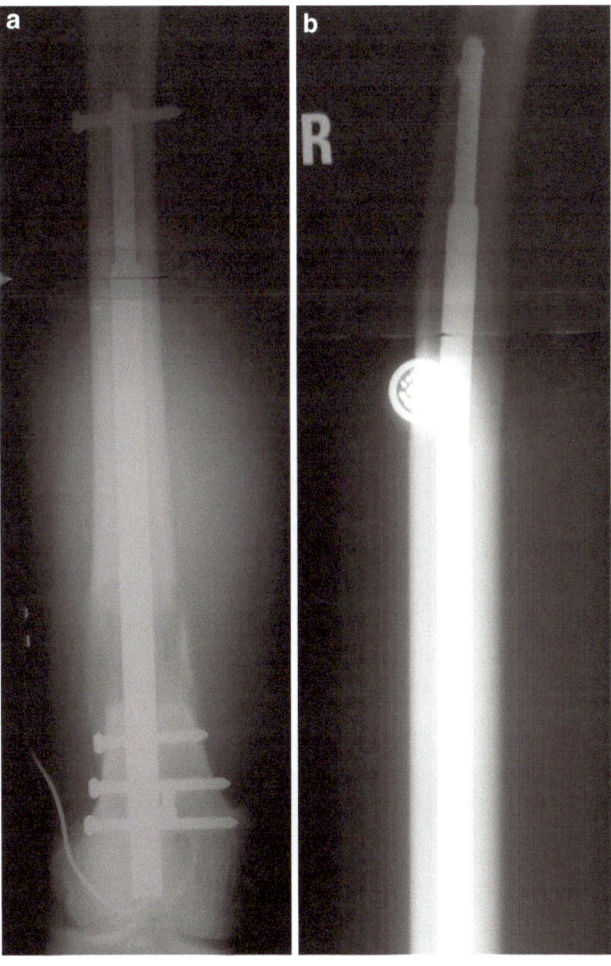

Fig. 4.32 Posttraumatic shortening and flexion deformity of the right femur due to partial growth arrest. Fitbone in situ with lengthening achieved. Correction of distal femoral malalignment performed using the placement of two bollar screws to achieve deformity correction. (**a**) AP projection. (**b**) Lateral projection

Obstacles in Limb Lengthening

Limb lengthening is a demanding surgical procedure and should be performed by experienced orthopaedic surgeons. As the entire treatment may take several weeks or even months, a number of minor or major complications may occur [112].

Minor Complications

Proper pin care is essential. The pin sites must be cleaned and disinfected on a daily basis; a regular shower is recommended. Pin site infections are usually painful as long as bone lengthening is in progress.

In case of early osseous consolidation of the bone regenerate, the osteotomy has to be repeated.

Major Complications

Severe stiffness as well as dislocation of the hip and knee joints may occur and may be difficult to treat.

Equinus deformity is common when physiotherapy is not performed on a regular basis. Support for the foot during distraction may be of value.

Nerve lesions, particularly those of the peroneal nerve, are a risk during treatment of congenital deficiencies and valgus deformities of the knee.

During lengthening, fractures may occur proximal or distal to the external fixator. After removal of the fixator, fractures may occur through the lengthened segment. Therefore, particularly in dysplastic bone and poor bone regenerate, it is advisable to protect the lengthened bone from fracture by inserting a Rush pin or Kirschner wire.

Axis deviation should not be overlooked and must be corrected prior to consolidation of the lengthened segment. The deviation can be corrected by new data input and an adjusted program for deformity correction using the Taylor spatial frame, or by hinge adjustment when Ilizarov frame distraction is in progress.

Prostheses

In congenital deficiencies with an anticipated LLD of more than 25 cm at maturity, equalization by surgery is not advisable because the patient may require repeated operations and prolonged hospitalization and because of the high risk of complications such as joint dislocation, stiffness, bone regenerate fracture, and psychological problems.

Treatment should be orientated toward maintaining a good function during childhood. This should be achieved by a combination of surgical procedures which allow optimal fitting of the prosthesis. Amputation may be an option in some instances, but leads to loss of proprioception, sensitivity and function. Modern orthoprosthetic technology increasingly provides nearly normal function and quality of life, and children usually tolerate prostheses well.

References

1. Frantz CH, O'Rahilly R. Congenital skeletal limb deficiencies. J Bone Joint Surg 1961; 43A:1202–1224.
2. Day HJB. The ISPO/ISO classification of congenital limb deficiency. Prosthetics Orthotics International 1991; 15:67–69.
3. Fixsen JA. Major limb congenital shortening: a mini review. J Pediatr Orthop B 2003; 12:1–12.
4. Morgan JD, Somerville EW. Normal and abnormal growth at the upper end of the femur. J Bone Joint Surg 1960; 42B:264–272.
5. Hootnick DR, Levinsohn EM, Randall PA, Packard DS Jr. Vascular dysgenesis associated with skeletal dysplasias of the lower limb. J Bone Joint Surg 1980; 62A:1123–1129.
6. Szeizel AE, Codaj I, Lenz W. Smoking during pregnancy and congenital limb deficiency. Brit Med J 1994; 308:1473–1476.
7. Amputee Medical Rehabilitation Society. Congenital Limb Deficiency. Recommended Standards of Care. A report by the working party of the Amputee Medical Rehabilitation Society published December 1997. Available from the Amputee Medical Rehabilitation Society c/o of the Royal College of Physicians, 11 St Andrew's Place, Regents Park, London NW1 4LE, UK.
8. Kim MT, Chambers HG, Mubarak SJ, Wenger DR. Congenital coxa vara: Computed tomographic analysis of femoral retroversion and the triangular metaphyseal fragment. J Pediatric Orthop 2000; 20:551–556.
9. Subharwal S, Muttal R, Cox G. Percutaneous triplantar femoral osteotomy correction for developmental coxa vara: A new technique. J Pediatr Orthop 2005; 25:28–33.
10. Hamanishi C. Congenital short femur: clinical, genetic and epidemiological comparison of the naturally occurring condition with that caused by thalidomide. J Bone Joint Surg 1980; 62B:307–320.
11. Amstutz HC, Wilson PD Jr. Dysgenesis of the proximal femur (coxa vara) and its surgical management. J Bone Joint Surg 1962; 44A:1.
12. Aitken GT. Proximal femoral focal deficiency. A congenital anomaly. Symposium held in Washington, 3 June 1968. Washington DC: National Academy of Sciences; 1969:1–22.
13. Pappas AM. Congenital abnormalities of the femur and related lower extremity malfunction: classification and treatment. J Pediatr Orthop 1983; 3:45–60.
14. Fixsen JA, Lloyd-Roberts GC. The natural history and early treatment of proximal femoral dysplasia. J Bone Joint Surg 56B; 1974 86–95.
15. Gillespie R. Classification of congenital abnormality of the femur. In: Herring JA, Birch JG, eds. The Child with a Limb Deficiency. Rosemont IL: American Academy of Orthopaedic Surgeons; 1998:63–72.
16. Paley D. Lengthening reconstruction surgery for congenital femoral deficiency. In: Herring JA, Birch JG, eds. The Child with a Limb Deficiency. Rosemont IL: American Academy of Orthopaedic Surgeons; 1998:113–132.

17. Gillespie R, Torode IP. Rotationplasty of the lower limb for congenital defects of the femur. J Bone Joint Surg 1983; 65B: 569–573.

18. Ring PA. Congenital short femur. J Bone Joint Surg 1959; 41B:73–77.

19. Ring PA. Congenital abnormalities of the femur. Arch Dis Child 1961; 36:410.

20. Paley D, Bhave A, Hertzenberg JE, Bowen JR. Multiplier method for predicting limb-length discrepancy. J Bone Joint Surg 2000; 82A:1432–1446.

21. Thomas MP, Jackson AM, Aichroth PM. Congenital absence of the anterior cruciate ligaments. J Bone Joint Surg 1985; 67B: 572–575.

22. Sanpera I Jr, Fixsen JA, Hill RA. The knee in congenital short femur. J Pediatr Orthop B 1995; 4:159–163.

23. Hosalkar HS, Jones S, Chowdhury M, et al. Quadricepsplasty for knee stiffness after lengthening in congenital short femur. J Bone Joint Surg 2003; 85B:261–264.

24. Goddard NJ, Hashemi-Nejad A, Fixsen JA. Natural history and treatment of instability of the hip in proximal femoral focal deficiency. J Pediatr Orthop B 1995; 4:145–149.

25. Damsin JB, Pous JG, Ghanem I. Therapeutic approach to severe congenital lower limb length discrepancies, surgical treatment versus prosthetic management. J Pediatr Orthop B 1995; 4: 164–170.

26. Panting AL, Williams PF. Proximal femoral focal deficiency. J Bone Joint Surg 1978; 60B:46–52.

27. Borggreve J. Kniegelenkersatz durch das in der Beinlangsachse um 180 Grad gedrehte Fussgelenk. Archiv der orthopadischen und Unfallchirurgie 1930; 28:175–178.

28. King RE. Some concepts of proximal femoral focal deficiency. In: Aitken GT, ed. Proximal femoral focal deficiency. A congenital anomaly. Symposium held in Washington, 3 June 1968. Washington DC: National Academy of Sciences; 1969: 23–49.

29. Achterman C, Kalamchi A. Congenital deficiency of the fibula J Bone Joint Surg Br 1979; 61B:133–137.

30. Birch JG, Lincoln TL, Mack PW. Functional classification of fibular deficiency. In: Herring JA, Birch JG, eds. The child with a limb deficiency. Rosemont IL: American Academy of Orthopaedic Surgeons; 1998:161–171.

31. Stanitski DF, Stanitski CL .Fibular hemimelia: A new classification. J Pediatr Orthop 2003; 23:30–34.

32. Hootnick DR, Boyd NA, Fixsen JA, Lloyd-Roberts GC. The natural history and management of congenital short tibia with dysplasia or absence of the fibula. A preliminary report. J Bone and Joint Surg 1977; 59B:267–271.

33. Maffuli N, Fixsen JA. Fibular hypoplasia with absent lateral rays of the foot. J Bone Joint Surg 1991; 73B:1002–1004.

34. Jones D, Barnes J, Lloyd-Roberts GC. Congenital aplasia and dysplasia of the tibia with intact fibula. J Bone Joint Surg 1978; 60B:31–39.

35. Kalamchi A, Dawe RB. Congenital deficiency of the tibia. J Bone Joint Surg Br 1985; 67B:581–584.

36. Schoenecker PL, Kapelli AM, Miller EA, et al. Congenital longitudinal deficiency of the tibia. J Bone Joint Surg 1989; 71A:278–287.

37. Brown FW. Construction of a knee joint in congenital total absence of the tibia (paraxial hemimelia tibia)—a preliminary report. J Bone Joint Surg 1965 47A:695–704.

38. De Sanctis N, Nunziata Rega A. New rationale in management of tibial agenesis type II: a maturity review of its functional, psychological and economic value. J Pediatr Orthop B 1996; 5:1–5.

39. Boyd HB. Pathology and natural history of congenital pseduarthrosis of the tibia. Clin Orthop 1982; 166:5–13.

40. Choi T-J, Choi IH, Chung CY, et al. Isolated congenital pseudarthrosis of the fibula. J Pediatr Orthop 2006; 26: 449–454.

41. Murray HH, Lovell WW. Congenital pseudarthrosis of the tibia, a long term follow-up study. Clin Orthop 1982; 166: 14–20.

42. McFarland B. Pseudarthrosis of the tibia in children. J Bone Joint Surg 1951; 43B:36–46.

43. Lloyd-Roberts GC, Shaw NE. The prevention of pseudarthrosis of the tibia and congenital kyphosis of the tibia. J Bone Joint Surg 1969; 51B:100–105.

44. Strong ML, Wong-Chung J. Prophylactic bypass grafting of the prepseudarthrotic tibia in neurofibromatosis. J Pediatr Orthop 1991; 11:757–764.

45. Hardinge K. Congenital anterior bowing of the tibia. Ann Royal Coll Surg Engl 1972; 51:17–30.

46. Baker JK, Cain TE, Tullos HS. Intramedullary fixation for congenital pseudarthrosis of the tibia. J Bone Joint Surg 1992; 74A:169–178.

47. Charnley J. Congenital pseudarthrosis of the tibia treated by the intramedullary nail. J Bone Joint Surg 1965; 38A:283–290.

48. Anderson DJ, Schoenecker PL, Sheridan JJ, Rich MM. Use of an intramedullary rod for treatment of congenital pseudarthrosis of the tibia. J Bone Joint Surg 1992; 74A:161–168.

49. Paterson DC, Simonis RB. Electrical stimulation in the treatment of congenital pseduarthrosis of the tibia. J Bone Joint Surg 1985; 67B:454–462.

50. Gilbert A. Vacularised fibular transfer for treatment of congenital pseudarthrosis. Annual Meeting of the American Academy of Orthopaedic Surgeons, Anaheim, California, 14 March 1983.

51. Pho RWH, Levack B, Satku K, Patradul A. Free vascularised fibulograft in the treatment of congenital pseudarthrosis of the tibia. J Bone Joint Surg 1985; 67B:64–70.

52. Simonis RB, Seirali HR, Mayou B. Free vascularised fibular grafts for congenital pseudoarthrosis of the tibia. J Bone Joint Surg 1991; 73B:211–215.

53. Grill F. Treatment of congenital pseudarthrosis of tibia with the circular frame technique. J Pediatr Orthop B 1996; 5:6–16.

54. Ilizarov GA. Basic principles of transosseous compression and distraction osteosynthesis. Ortopedia Travmatologiial i Protezirovanie 1971; 32:7–15.

55. Grill F, et al. Results of the EPOS multicentre study of congenital pseudarthrosis of the tibia. J Pediatr Orthop B 2000; 9:1–15, 69–102.

56. Muharrem I, El-Rasi G, Riddle EC, Kumar SJ. Residual deformities following successful initial bone union in congenital pseudarthrosis of the tibia J Pediatr Orthop 2006; 26:393–399.

57. Pappas AM. Congenital posteromedial bowing of the tibia and fibula. J Pediatr Orthop 1984; 4:525–531.

58. Heyman CH, Herndon CH, Keiple KG. Congenital posterior angulation of the tibia with talipes calcaneus. J Bone Joint Surg 1959; 41A:476–488.

59. Knutson GA. Anatomic and functional leg-length inequality: A review and recommendation for clinical decision-making. Part I, anatomic leg length inequality: prevalence, magnitude, effects and clinical significance. Chiropractic Ostopath 2005; 13:11.

60. O'Toole GC, Makwana NK, Lunn J, et al. The effect of leg length discrepancy on foot loading patterns and contact times. Foot Ankle Int 2003; 24:256–259.

61. Gurney B. Leg length discrepancy, Gait Posture 2002; 15: 195–206.

62. Kakushima M, Miyamoto K. The effect of leg length discrepancy on spinal motion during gait: three-dimensional analysis in healthy volunteers. Spine 2003; 28(21):2472–2476.

63. Song KM, Halliday SE. The effect of limb-length discrepancy on gait. J Bone Joint Surg Am 1997; 79(11):1690–1698.

64. Goel A, Loudon J, Nazare A, et al. Joint moments in minor limb length discrepancy: a pilot study Am J Orthop 1997; 26(12): 852–856.

65. Walsh M, Connolly P, Jenkinson A, O'Brien T. Leg length discrepancy—an experimental study of compensatory changes in three dimensions using gait analysis. Gait Posture 2000; 12(2):156–161.

66. Friberg O. Clinical symptoms and biomechanics of lumbar spine and hip joint in leg length inequality. Spine 1983; 8(6): 643–651.

67. Tallroth K, Ylikoski M, Lamminen H, Ruohoncn K. Preoperative leg length inequality and hip osteoarthrosis: a radiographic study of 100 conservative arthroplasty patients. Skeletal Radiol 2005; 34:136–139.

68. Gofton JP, Trueman GE. Studies in osteoarthritis of the hip: Part II. Osteoarthritis of the hip and leg length disparity. C M A J 1971; 104:791–799.

69. Golightly PT, Allen KD, Renner JB, et al. Relationship of limb length inequality with radiographic knee and hip osteoarthritis, Osteoarthritis Cartilage 2007; 15:824–829.

70. Kujala UM, Osterman K, Kvist M, et al. Factors predisposing to patellar chondropathy and patellar apicitis in athletes. Int Orthop 1986; 10(3):195–200.

71. Pritchett JW. Longitudinal growth and growth-plate activity in the lower extremity. Clin Orthop 1992; 275:274–279.

72. Paley D. Principles of Deformity Correction. Berlin: Springer; 2003.

73. Green WT, Anderson M. Epiphyseal arrest for the correction of discrepancies in length of the lower extremities. J Bone Joint Surg 1957; 39A:853–872.

74. Green WT, Anderson M. Experiences with epiphyseal arrest in correcting discrepancies in length of the lower extremities in infantile paralysis: A method of predicting the effect. J Bone Joint Surg Am 1947; 29:659–678.

75. Herzenberg JE, Paley D. Leg lengthening in children (Review). Curr Opin Pediatr 1998; 10(1):95–97.

76. Paley D, Tetsworth K. Mechanical axis deviation of the lower limbs. Preoperative planning of uniapical angular deformities of the tibia or femur. Clin Orthop Relat Res 1992; 280: 48–64.

77. Paley D, Herzenberg JE, Tetsworth K, et al. Deformity planning for frontal and sagittal plane corrective osteotomies. Orthop Clin North Am 1994; 25(3):425–465.

78. Greulich WW, Pyle SI. Radiographic atlas of skeletal development of the hand and wrist, 2nd ed. Stanford CA: Stanford University Press; 1959.

79. Sempé M, Pavia C. Atlas de la maturation squelettique: ossification séquentielle du poignet et de la main. Paris: SIMEP; 1979.

80. Diméglio A, Charles YP, Daures JP, et al. Accuracy of the Sauvegrain method in determining skeletal age during puberty. J Bone Joint Surg Am 2005; 87(8):1689–1696.

81. Greulich JW, Pyle SI. Radiographic Atlas of Skeletal Development of the Hand and Wrist, 2nd ed. Stanford: Stanford University Press; 1959.

82. Tanner JM, Whitehouse RH. Clinical longitudinal standards for height, weight, height velocity, weight velocity and stages of puberty. Arch Dis Child 1976; 51(3):170–179.

83. Moseley CF. A straight line graph for leg length discrepancies. J Bone Joint Surg Am 1977; 59:174–179.

84. Westh RN, Menelaus MB. A simple calculation for the timing of epiphysial arrest: a further report. Bone Joint Surg Br 1981; 63-B(1):117–119.

85. Bailey N, Pinneau SR. Tables for predicting adult height from skeletal age, revised for Greulich and Pyle hand standards. J. Pediatr 1952; 40:423–441.

86. Little DG, Nigo L, Aiona MD. Deficiencies of current methods for the timing of epiphysiodesis. J Pediatr Orthop 1996; 16: 173–179.

87. Anderson M, Green WT, Messner MB. Growth and predictions of growth in the lower extremities. J Bone Joint Surg Am 1963; 45:1–14.2.

88. Timperlake RW, Bowen JR, Guille JT, Choi IH. Prospective evaluation of fifty-three consecutive percutaneous epiphysiodeses of the distal femur and proximal tibia and fibula. J Pediatr Orthop 1991; 11:350–357.

89. Canale ST, Christian CA. Techniques for epiphysiodesis about the knee. Clin Orthop Rel Res 1990; 255:81–85.

90. Macnicol MF, Gupta M. Epiphysiodesis using a cannulated tube-saw. J Bone Joint Surg Br 1997; 97B:307–309.

91. Macnicol MF. Tubesaw epiphysiodesis. In: Tachdjian MO, ed. Atlas of Pediatric Orthopaedic Surgery. Philadelphia: WB Saunders; 1994.

92. Phemister DB. Epiphysiodesis for equalizing the length of the lower extremities and for correcting other deformities of the skeleton. Mem Acad Chir Paris 1950; 76(26–27): 758–763.

93. Codivilla A. On the means of lengthening in the lower limbs, the muscles and the tissues which are shortened through deformity. Am J Orthop Surg 1905; 2:353–369.

94. Bastiani G, Aldegheri R, Renzi-Brivio L, Trivella G. Chondrodiatalsis—controlled symmetrical distraction of the epiphyseal plate: limb lengthening in children. J Bone Joint Surg 1986; 688:550–556.

95. De Bastiani G, Aldegheri R, Renzio-Vrivio L, Trivella G. Limb lengthening by callus distraction (callotasis). J Pediatr Orthop 1987; 7:129–134.

96. Ilizarov GA. Clinical application of the tension-stress effect for limb lengthening. Clin Orthop Rel Res 1980; 258:8.

97. Ilizarov GA, Deviatov A. Operative elongation of the leg. Ortopedica Travmatologiia Prptezirovanie 1971; 32:20–25.

98. Taylor JC. Taylor spatial frame. In: Rozbruch SR, Ilizarov S, eds. Limb Lengthening and Reconstruction Surgery. Informa Healthcare USA; 2007: 613–637.

99. Baumgart R, Betz A, Schweiberer L. A fully implantable motor-ized intramedullary nail for limb lengthening and bone transport. Clin Orthop Rel Res 1977; 343:135–143.

100. Ilizarov GA. The tension-stress effect on the genesis and growth of tissues. Part I: The influence of stability of fixation and soft-tissue preservation. Clin Orthop Rel Res 1989; 238: 249–281.

101. Ilizarov GA. The tension-stress effect on the genesis and growth of tissues. Part II: The influence of the rate and frequency of distraction. Clin Orthop Rel Res 1989; 239: 263–285.

102. Baig MR, Rajan M. Effects of smoking on the outcome of implant treatment: a literature review. Indian J Dent Res 2007 Oct-Dec, 18(4):190–5.

103. Götz J, Schellmann WD. Continuous lengthening of the femur with intramedullary stabilisation. Arch Orthop Unfallchir 1975; 82(4):305–310.

104. Baumann F, Harms J. The extension nail. A new method of the femur and tibia. Arch Orthop Unfallchir 1977; 90(2):139–146.

105. Witt AN, Jäger M. Results of animal experiments with an implantable femur distractor for operative leg lengthening. Arch Orthop Unfallchir 1977; 88(3):273–279.

106. Bliskunov AI. Implantable devices for lengthening the femur without external drive mechanisms. Med Tekh 1984; (2): 44–49.

107. Bliskunov AI. Lengthening of the femur using implantable appliances. Acta Chir Orthop Traumatol Cech 1984; 51(6): 454–466.

108. Bliskunov AI. Intramedullary distraction of the femur (preliminary report). Ortop Travmatol Protez 1983; 10:59–62.

109. Guichet J, Deromedis B, Donnan L, et al. Gradual femoral length-
     ening with the Albizzia intramedullary nail. J Bone Joint Surg Am
     2003; 85-A:838–848.
110. Cole J, Justin D, Kasparis T, et al. The intramedullary skeletal
     kinetic distractor: first clinical results of a new intramedullary
     nail for lengthening of the femur and tibia. Injury 2001; 32 Suppl
     4:SD1229–1239.
111. Baumgart R, Zeiler C, Kettler M, Weiss S, Schweiberer
     L (1999) Der voll implantierbare Distraktionsmarknagel
     bei Verkürzungen, Deformitäten und Knochendefekten.
     Indikationsspektrum. Orthopäde 28: 1058–65.
112. Paley D. Problems, obstacles, and complications of limb length-
     ening by the Ilizarov technique. Clin Orthop 1990; 250:
     81–104.

Chapter 5

Developmental Dysplasia of the Hip

Michael K.D. Benson and Malcolm F. Macnicol

Introduction

This common disorder, which ranges from mild, spontaneously resolving instability in the newborn to complete dislocation with secondary acetabular and proximal femoral deformity, continues to provoke debate about its assessment and management.

Embryology and Development

An understanding of development of the hip joint allows an insight into the dysplasias and vascular insults to which it is vulnerable.

Three weeks after fertilization primitive limb buds are already beginning to form in the embryo. Strayer demonstrated that these are initially filled with mesenchyme which differentiates in time to form all joint components except for the blood vessels and nerves [1].

The *6-week* embryo is 12-mm long. Areas within the mesenchyme have condensed to outline the ilium, ischium, pubis, and femoral shaft. Rapid differentiation follows. The femoral head appears slightly later than the femoral shaft but by *7 weeks,* when the embryo is 17-mm long, an inter-zone develops between the femoral head and the acetabulum. Three separate layers develop within this inter-zone and come to form the perichondrium of the acetabulum and the femoral head together with the synovial membrane.

By 8 *weeks* the embryo is 30-mm long and blood vessels have grown into the ligamentum teres. There is the beginning of angulation of the femoral neck upon the femoral shaft. The cleft which heralds the true joint cavity begins to develop by apoptosis and the acetabular labrum is identifiable as a separate entity.

At 11 *weeks* the embryo is 50-mm long. The femoral head is spherical and 2 mm in diameter. It is clearly separate from the acetabulum and Watanabe [2] showed that it was possible experimentally to dislocate the hip for the first time at this age. The neck–shaft angle now measures 130–150°; it is already possible to detect femoral anteversion of between 5 and 10°; the vascular supply to the hip is established.

The *16-week* fetus is 120-mm long. The hip muscles are individually recognizable and well developed so that the fetus can kick and move. The femoral shaft shows early ossification within its cartilage anlage but the femoral head and trochanters remain cartilaginous until well after birth (Fig. 5.1). In utero fetal hips lie typically in flexion, abduction, and external rotation, with the left hip usually being the more rotated. The blood supply to the femoral head is predominantly through the epiphyseal and metaphyseal vessels. The vessels in the ligamentum teres are insignificant at this stage but contribute more to the femoral head blood supply later in gestation.

During the *last 20 weeks* of intra-uterine life the hip joint enlarges and matures. In 1912, Le Damany [3] showed neatly that the capacity of the acetabulum relative to the femoral head decreases in the last 3 months of gestation; the studies of Ralis and McKibbin in 1973 [4] confirmed that the acetabular capacity and depth are least at birth and the femoral head therefore most vulnerable to displacement. Neck–shaft angulation, femoral neck anteversion, and acetabular orientation have been interpreted very differently by different authors. The flexed position of the pelvis upon the lumbar spine and the tightly flexed hips contribute to this confusion because the anatomical position is not achieved until the neonatal lumbar kyphosis and the fixed hip flexion present at birth are lost. Most believe that femoral neck anteversion increases during the second half of fetal life reaching an average of 35° at birth. The neck–shaft angle probably changes little: it averages 135–140° at birth.

At birth the femoral shaft has usually ossified to just above the lesser trochanter. The femoral head and greater trochanter combine in a common proximal chondro-epiphysis (Fig. 5.1). The ossific nucleus is occasionally

M.K.D. Benson (✉)
Nuffield Orthopaedic Centre Oxford, UK

Fig. 5.1 Maturation of the femoral head in the first 5 years

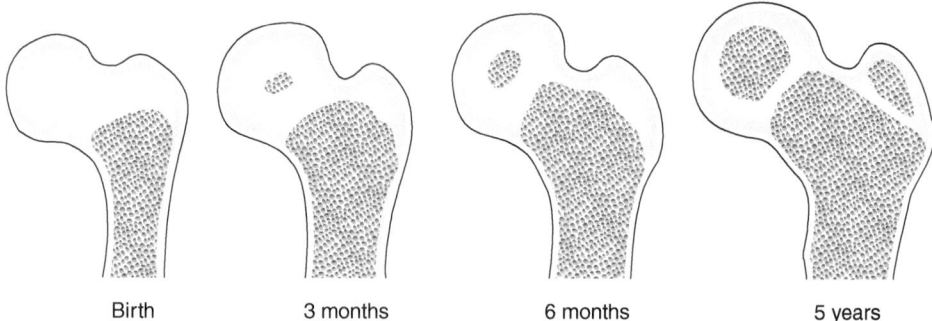

Birth   3 months   6 months   5 years

present within the femoral head at birth but usually does not appear for 3–6 months. In black Africans ossification is often present at birth but this is rare in Caucasians. Ossification of the pelvis is well advanced although the pubis lags behind the ischium and ilium.

Hip Growth After Birth

Acetabular growth is complex: the triradiate cartilage contributes 70%, enlarging both in diameter and depth. At the interface between the pelvic bones and the triradiate cartilage double growth plates allow the circumferential enlargement of the cavity to accommodate the growing femoral head. Growth plates extend also beneath the articular surface of each pelvic bone [5]. The acetabular ring epiphysis which surrounds the acetabular margin contributes nearly 30% to acetabular depth. Small centers of ossification appear in the ring epiphysis between 11 and 14 years. It usually fuses to the acetabular margin in mid-adolescence. Persistent hip instability may lead to failure of fusion and is an indicator of this instability. The triradiate cartilage closes at about 11 years in girls and a year later in boys.

At birth the femoral neck is short and the greater trochanter only slightly distal to the femoral head (Fig. 5.1). Differential growth in the proximal chondro-epiphysis allows the neck to lengthen and the trochanter to lateralize. Although the ossific nucleus in the femoral head should be seen radiologically by 6 months its appearance is often delayed for several months if the hip is dislocated. The greater trochanter starts to ossify by the fourth and the lesser trochanter by the eighth year. The proximal femoral physeal plate contributes about 30% to the eventual length of the femur.

Blood Supply

Despite its rich blood supply, the femoral head is vulnerable to infarction. This is the consequence partly of its deformable cartilaginous structure and partly of its end-arterial blood supply. The two main sources of blood supply

to the proximal femur arise from the medial and lateral circumflex vessels, each of which arises typically from the profunda femoris artery (Fig. 5.2). The lateral circumflex artery and its ramifications supply the lateral and anterior part of the chondro-epiphysis, largely the greater trochanter. The postero-superior branch of the medial circumflex artery supplies the bulk of the intracapsular blood supply to the femoral head. At birth the artery of the ligamentum teres supplies only a small area around the fovea. Although each supplying vessel branches extensively in the proximal epiphysis Trueta [6] demonstrated that there is no intercommunication between the systems as each is end arterial. There is then a vascular ring around the hip joint arising predominantly from the medial and lateral circumflex arteries. Additional contributions come from the superior gluteal artery and an ascending branch from the first perforating artery. There is a second, often smaller and incomplete, subsynovial vascular anastomosis. The dominant posterior supply perforates the capsule posteriorly and passes proximally with the synovial reflection to the femoral head. The vessels are bound firmly to the femoral neck by the reflected retinacular portion of the capsule and the periosteum. The epiphyseal and metaphyseal arteries arise directly from these posterior vessels. Chung [7] showed in elegant post-natal perfusion studies that the epiphyseal plate acts as an absolute barrier between the epiphyseal and metaphyseal blood supplies, although there may be a limited and incomplete anastomosis at the periphery.

An extensive cartilage canal vascular network ramifies through the femoral head. These canaliculi may be occluded by pressure. If the hip is forced into extreme flexion and abduction the posterior vessels may be compressed between the short femoral neck and the acetabular margin. Full extension and internal rotation may also "ring out" the retinacular vessels and lead to avascular necrosis.

Displacement and Dysplasia of the Hip

In 1989 Klisic [8] suggested that the umbrella term "developmental dysplasia of the hip" (DDH) should replace "congenital dislocation of the hip" (CDH) as it embraced the concepts of instability and imperfect formation but had the further

Fig. 5.2 The vascular supply of the infant's hip at 6 months. Note that the femoral head is supplied predominantly by the ascending branches of the medial circumflex artery

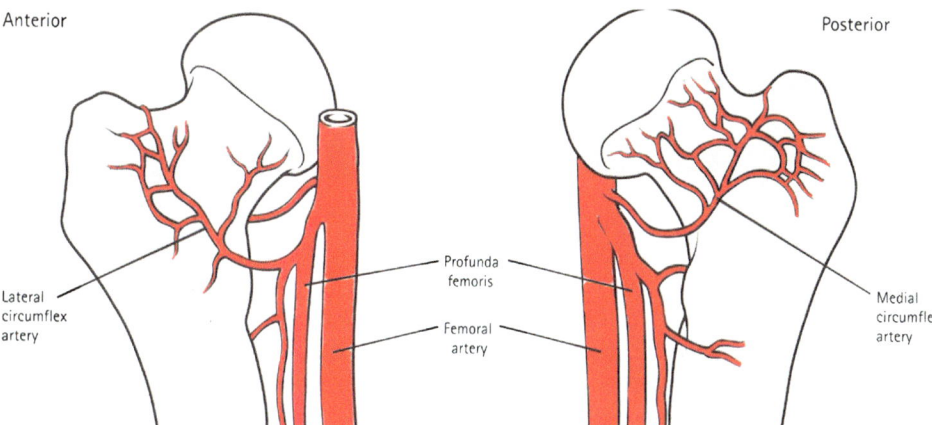

advantage of not specifying *when* the displacement or dysplasia occurred. This may have medico-legal consequences. It is nonetheless accepted that congenital factors contribute to developmental abnormalities.

The hip joint during early infancy is vulnerable to displacement. Although the clinical signs of instability may be subtle, they are usually detectable by careful examination. Early recognition and treatment in the neonatal period may prevent progressive subluxation or dislocation. Early treatment encourages the hip joint to grow normally and makes dysplasia less likely. It limits the otherwise inevitable progression to deformation, lost function, and eventual osteoarthritis.

Etiology

Genetic, gender, environmental, hormonal, and mechanical factors may predispose the hip to displace.

Genetics and Gender

The inheritance of DDH is multifactorial. Hip dysplasia is approximately nine times more common in females than males. If one child is born with hip dysplasia there is a 6% likelihood that a second child will have dysplasia also. In identical twins if one has DDH the second has a 34% chance of having displacement also. It is not clear, however, what the inherited factors are: these may, for example, reflect joint laxity or an abnormality of uterine shape. Ethnic background is important. Congenital dislocation is almost unknown in black Africans but is common in Japan and the Middle East.

Environmental and Mechanical Factors

So-called packaging anomalies in utero are important. In association with oligohydramnios or an eccentric uterine shape, the fetus may be squashed in utero. When cramped, freedom of movement is limited and the fetus cannot move around by kicking. Breech presentation is more common which independently makes displacement of the hip more likely. The infant with packaging abnormality may have an eccentric head shape (plagiocephaly), postural scoliosis, torticollis, eccentric hip movement (with greater abduction at one hip and greater adduction at the other), or calcaneovalgus foot positioning. As first-born children appear more vulnerable to hip displacement presumably uterine and abdominal muscular tone are greatest in a first pregnancy and hence the fetus has less freedom to move.

While club foot had been considered to increase the likelihood of associated DDH, Chan et al. [9] found that it did not predispose to hip displacement. They reviewed 1127 isolated DDH hips and reported that breech presentation, oligohydramnios, female sex, and primiparity were confirmed as major risk factors. There appeared to be an increased risk when a breech-presenting child was delivered vaginally rather than by caesarean section. High birth weight, post-maturity, and older maternal age slightly increased the risk of DDH. Breech presentation led to DDH in 2.7% of girls and 0.8% of boys. The left hip is up to four times more likely to dislocate than the right. This reflects the predominant left occiput anterior position of the fetus in utero in which the left hip is relatively adducted. Knee dislocation, almost invariably associated with breech presentation, was very likely to occur together with DDH.

Hormones

Carter and Wilkinson in 1960 [10] suggested that increased maternal hormone concentrations may cause pathologically lax tissues in some newborn infants. Although other studies failed to demonstrate consistently high levels of maternal hormones it is not possible to measure end organ sensitivity. The hips of girls and boys are anatomically identical at birth and this suggests that girls are more susceptible to female hormones than boys and hence at greater risk of hip displacement. Vogel et al. [11] found no relationship between serum levels of the polypeptide relaxin and hip instability in 21,865 newborns.

Syndromic Dislocations

It is important to remember that neonatal hip anomalies may be part of many syndromes and one abnormality should always prompt a careful search for others. Neuromuscular imbalance may cause the atypical congenital hip displacement seen in association with arthrogryposis and spina bifida, severe joint laxity, major chromosome defects, and a wide variety of other syndromes such as Down's and the thrombocytopenia-absent radius (TAR) syndrome.

When atypical "teratological" dislocations occur they are characterized by being irreducible at birth. Such hips need a different therapeutic approach. Standard neonatal splintage may be both fruitless and dangerous; it is often wise to wait until later in the first year of life before considering surgical treatment.

Patho-anatomy

In the typical hip displacement of the newborn, the only anatomical abnormalities appear to be stretching of the hip capsule and elongation of the ligamentum teres. McKibbin [12] showed the acetabulum and its labrum, the femoral head, and the orientation of femur and acetabulum appear essentially normal. At birth, the tight fit between femoral head and acetabulum is maintained by the surface tension created by the synovial fluid. It is very difficult to dislocate the normal neonatal hip in a postmortem specimen.

If the displaced hip is not reduced it may become permanently subluxated or dislocated. Eccentric pressure upon the head leads to segmental flattening, uneven growth, and increased femoral neck anteversion. The acetabulum, lacking the normal stimulus of a spherical contained femoral head, fails to develop anterosuperiorly, particularly if the rim is directly compressed by the displaced femoral head. This leads to loss of sphericity, a shallow, oval shape, and apparent anteversion. The labrum of the subluxating hip is typically stretched and everted. As the labrum stretches it takes with it part of the pre-osseous cartilage of the acetabular margin. The enveloping hip capsule is invaginated in front and below by the ilio-psoas tendon, adaptively shortening with time. Indentation of the capsule may produce the so-called hourglass capsular deformity. In time a secondary acetabulum develops: with subluxation this forms in the anterosuperior

part of the roof of the true acetabulum; with dislocation it develops in the iliac wing above the true acetabulum.

Subluxation blends almost imperceptibly into dislocation. The everted labrum may become squashed and distorted and folded into the joint, carrying with it part of the acetabular ring epiphysis and a sleeve of capsule. This complex is called the "limbus" and may prevent reduction (Figs. 5.3 and 5.4). When the head is not contained within the acetabulum the acetabular floor thickens and this contributes to the increasingly shallow acetabulum. The fibro-fatty pulvinar and the transverse acetabular ligament hypertrophy may encroach on the entrance to the acetabulum. The superior, elongated hip capsule may adhere to the outer iliac wing. The muscles that span the hip, particularly the ilio-psoas but also the adductors and hamstrings, shorten and contribute to the maintenance of hip displacement (Fig. 5.4).

Avascular necrosis does not occur spontaneously in the subluxated or dislocated hip. When it does occur it is iatrogenic. The growth and shape of the acetabulum are dependent upon the contained femoral head. Experimentally, if a square block is placed in the hip joint the acetabulum will grow square. The capacity for remodeling of the femoral

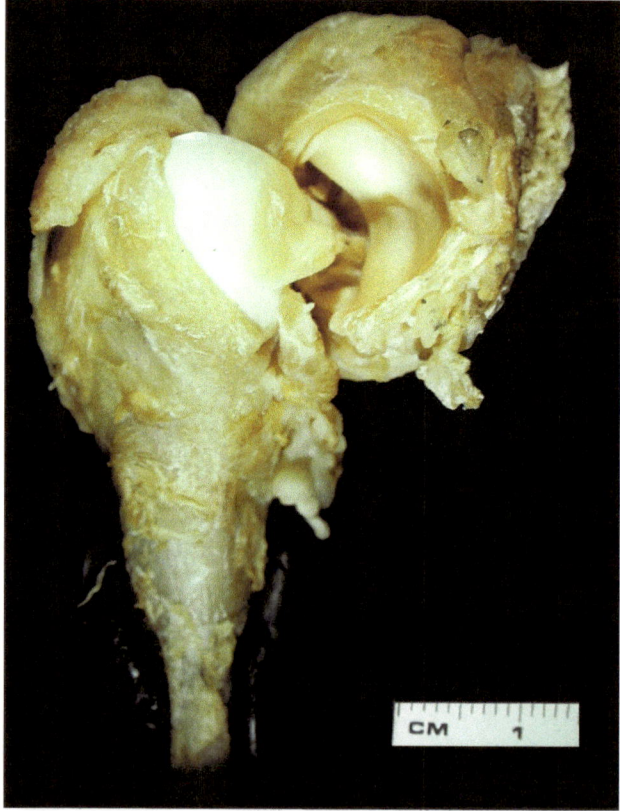

Fig. 5.3 Pathological specimen of an infant's dislocated hip. Note the oval femoral head, the hypertrophic ligamentum teres, the inverted limbus, and the eccentric position the femoral head occupied in the acetabulum

Fig. 5.4 (**a**) Anatomy of the normal hip: the labrum envelops the head and deepens the acetabulum. (**b**) In the subluxating hip the labrum everts; the head lies eccentrically in the acetabulum which deforms. (**c**) In the dislocated hip the cartilaginous acetabular margin deforms and the labrum may invert and obstruct reduction. (**d**) The ilio-psoas tendon may invaginate the capsule anteriorly and inferiorly

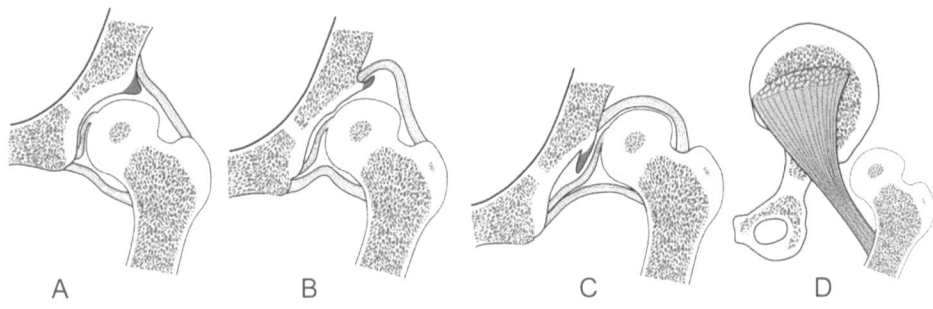

head and acetabulum when correctly relocated is excellent for the first few months but slowly decreases thereafter. From the age of 3 years this spontaneous remodeling capacity decreases relentlessly.

Incidence

There remain problems with assessing hip dysplasia and displacement. Before neonatal clinical screening was implemented the figures represented only late presenters; when clinical screening was introduced widely in the 1950s the incidence appeared to rise and ultrasound screening in the 1980s heralded a further upturn. If we simply consider neonatal instability, Barlow showed in 1962 [13] that 1 in 60 neonates had hip instability demonstrable by clinical examination alone. He noted that the capsular laxity causing instability usually tightened without treatment and that in 80% the instability resolved. With ultrasonographic techniques the neonatal incidence of instability may appear substantially higher with some estimates up to 6%. In the UK, Macnicol's value of 1 in 400 children [14] is probably close to the overall British incidence. In the native North American, instability has been reported to be as high as 1 in 5, but the condition is virtually absent in the black African. The left hip is displaced three times more often than the right at birth and in 20% the displacement is bilateral.

Although most neonatal instability resolves spontaneously, should it fail to do so children may present at walking age with a painless limp and leg shortening. Some, with partially displaced hips, will present as painful dysplasias in adolescence or early adult life. It should be noted that unrecognized or untreated dysplasia is responsible for up to 30% of those adults under the age of 45 years who develop degenerative hip arthritis.

Screening

Roser noted in 1879 [15] that some children's hips could be "dislocated by adduction of the leg and then reduced again by abduction." Little was made of this observation until 1937 when Ortolani [16] described the test named after him and the "snap of entry" of the dislocated hip as it reduced. Von Rosen [17] introduced routine clinical screening of newborns in Sweden in 1957. This dramatically reduced the incidence of late presentation. Palmén's [18] ground-breaking Swedish study led many to believe that the specter of the late-presenting hip dislocation could be avoided.

Preventing late-presenting dislocation remains the goal of neonatal screening programs. When the clinical tests of von Rosen and Barlow (v.i.) were introduced it was believed initially that clinical examination alone would avoid late-presenting DDH. This has proved not to be the case. There seems little doubt that clinical screening is more reliable when performed by experienced and dedicated staff. Without these the likelihood of clinical diagnosis is probably less than 50% [19]. Recognizing that not all dysplastic hips could be clinically diagnosed led to the concept of secondary screening: in the UK statutory guidelines ensured that babies' hips should be re-examined at 6 weeks and at 6–9 months. The guidelines stopped short of specifying the qualifications and experience needed to examine: typically a junior doctor performed the neonatal examination, a general practitioner the 6-week examination, and a nurse or health visitor the last screening. It was a recipe which ensured that children with DDH would continue to be diagnosed late.

Over 25 years ago Graf introduced the technique of ultrasonographic (US) screening of the infant's hip [20]. This radically changed our understanding of hip problems in infancy as the anatomy of the child's hip could be better understood non-invasively. As US screening was refined and developed its use became widespread and in some European countries it became routine for all neonates to have their hips examined by ultrasound. In other countries ultrasonography was reserved for those felt to be at special risk of dysplasia. Analyses of risk and cost–benefit around the world drew different conclusions. In Austria, Germany, and Italy all infants are screened with US. In the United States, Canada, the UK, and Scandinavia only those with at-risk factors or clinical abnormality undergo US examination.

Lehmann et al. [21] were not convinced from their meta-analysis that universal screening could be recommended. Conversely, Clegg [22] believed that cost analysis showed that it should be. He believed that many analyses failed to account fully for the heavy costs associated with late diagnosis, complex treatment, and the premature arthritis that stems from imperfect reduction and persisting dysplasia.

Why should there be doubt? If infants are screened by ultrasound shortly after delivery up to 6% may show instability. If rescreened at 4 weeks most instability has resolved so if routine screening is undertaken it should not be earlier than 3 weeks. Since splintage carries small but finite risks of avascular necrosis it is important that infants should not be over-treated.

Risk Factors for DDH

- Breech presentation either before or during delivery.
- Family history of hip dysplasia in a first-degree relative.
- Evidence of "packaging" anomaly such as torticollis or calcaneovalgus feet.
- Oligohydramnios and/or maternal hypertension.
- Dislocated knees.
- First-born children.
- Girls (who are up to nine times more likely to be affected by hip displacement than boys).
- Syndromes associated with hip anomalies.
- Increased birth weight (over 4.5 kg).

Where selective US screening is performed only some of these risk factors are usually considered. These include a positive family history, breech presentation, associated musculo-skeletal anomaly, and evidence of a cramped intra-uterine position. Clearly if there is any suggestion clinically of hip instability this is the prime reason for ultrasound scanning.

Clinical Examination

Ideally the baby should be relaxed and warm. All clothing, including the nappy, should be removed and the baby placed on a firm surface that allows easy access. General examination of the skull, trunk, arms, and legs should be swift and gentle. Asymmetry or malformation should be looked for. When examining the hip it must be remembered that all newborns have a physiological flexion deformity of 30–40° which may take several months to resolve.

It is important to establish a routine hip examination. The following is recommended:

1. Look for thigh asymmetry. Is one leg shorter? Is one leg more externally rotated than the other? Is there thigh crease asymmetry; in particular is there a deeper groin crease on one side than the other? Does the perineum look too wide? A dislocated hip may look no different from the normal hip, although with the hips flexed one knee may appear lower than the other (Galeazzi's sign).
2. Palpation of bony landmarks may help. Does one trochanter lie higher than the other in relationship to the anterior superior spine? When palpating deep to the femoral artery does one socket feel empty by comparison with the other? When palpating the buttock the greater trochanter may be mistaken for a displaced femoral head.
3. (a) Ortolani's test [16] is key in deciding if the hip is dislocated. With the baby's hip and knee flexed, the thumb in the groin, and the fingers over the greater trochanter, gently abduct the hip (Fig. 5.5a). In the first few weeks of life it should be possible to abduct the hip 90° until the knee is flat on the table. If abduction is restricted gently lift the leg forward and repeat the abduction maneuver. If the hip is dislocated this may allow the femoral head to slide into the acetabulum. Ortolani described the "jerk of entry" or clunk associated with this reduction, which shows that the hip is habitually dislocated at rest but reducible. If abduction is limited and cannot be completed it should be assumed, until proven otherwise, that the hip is dislocated and irreducible.
3. (b) Barlow's test [13] is performed when the Ortolani test is negative. The hip is therefore in joint. It is a provocative test to see if the hip will subluxate or dislocate out of the acetabulum. With the hips and knees flexed and in slight adduction, the thumb on the inner proximal thigh pushes gently backward and laterally (Fig. 5.5b). When capsular laxity or instability is present the femoral head may be felt to jump over the posterior acetabular border and reduce either spontaneously or by Ortolani's maneuver. The test therefore demonstrates whether the normally located hip is unstable.

Asymmetry or limited abduction should alert the examiner as much as the clunk of reduction or displacement. The "click" is usually of little significance and represents a transient vacuum phenomenon or a tendon snap at hip or knee. The tests should therefore be conducted with the knee fully flexed in order to remove this artifact. The pathological clunk is usually not audible but palpable. In any clinical screening program the infant who causes concern should be re-examined, preferably by an experienced examiner with access to US testing.

Fig. 5.5 (**a**) Ortolani's test: when the hip is normally located, full abduction of the flexed hip is possible. Note the reduced abduction of the left hip. (**b**) Barlow's test: with the hip flexed and adducted, posterior and lateral pressure from the thumb on the proximal femur will demonstrate if instability is present

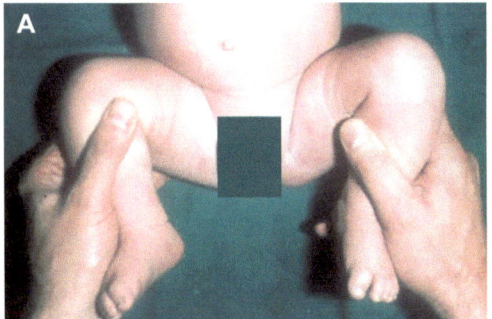
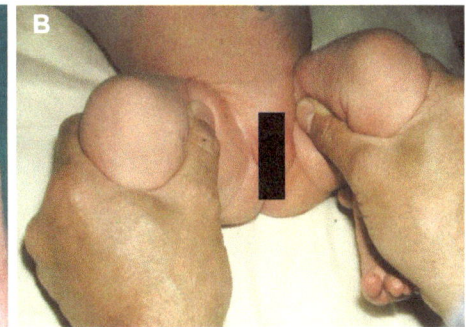

Investigations

Ultrasound

Although careful clinical examination of the infant should detect instability, it is clear that a proportion of children are not diagnosed by the initial clinical screening. This may reflect inexperience of the examiner, an inadequate screening program, or a hip in which the abnormality is not physically detectable at birth.

The neonatal hip is largely cartilaginous and although a pelvic radiograph may help, it is difficult to interpret. In 1984, Graf [19] delineated the different appearances of the infant's hip as "seen" ultrasonographically. The investigation is non-invasive and gives both a static and a potentially dynamic portrayal of the hip joint and any soft tissue distortions. A linear scanner should be used, and the images are produced graphically upon a screen or as hard copies. A variety of different projections and views have been defined.

Graf has shown that a mid-sagittal scan of the hip allows the contour of the femoral head and acetabulum to be gauged. Figure 5.6 illustrates his technique for measuring the bony (α[alpha]) and cartilaginous (β[beta]) angles upon the scan. An analysis of these angles allows quantification of the maturity of the hip and the severity of any dysplasia. Figure 5.7 illustrates a normal and a dislocated hip and Table 5.1 lists Graf's classification. He recognized immaturity and advised splintage for all hips worse than type IIc, with careful review of all but type I normal hips.

Other systems for classifying the US appearances have evolved. The Morin [23] classification assesses acetabular depth relative to head size: this gives a measure of head coverage. It is simpler than Graf's technique. The Suzuki method [24] scans from the front, but the images obtained are more difficult to interpret. Adequate statistical comparison of the systems has not been made.

US has increased considerably our understanding of the morphology of hip development. The natural history of each

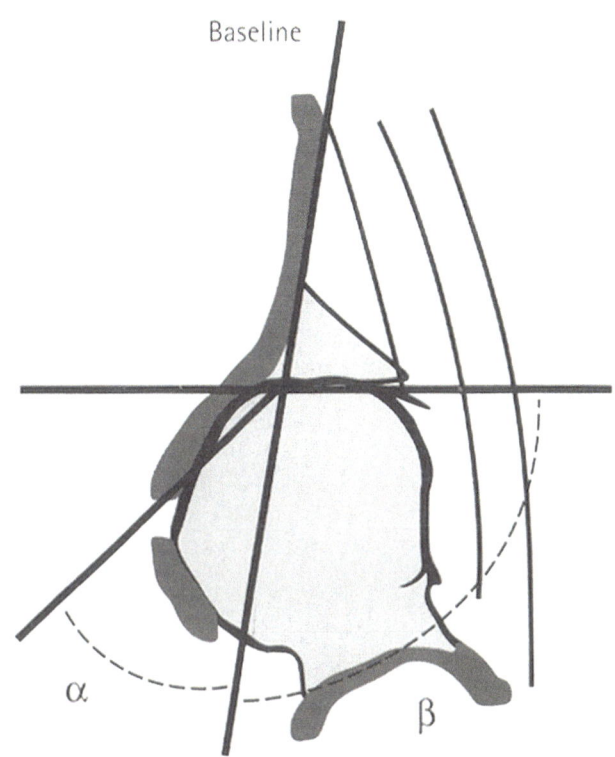

Fig. 5.6 Diagram of the US appearance of a reduced but dysplastic hip. An α [alpha] angle under 60° suggests a poor bony acetabular roof. A large β [beta] angle, as here, shows a poor cartilage roof cover

type of hip appearance is, however, difficult to evaluate. Not surprisingly, investigators have been tempted to treat hips that appear to be morphologically dysplastic. It is not always clear whether treatment or simple maturation has allowed such hips to improve.

US may be used not only statically but also dynamically. If the examiner attempts to displace the hip by Barlow's test, graphic images of the maneuver are easily obtained. Clarke et al. [25] focused attention on this hip instability and Engesaeter et al. [26] suggested that dynamic instability was of greater prognostic significance than morphological appearance.

Fig. 5.7 (**a**) US of normal hip and (**b**) its graphic interpretation. (**c**) US of dislocated hip and (**d**) its graphic interpretation

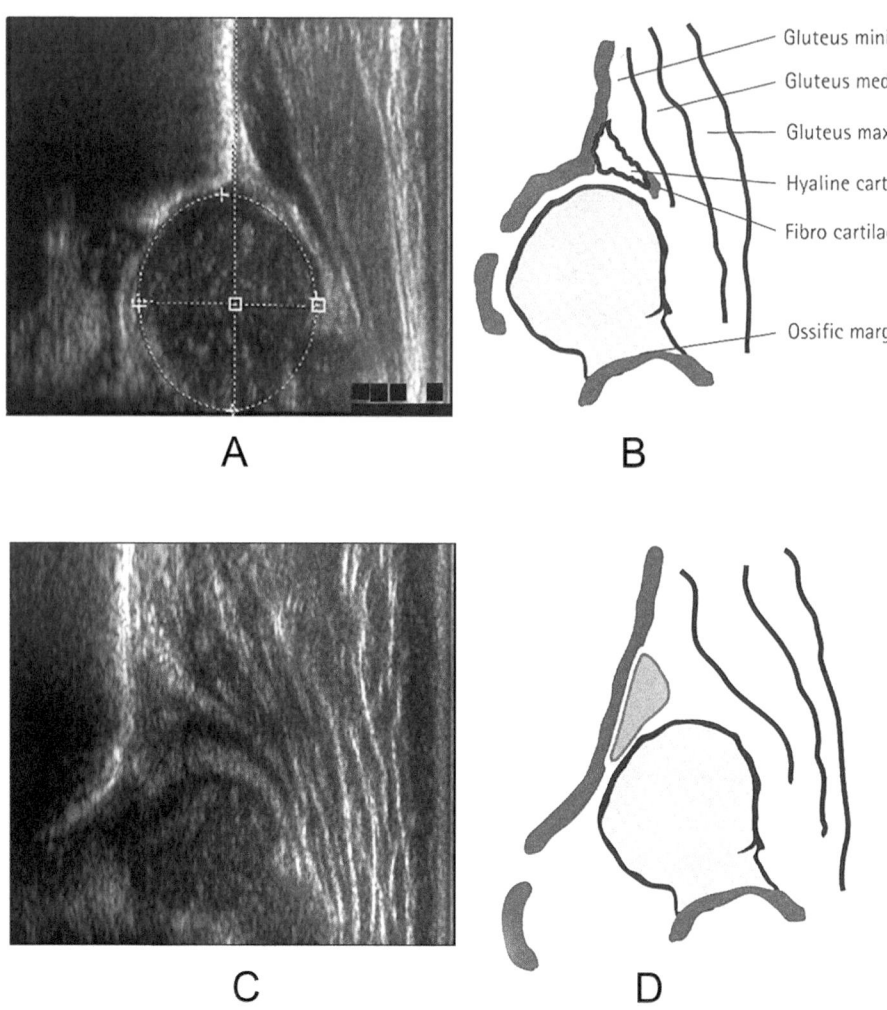

Table 5.1 Graf'S Ultrasonographic Classification of Hip Dysplasia

Hip type	Bony roof	Bony rim	Cartilage rim	α [alpha]: bony roof angle (°)	β [beta]: cartilage roof angle (°)
Ia	Good	Angular	Narrow; covers head	60	<55
Ib	Good	Sl. Rounded	Wide; short; covers head	60	<55
IIa + delay in ossification ≈ age	Adequate	Round	Wide; covers head	50–59	>55
IIa – delay; immature	Deficient	Round	Wide; covers head	50–59	>55
IIb delay ossification > 3 months	Deficient	Round	Wide; covers head	50–59	>55
IIc: critical (any age)	Deficient	Round to flat	Wide; covers head	50–59	70–77
D: decentered (any age)	Deficiency severe	Round to flat	Displaced	43–49	70–77
IIIa	Poor	Flat	Displaced with no structural alteration	<43	>77
IIIb	Poor	Flat	Displaced with structural alternation	<43	>77
IV	Poor	Flat	Displaced infero-medial	<43	>77

In Austria, Italy, and Germany, it has become a national requirement that all babies should undergo US examination after birth. In Britain and the United States, US examination is reserved for those children who are suspected of a clinical anomaly or to be at high risk by virtue of family history or breech presentation. Clegg et al. [22] have shown that universal US screening may prove cheaper than treating late those children with a missed diagnosis of DDH. It remains to be seen whether the routine neonatal use of US will become the norm.

US has established a secure role for monitoring the progress of treatment. In the first few months of life, before the developing ossific nucleus develops in the femoral head, it allows the surgeon to assess the quality of reduction and to monitor acetabular depth. It has the great advantage over other imaging techniques that it is non-invasive and is relatively inexpensive. The danger is that it may lead the unwary to over-treat a condition that often resolves.

Radiography

Where US equipment is not available a standardized antero-posterior pelvic radiograph is of value. Clearly, it is impractical to investigate all babies in this manner, but in suspicious cases, particularly if there is a suggestion of skeletal deformation or asymmetry [27], Bertol and Macnicol highlighted how a carefully taken film adds to the precision of neonatal diagnosis [28].

It should be remembered that the *bony* contours demonstrable radiographically give an imperfect indication of the quality of the *cartilaginous* acetabular roof. Nonetheless, the bony acetabular contour may be assessed by the acetabular index (Fig. 5.8). While this is prone to some measurement error it should be compared, as shown by Tönnis [29], with the angle expected at the child's age. The "medial gap" [27] between ischium and its closest femoral landmark should not

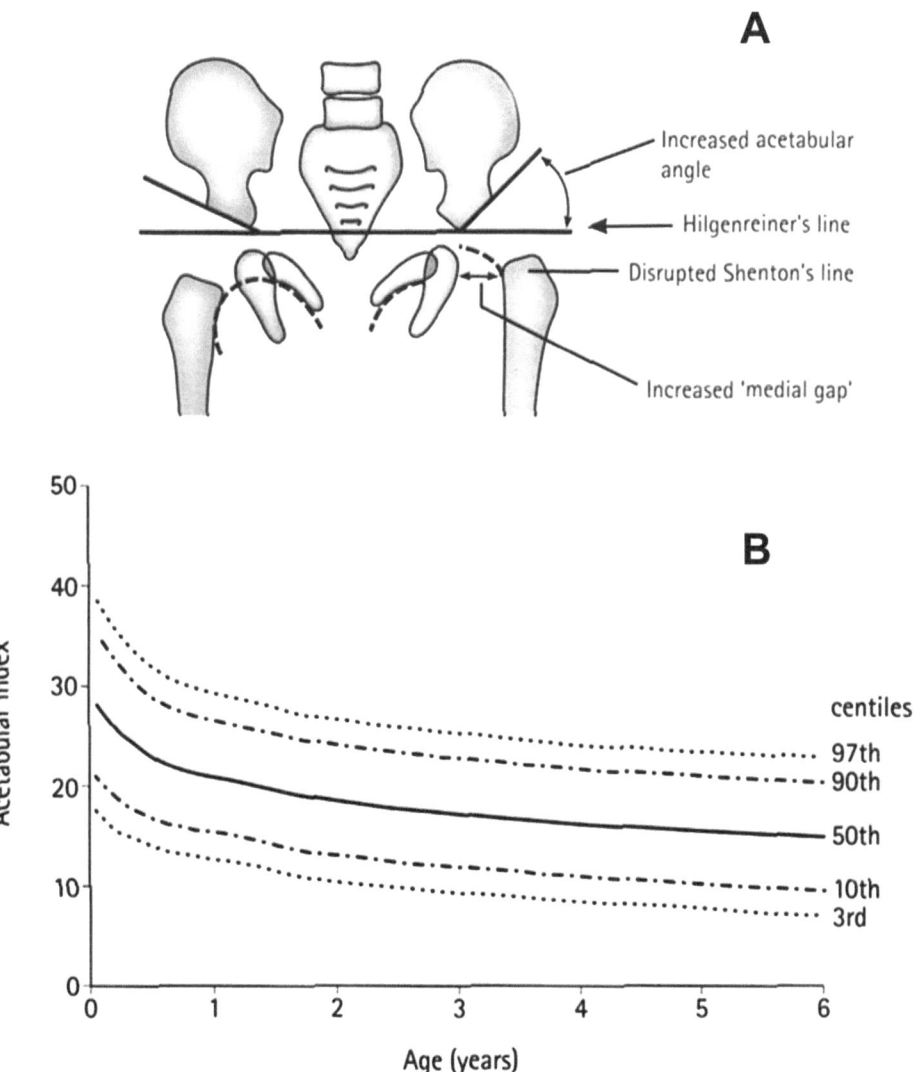

Fig. 5.8 (a) The features of an infant's radiograph that are used to determine the acetabular index. Note also Shenton's line and its disruption; the increased "medial gap" when the hip is displaced. (b) Graph (after Tönnis) demonstrating the change in acetabular angle with time

measure more than 5 mm on a standardized radiograph. A smoothly curved line produced along the lower border of the superior public ramus should follow the curve of the lower border of the medial femoral neck (Shenton's line). Once the ossific nucleus appears in the femoral head (between 3 and 6 months), radiological assessment becomes easier. The ossific nucleus should lie wholly beneath the triradiate cartilage in infancy and early childhood and medial to the perpendicular dropped from the lateral acetabular margin.

After a child has been treated for hip instability, sequential review with serial ultrasonograms and later radiographs is important to ensure that the hip develops normally. When it becomes possible, the child should stand for a weight-bearing film. In the younger child, the acetabular index should be measured at each review and compared with expected development (Fig. 5.8).

Hip displacement causes the ossific nucleus of the femoral head to appear later and smaller than its normal counterpart. Furthermore, the ossific nucleus may be eccentric within the femoral head. As the child grows older and the ossific nucleus enlarges, the center of the femoral head and its sphericity may be estimated by using Mose's concentric rings (Fig. 5.9). Once the center of the femoral head is known, the acetabular cover of the femoral head, the so-called center-edge angle of Wiberg [30], may be measured. In the child this should measure at least 15°; in the adult it should be more than 25°. Severin [31] produced a scheme of classification of later hip dysplasia based upon its radiological appearance and the center-edge angle (Table 5.2). Although imperfectly reproducible, it remains the most widely used system for judging outcomes of treatment.

Table 5.2 Severin's radiographic classification of hip dysplasia

Classification	Radiographic appearance	Center-edge angle (after Wiberg)
Class I	Normal	
Ia		6–13 years: > 19°
		Over 14 years: > 25°
Ib		6–13 years: > 15–19°
		Over 14 years: 20–25°
Class II	Moderate deformity of head, neck, or socket	
IIa		6–13 years: > 19°
		Over 14 years: > 25°
IIb		6–13 years: 15–19°
		Over 14 years: 20–25°
Class III	Dysplasia without subluxation	6–13 years: < 15°
		Over 14 years: < 20°
Class IV		
IVa	Moderate subluxation	>0°
IVb	Severe subluxation	<0°
Class V	Head lies in false socket in upper true acetabulum	
Class VI	Re-dislocation	

When a decision is being taken as to whether additional radiographs of the child's hip should be taken, the risk of irradiation should not be forgotten. Gonadal shields should be used and unnecessary films avoided.

Avascular Necrosis

Idiopathic necrosis is very rare in infancy and young childhood. When it occurs in children with DDH it is almost always iatrogenic. We have seen how the cartilaginous femoral head of infancy is vulnerable to pressure which flattens the canaliculi and obliterates the end-arterial blood supply. The short femoral neck makes compression of the posterior retinacular vessels between acetabular margin and neck all too easy if the hip is held in extreme abduction and flexion. Equally, the vessels may be stretched and wrung out by forced internal rotation. The head is particularly vulnerable if it remains dislocated or subluxed.

If the epiphysis alone is injured, the ossific nucleus may be late in appearing and mottled or fragmented when it does. Salter et al. [32] showed that if the nucleus had not ossified by 1 year it had probably been damaged. The epiphyseal injury may lead to coxa plana or magna and secondary acetabular dysplasia. Occasionally, of course, other disorders such as thyroid deficiency or epiphyseal dysplasia may delay ossification.

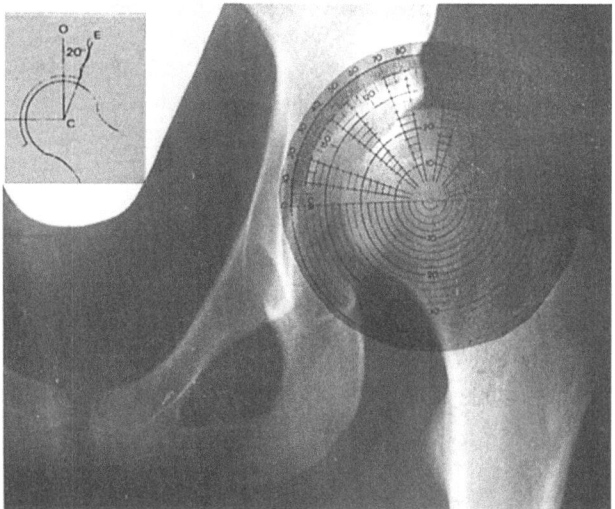

Fig. 5.9 Radiograph with Mose's rings superimposed. The center of the femoral head and the center-edge angle are readily measured. In the insert the angle is 20° and on the radiograph 0°

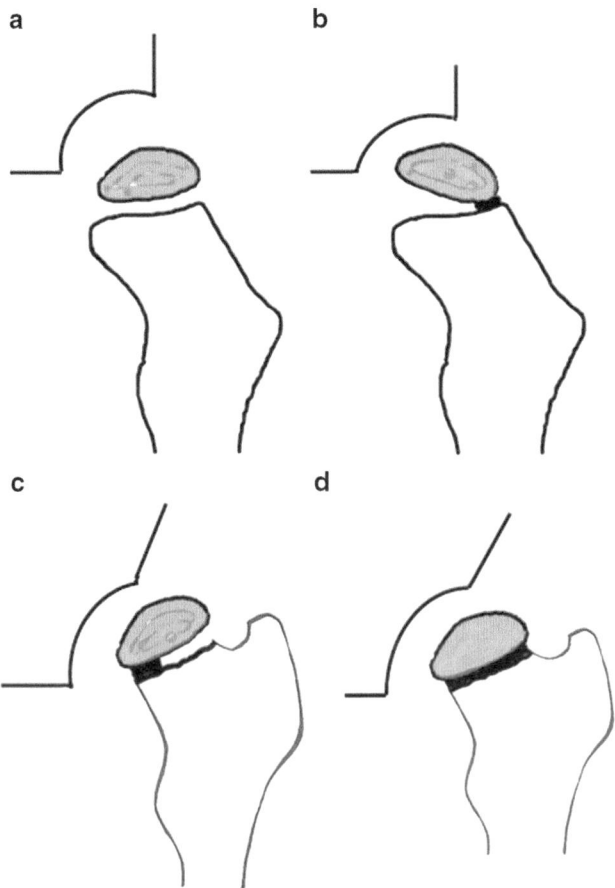

Fig. 5.10 Kalamchi and McEwan's avascular necrosis classification: (**a**) Type I: changes in the ossific nucleus only—mottling or late appearance. (**b**) Type II: ossific nucleus injury and lateral growth plate early closure—valgus tilt. (**c**) Type III: epiphyseal and medial growth plate injury—progressive varus; some trochanteric overgrowth; modest acetabular dysplasia. (**d**) Type IV: epiphyseal and whole growth plate injury—short neck; major trochanteric overgrowth; subluxation with marked dysplasia

The avascular insult may affect not only the epiphysis but also the growth plate. When it does, part or all of the plate may be affected. Kalamchi and MacEwan [33] described lateral, central, and complete injuries to the physis (Fig. 5.10). These produce deformities of the head and neck which become more apparent with growth. The head and neck deformity leads to secondary adaptive acetabular changes, many of which lead in turn to poor head cover and subluxation (Fig. 5.11). Leg length may be severely affected.

The risk of ischemia varies with age, treatment modality, surgical experience, and the form of splintage. It concerns all who treat children and dictates the need for careful splint supervision, avoidance of extreme positions of the leg, and the importance of long-term review.

Treatment

At Birth

We have seen how most neonatally unstable hips resolve spontaneously. Sadly there remains no clear indicator for those that need treatment. The hip that is dislocated rather than dislocatable may be less likely to recover. The hip that is irreducible at birth, the so-called teratological hip, is least likely to reduce.

The dislocatable hip: When the hip is loosely in joint no treatment should be given from birth. The situation should be carefully explained to the family and the infant reviewed in 3–4 weeks for further clinical and US evaluation. If instability persists or there is US evidence of acetabular dysplasia the hips should be splinted in flexion and abduction.

The dislocated but reducible hip: Such hips should have prompt US assessment. Some would observe for 3 weeks to see if spontaneous reduction occurs. Some would splint from birth. The evidence is not there to decide but a clear local policy should be established.

The irreducibly dislocated hip: Early confirmation by US is important to distinguish the irreducible dislocation from the "skew" baby. Marked molding may cause the infant to have one or several findings: plagiocephaly, correctable scoliosis, calcaneovalgus feet, or asymmetry of hip abduction and adduction. It seems sensible to undertake a trial of reduction. Rigid abduction splintage should never be applied but flexible splints such as the Pavlik harness are effective, applied as soon as possible after birth. The infant is monitored carefully both clinically and by US. If the hip reduces within 2 weeks splintage is continued until stability and acetabular maturation develop. If the hip does not reduce progressively within 2 or 3 weeks splintage should be discarded and the child left free until older.

The "at risk" infant: Infants with a recognized risk such as breech presentation or affected family member should be reviewed clinically and with US within 6 weeks of delivery. If they are found to be normal they may safely be discharged from further review. If there is any evidence of instability, displacement, or dysplasia they too should be splinted and serially reviewed. Figure 5.12 outlines the treatment algorithm used in Oxford.

Splintage: It may be asked why all infants are not splinted. Programs have indeed been recommended where all newborns are treated with double nappies or simple abduction splints. There is some evidence that late-presenting problems may be fewer but all splints carry a small but finite risk of avascular necrosis, a complication which imperils the future of the hip. This danger has modified our approach to US. In the early heady days of the new technique subtle immaturity

Fig. 5.11 (**a**) An 8-month-old girl with right DDH. (**b**) Position after 3 months splintage. (**c**) The right ossific nucleus has grown imperfectly, with a fragmented ossific nucleus. (**d**) At 5 years there is loss of epiphyseal height and modest residual dysplasia

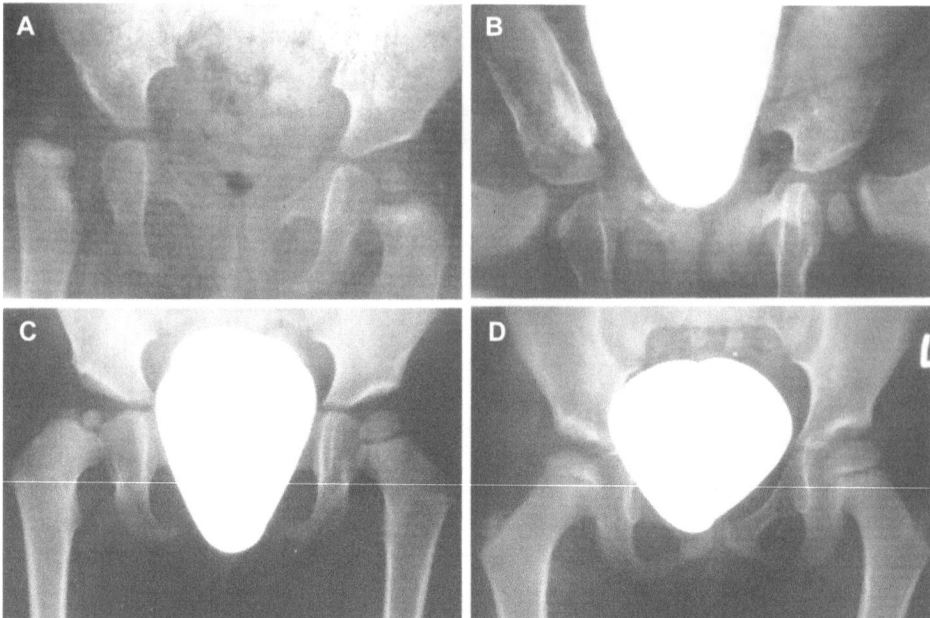

and instability of the neonatal hips led to splintage rates of up to 10%. While the great majority came to no harm a few developed avascular necrosis not only in the affected but also in the contralateral normal hip. Most centers now splint 4–6 infants per 1000. It is difficult to compare splintage rates as DDH incidence varies so widely around the world but each country should have an expected norm. If selection for splintage is not carefully evaluated it will call into question the local screening process.

Types of splint: The principle of any splint is to reduce the hip and maintain reduction safely while the capsule tightens and the acetabulum molds to its proper shape around the femoral head. The Malmö or von Rosen splint was the first widely used. It was pioneered in Sweden and remains in common use. It is H shaped, made of a malleable metal core, padded and encased in a waterproof shell (Fig. 5.13). The splint hooks over the shoulders and under the flexed and abducted thighs. It is essential that some freedom of movement be retained: 30° of flexion and 30° of abduction must be left to avoid compression of the head in the acetabulum and to minimize the risk of avascular necrosis. It is applied next to the skin and should not be removed by the family. Careful, regular supervision is needed to ensure it is used properly and does not tighten as the baby grows.

The Pavlik harness has gained widespread popularity (Fig. 5.13). A simple harness is fitted over the shoulders and around the chest. Front- and back-legging straps are attached to this and hooked under the feet. This ensures the hips are flexed to at least 90°. The straps are so adjusted that, with hips and knees flexed to a right angle, the knees just meet in

the midline. Just as with the von Rosen splint it is essential the harness is not too tight. It was believed at one time that the infant "kicked" the displaced hip into joint. Suzuki et al. [24], however, demonstrated that reduction occurs when the infant relaxes or sleeps.

Both Malmö and Pavlik splints demand some restrictions on bathing and clothing. A variety of other splints are available. Examples include the Craig splint and the Frejka pillow. These are positioned over the nappy and regularly removed. Help from trained support staff, health visitor, or "mothers' club" is essential. We should remember that new mothers are upset when their children need treatment, and care and tact are very important. Fortunately splintage rarely affects bonding between mother and child.

All splints carry the risk of complications: the most serious are avascular necrosis and failure to reduce and stabilize the hip. Bradley et al. [34] noted in addition that skin rashes, temporary femoral nerve palsy, inferior subluxation of the hip, and cavus foot deformity may be occasional complications. Early advice to nurse children prone in splints was set aside when it was recognized that prone lying may increase susceptibility to cot death. It is thought that children are safer lying supine or on their sides.

Splintage does not always succeed. There has been a general trend to prefer Pavlik harnessing to more rigid splintage. The European multicenter trial of 1988 [35] showed a success rate of 92% for those without irreducible dislocation and an avascular necrosis rate of 2.4%. In a small series comparing children splinted with Pavlik harness, von Rosen, and Craig splints the von Rosen was found to be the most reliable [36].

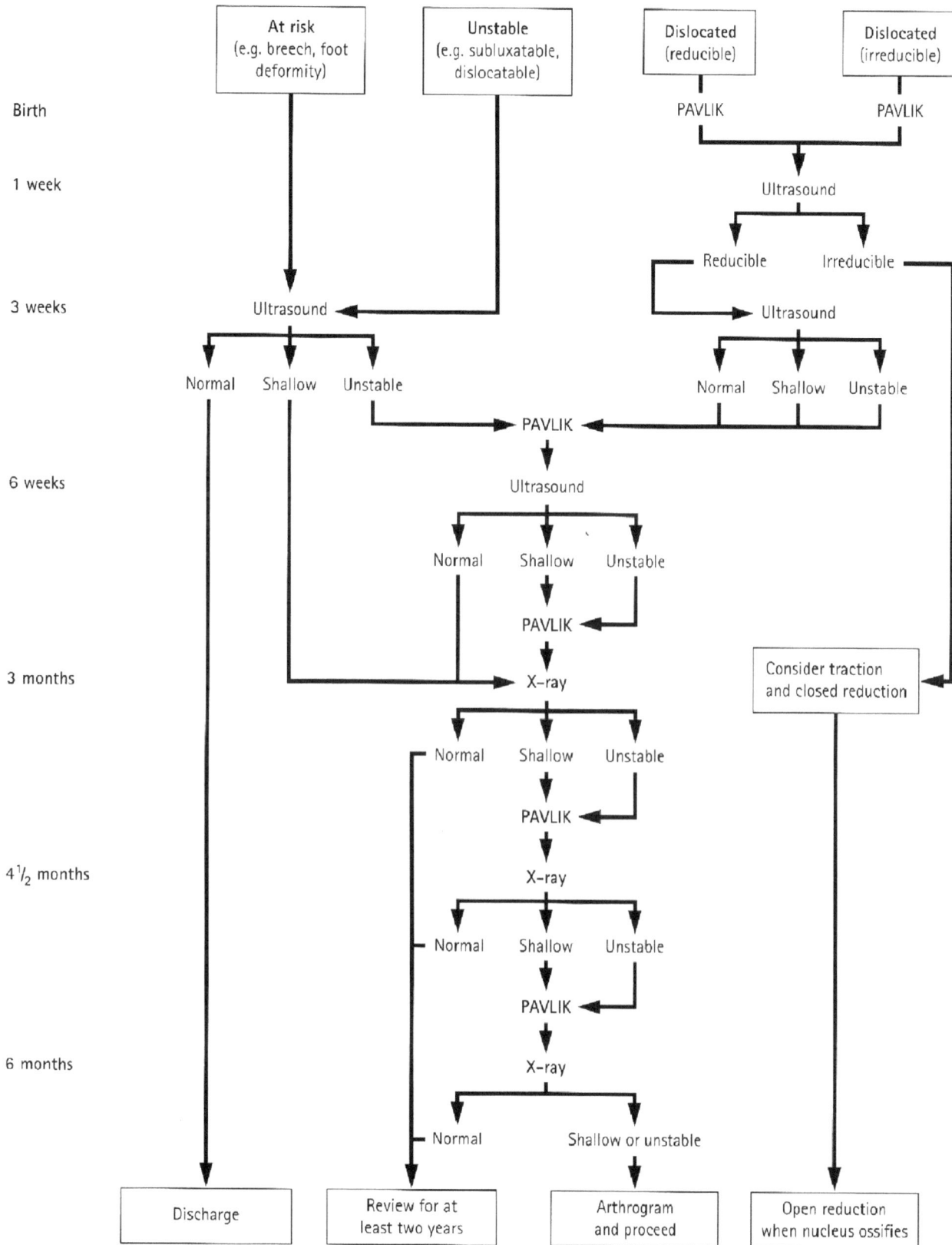

Fig. 5.12   Treatment algorithm for developmental dysplasia of the hip in the first 6 months

Fig. 5.13 Abduction splints in infancy. (**a**) The von Rosen splint. Flexion and abduction are readily obtained but care is needed to avoid extreme abduction. (**b**) The Pavlik harness maintains hip flexion and abduction but allows more freedom of movement

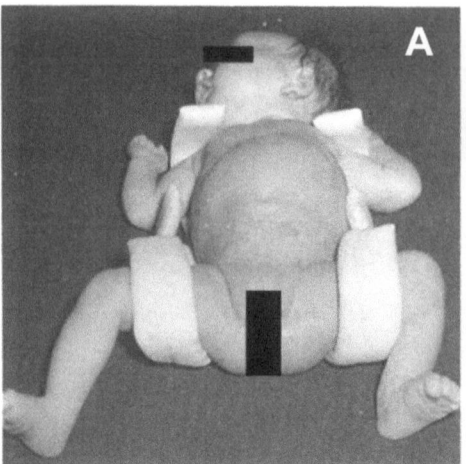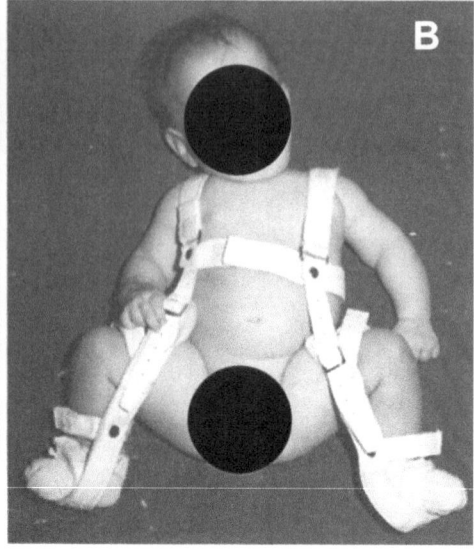

Treatment in the First Few Months

The best time to treat babies with unstable hips is in the first few weeks of life. Failed primary screening, failed primary splintage, and secondary screening still lead to an appreciable number of infants presenting with dislocation later in their first year. In the first few months children with hip subluxation or dislocation may still be treated in simple splintage, and the Pavlik harness is used widely. Nakamura et al. [37], who used the harness for slightly older children (1–12 months: mean 4.8), found it successful in 83% with an avascular necrosis rate of 12%. Once again, careful supervision and repeated US are needed to ensure reduction and compliance. In general, the later the diagnosis, the longer the period of splintage needed. As a rule of thumb children at birth need 6 weeks and those of age 3 months need 3 months. Satisfactory acetabular maturation and stability must be demonstrated before splintage is discontinued. Furthermore, children should be regularly reviewed clinically and radiographically until at least the age of 2 years to ensure their hips develop normally with no evidence of ischemic change.

Treatment Before 12 Months

When the hip has been displacing or displaced for several months the clinical findings change. While in early infancy most unstable hips are readily reducible, this becomes less likely after 3 or 4 months. The abnormal hip tends to become irreducibly subluxated or dislocated. The clinical signs also change. The affected leg may look shorter and lie more clearly in external rotation. Thigh creases, although notoriously unreliable as a diagnostic aid, may show a deep

unmatched groin crease on the affected side posteriorly. Galeazzi's sign of the lower-lying knee when hips and knees are flexed may be more apparent. *The cardinal finding, however, is restricted abduction of the flexed hip.* It is, not surprisingly, more difficult to recognize this lost abduction when both hips are displaced as there is no normal hip for comparison. The loss of abduction may be subtle, only 15–20°. While many surgeons continue to rely on US for diagnosis, many prefer radiographs after the age of 3–4 months.

It may be reasonable to undertake a trial of Pavlik harnessing for infants up to 8 months old with subluxation only but it is fruitless and potentially dangerous for children older than this. If the hip fails to show progressive reduction over the course of the first 2 weeks the harness should be discarded as the postero-superior acetabulum may be flattened by the pressure of an eccentrically lying femoral head. Furthermore, the risk of avascular necrosis of the femoral head increases.

If the hip is reducible in a harness it may need to be used full time for several months to allow the acetabulum to mature properly. There has been argument as to whether splintage should be discarded promptly or weaned. While most surgeons have practiced weaning there is evidence to suggest that, once the hip is stable and the acetabulum well formed, splintage may be discarded without.

Macnicol [38] highlighted the postural asymmetry, "infantile skeletal skew," which may develop when the child lies exclusively on one side. On the habitually dependent side hip abduction is greater and adduction less than the opposite side. By contrast the upper hip, which falls into adduction, has increased adduction but decreased abduction (Fig. 5.14). Radiographically the pelvis seems to be tilted and the appearance of the ossific nucleus on the adducted side may be delayed. Simple stretching and alternate positioning may be

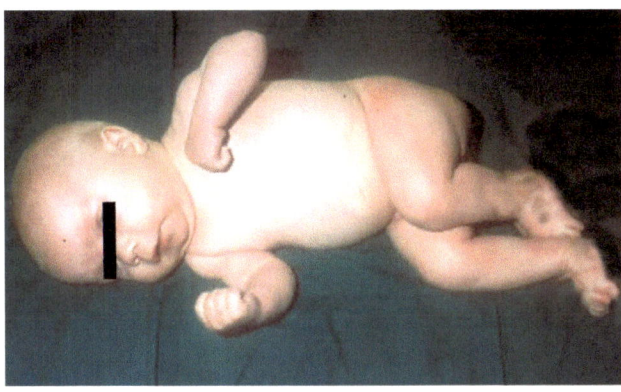

Fig. 5.14 Postural asymmetry in the side-lying child. Note the plagiocephaly, the dependent abdomen encouraging scoliosis and the asymmetric hip position

sufficient to allow such hips to develop normally without formal splintage. If splintage is used the hip must never be abducted forcibly.

It is debatable how the young infant over 3 months old with an irreducible dislocation should be treated. Some suggest treatment should be deferred until ossification begins within the femoral head, believing that this increases stability of the femoral head, making it less vulnerable to pressure and avascular necrosis. Segal et al. [39] showed experimentally in a porcine model that the presence of the ossific nucleus appears to protect the cartilaginous femoral head from compressive ischemic injury. The presence of the ossific nucleus before reduction was statistically significant in avoiding avascular necrosis, which was more frequent when children were treated by open or closed reduction in the first year of life. Luhmann et al. [40], however, found in their series that the ossific nucleus appeared not to be protective against avascular necrosis and believe that the displaced hip should be reduced at diagnosis rather than waiting for nuclear ossification. There is no consensus about this matter.

Closed Hip Reduction

When simple abduction splintage fails alternative treatment is necessary. Children were commonly treated by skin traction for a period ranging from a few days to several weeks. The theoretical aim of such traction was to stretch the soft tissues and to minimize the likelihood of pressure necrosis when the hip was reduced. The Morin School in France continues to use such traction for several weeks and has an excellent record of successful closed reduction with satisfactory long-term outcomes. Their latest results are awaited. This has not always been matched by others. Traction was widely discontinued in the United States, partly because of the cost–benefit aspect and partly because there was some

evidence to suggest that it conferred no benefit either on the reduction itself or on the risk of avascular necrosis. Many centers throughout the world have now abandoned traction as a consequence. Weinstein and Ponseti [41] also suggested that traction may allow the labrum and part of the pre-osseous acetabular rim cartilage (the limbus) to become incarcerated in the hip joint and make subsequent reduction more difficult.

For the 3- to 9-month-old infant whose displaced hip shows no femoral head ossification it is sensible to examine the hip under anesthesia. This also offers the opportunity to carry out an arthrogram.

Arthrography

Injecting contrast medium into the hip joint outlines the femoral head and acetabulum and demonstrates whether the hip will reduce satisfactorily. Any obstacles to reduction can be assessed and a decision taken as to whether closed reduction is possible. Injection into the joint may be made anterolaterally, anteriorly, laterally over the greater trochanter, or infero-medially. The needle should be inserted into the joint under image intensifier control. The joint should not be overdistended with contrast medium as this may obscure the features one hopes to demonstrate. It is best if the contrast medium is diluted 50%. The arthrogram allows the surgeon to examine the hip in a variety of positions, judging the one that allows the best "fit."

In the normal hip the spherical femoral head sits within a spherical acetabulum. The cartilaginous acetabular roof "covers" the femoral head and the labrum extends clearly beyond this. The limbic "thorn," the interval between labrum and capsular reflection, suggests the labrum is correctly located and the acetabular margin not deformed. The so-called zona orbicularis is produced by slight out-pouching of the synovium between the limbs of the Y-shaped ligament of Bigelow. The acetabular fossa and the transverse ligament indentation should be identified. The contrast medium should extend far enough down the neck to delineate the normal capsular attachments and should assess its capacity (Fig. 5.15).

With subluxation a crescent of the contrast may be seen centrally. When, as often happens, subluxation is associated with acetabular insufficiency, this crescent may shift from central to superior when longitudinal traction is applied to the leg and the head centralizes more normally into the acetabulum.

Progressive degrees of subluxation and dislocation may deform and entrap the limbus (the labrum, deformed pre-osseous rim cartilage, and a capsular fold) within the joint. The ligamentum teres is often hypertrophic and may be seen as an obstacle to reduction; the transverse ligament may

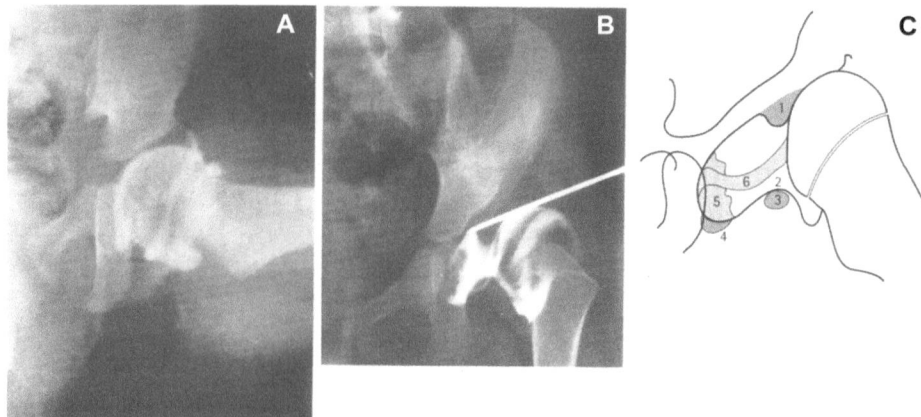

Fig. 5.15 (**a**) Arthrogram of a reduced hip in the frog lateral position. Although the bony acetabulum is deficient, the cartilaginous roof is satisfactory and the labrum normally located. The prognosis is good with simple abduction splinting. (**b**) Arthrogram of dislocated hip in neutral. The injecting needle is superolateral. The infolded labrum and deformed cartilaginous acetabular margin are clearly seen. The deep inferior indentation is made by the ilio-psoas. (**c**) Line diagram of arthrogram findings: (1) deformed acetabular rim and infolded limbus; (2) capsular "waisting" by the invaginating ilio-psoas (3); (4) inferior transverse acetabular ligament; (5) fibro-fatty pulvinar; (6) ligamentum teres

encroach upon the inferior aspect of the hip joint. When the hip is displaced the ilio-psoas tendon may indent the anterior-inferior capsule creating an hourglass constriction.

The arthrogram defines the hip as

- Normal.
- Subluxing with no block to reduction.
- Dislocated or dislocatable but fully reducible.
- Dislocated with an obstacle to reduction.
- Subluxated in a partially dislocated position that cannot be reversed.

Femoral anteversion may be assessed by the amount of rotation needed to align the femur optimally. The acetabulum may show varying severities of dysplasia or delayed ossification.

Management

Closed Reduction

If the child's hip is reducible, closed reduction should be undertaken. Almost invariably the hip needs to be held in flexion and abduction. Care is needed to assess the position of greatest stability and the position in which redisplacement occurs. Too little abduction and the hip dislocates; too much abduction and avascular necrosis follows. The safe zone of Ramsey [42] should be selected. It is a wise precaution to carry out a percutaneous tenotomy of the adductor longus tendon. This is performed simply by holding the flexed hip in abduction, identifying the tendon between finger and thumb, and dividing it with a small tenotome. The maneuver often adds an extra 20° of abduction and increases the safe zone in which a plaster cast may be applied.

Salter highlighted the importance of holding the leg in the right position. He advocated the "human" position in contradistinction to the "frog" position which he believed should be reserved for frogs. The treated hip should be flexed to at least a right angle and abducted to no more than 45–50°, allowing at least 30° of flexion and 30° of abduction beyond the position to be maintained. Unless care is taken there is a tendency for progressive abduction to occur as the hip spica is applied. It is important to not allow the hip to displace backward, careful molding over the greater trochanter restricting this (Fig. 5.16). The spica should extend to the lower thorax but allow the umbilicus to be visible. For hips with mild subluxation it is reasonable to keep the spica above the knee only; for severe subluxation or dislocation in general it is better to incorporate the knee in flexion to minimize hamstring tightness. The ankle and foot may be left free or incorporated in the plaster initially.

When the child wakes it is important to ensure that the hip does not subluxate or dislocate within the plaster cast. A plain radiograph in the plaster is not adequate for assessment: three-dimensional views are needed. While a computed tomography (CT) scan is entirely reasonable it carries the risk of significant gonadal irradiation and where possible a magnetic resonance imaging (MRI) scan is preferable [43]. As the child is incarcerated in plaster, movement artifact is usually not a problem (Fig. 5.17).

Hip spicas need to be changed after 4–6 weeks. The child should then be re-examined under anesthesia with the plaster

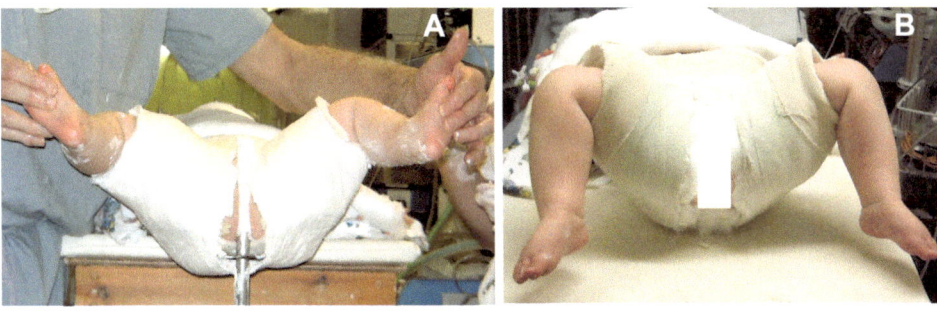

Fig. 5.16 (**a**) Hip spica maintaining reduction. At application care is taken to avoid excess abduction. Molding behind the trochanters makes posterior subluxation unlikely. (**b**) The completed double half hip spica

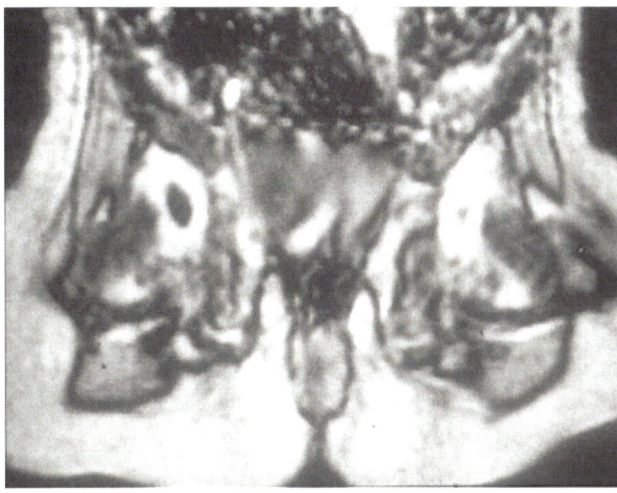

Fig. 5.17 MRI following closed reduction. The left hip acetabular roof is largely cartilaginous; the femoral head has a much smaller ossific nucleus but the head is well applied to the triradiate cartilage

removed and hip stability and alignment checked. At this stage a further 4–6 weeks in a hip spica is usually preferable to a removable abduction splint. After 3 months it is usually safe to remove the plaster cast and continue abduction splintage until satisfactory maturation has been radiologically confirmed. Careful follow-up until skeletal maturity is essential.

Open Reduction

If the arthrogram demonstrates that the hip is not reducible careful decision making is necessary. Some surgeons proceed directly to open reduction under the same anesthetic. Others prefer to wait until the ossific nucleus appears. Where the dislocation is clearly teratological and a well-formed false acetabulum has developed above the true acetabulum, it is advisable to wait for ossification as the risk of avascular necrosis is particularly high.

Open reduction is clearly necessary when closed reduction is not possible. It is also needed when teratological dislocation has delayed treatment until the ossific nucleus

has appeared in the cartilaginous femoral head. When there is a defined obstruction, such as an inverted limbus or an encroaching transverse acetabular ligament, surgical reduction is mandatory. The hip may be approached by the medial, anterolateral, or posterior approaches.

Medial approach: the incision is made parallel to adductor longus or transversely below the groin crease (Fig. 5.18); the transverse scar does not lengthen with growth and is cosmetically satisfactory. The femoral neurovascular bundle is retracted laterally. The lesser trochanter and its attached psoas tendon are approached from in front or behind adductor brevis. Care should be taken to protect the vessels adjacent to it. The psoas tendon is released from its insertion and allowed to retract proximally. This exposes the infero-medial hip capsule. Through a T incision, with its long limb along the femoral neck, the transverse acetabular ligament, the pulvinar, and the ligamentum teres may be inspected; the labrum is rarely seen because it lies posteriorly and superiorly. The approach allows release of the inferior capsule, division of the transverse ligament, and, if needed, excision of the ligamentum teres. This combination usually allows the femoral head to reduce deeply [41, 44].

Fig. 5.18 The medial adductor approach to the hip

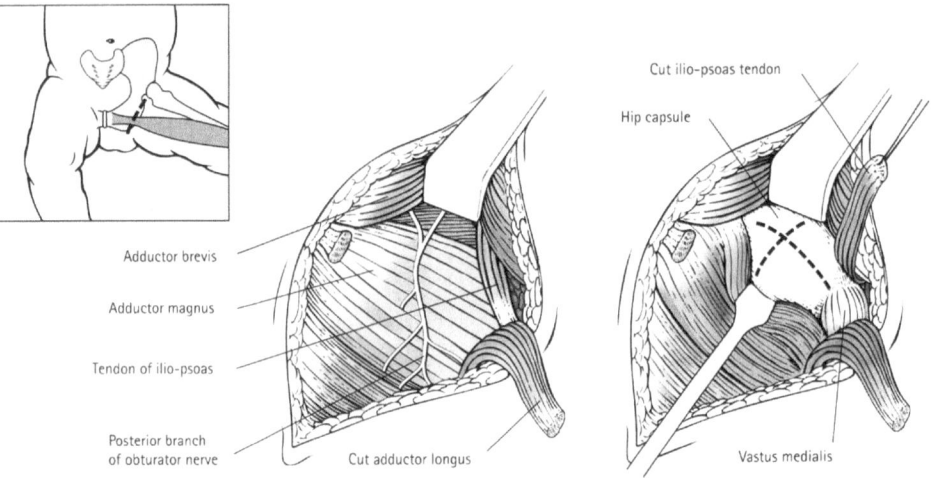

In general, the medial approach is appropriate only for the child under walking age. It is contraindicated when there is a large inverted limbus. A capsulorrhaphy cannot be performed and the medial circumflex artery may be damaged, causing avascular necrosis although its severity depends at least in part upon the preoperative management and the position in plaster. The approach is relatively bloodless, and the recovery of hip movement is usually excellent. Damage to the iliac apophysis is avoided.

Anterolateral approach: this was originally through a Smith-Petersen approach, but this leaves a cosmetically ugly scar. A "bikini" transverse incision below the iliac crest centered upon the anterior superior spine is preferred (Fig. 5.19). The space between sartorius and tensor fasciae latae is developed after identifying, protecting, and retracting the lateral femoral cutaneous nerve. The anterior one-third of the iliac apophysis is split by incising sharply through cartilage to bone. The apophysis with the abductor muscles and periosteum in one sheet are stripped from the outer surface of the ilium. The straight and reflected heads of rectus femoris are divided and reflected distally, exposing the

superior and anterior hip capsule. The psoas tendon within the iliacus at the pelvic brim is identified, rolled forward, and divided to provide muscle lengthening without loss of continuity.

A T-shaped incision is made in the hip capsule. The capsulotomy should skirt the capsular attachment to the pelvis, and the long arm of the T should pass along the anterior femoral neck. Hip dislocation is accomplished by adducting, extending, and externally rotating the leg. The femoral head is almost invariably slightly flattened and oval. Inspection of the acetabulum may be difficult. The ligamentum teres is the guide to the acetabular depth. It is usually excised as it is hypertrophic and contributes negligibly to capital epiphyseal blood supply after infancy. The transverse ligament, which blocks reduction inferiorly, should be divided. If a limbus is present and inverted, it should be preserved as it is composed partly of pre-osseous cartilage. It may be made more pliant by making one or two radial cuts, allowing it to be everted over the femoral head.

The acetabulum should be palpated to ensure that no other obstacle prevents reduction, as adhesions and capsular bands

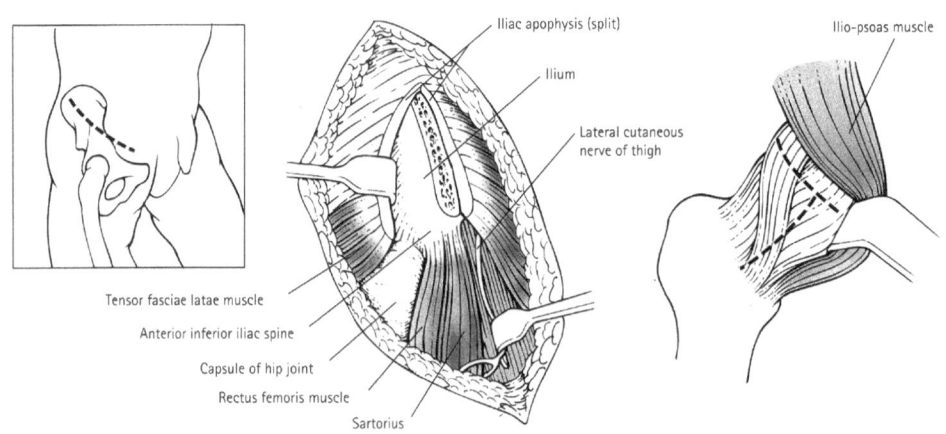

Fig. 5.19 The anterolateral approach to the hip

often extend below the femoral head. Image intensification helps to ensure the head is deeply reduced. Often, a thickened acetabular floor appears to "lateralize" the head. If in doubt, a small pledget soaked in radio-opaque dye may be inserted between head and socket to determine radiographically the adequacy of reduction.

As neither femoral head nor acetabulum is spherical, it is inaccurate to describe the reduction as "concentric" but the position of "best fit" must be estimated. Because of increased femoral anteversion this is usually with the hip flexed, abducted, and internally rotated, each by 30–40°. Capsulorrhaphy is performed by excising the redundant capsule superiorly (removing the superior triangle from the T-shaped incision) or by reefing the capsular margins. Rectus femoris is re-attached and the iliac apophysis is carefully repaired to ensure that it does not become deformed. The hip is maintained in a hip spica in sufficient flexion, abduction, and internal rotation for the head to be fully contained by the acetabulum but avoiding extreme positioning.

In the infant before walking age, it is unlikely that secondary femoral or acetabular procedures will be necessary, and 3 months of plaster immobilization is usually sufficient, followed by a period of abduction bracing if the acetabular response is slow. In the older child, secondary procedures become progressively more likely and it is often advisable to consider them coincidently with open reduction (Fig. 5.20).

Posterior approach: the hip may be approached posteriorly, either through a curved posterolateral or a simple transverse posterior incision. The approach has not gained wide popularity because, although theoretically attractive in giving good access to the limbus, it does not allow an effective capsulorrhaphy, psoas tenotomy has to be performed distally, and there is a significant risk of interfering with the posterior blood supply. Furthermore, if a later pelvic procedure is required, a second incision has to be made.

Treatment of the Toddler

The toddler with a hip dislocation presents typically with an abnormal gait. On average, children with a dislocated hip walk only 1–2 months later than their peers. Children walk with a combined short leg and Trendelenburg limp. The child walks on tiptoe on the affected side, with truncal asymmetry and external rotation of the leg. Clinical signs include elevation of the greater trochanter, flattening of the buttock, and hollowing below the femoral triangle. A groin lump may be palpable with the hip extended, where the femoral lies extruded anterosuperiorly. True shortening is demonstrable when the dislocation is unilateral. It is very rare to be able to reduce the dislocated hip of a child of walking age. Characteristically, abduction in flexion is markedly restricted. When both hips are dislocated, the child walks with a bilateral Trendelenburg lurch and develops hyperlordosis of the lumbar spine.

As in the younger infant, the principles of management in the toddler are straightforward: the hip should be reduced as atraumatically as possible. Reduction should be maintained for the minimum time necessary for stability to be assured.

Treatment of late-presenting congenital hip dislocation was once by forcible manipulation under anesthesia and splintage of the hip in the fully abducted and/or internally

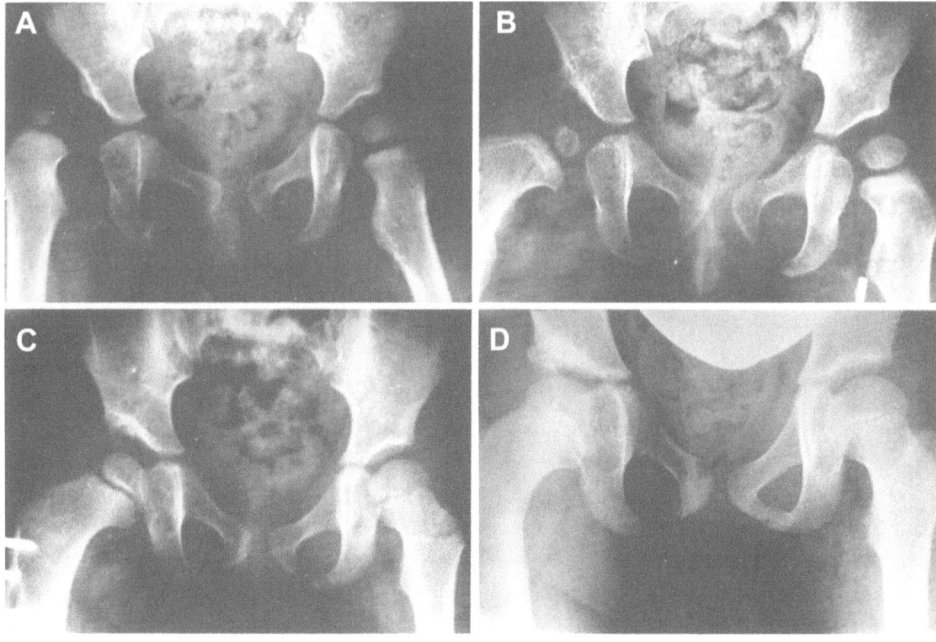

Fig. 5.20 (**a**) An 18-month-old girl with late-presenting right DDH: note the thick acetabular floor, the steeply sloping acetabular roof, and the smaller ossific femoral head nucleus. (**b**) Six weeks after open reduction. The lines of temporary growth arrest show symmetrical physeal growth. (**c**) One year after derotation femoral osteotomy.(**d**) At age 10 years the hip is stable. The acetabulum has improved and its ring epiphysis ossified but not yet united

rotated position, sometimes for up to 2 years. While many hips were successfully reduced by this technique, avascular necrosis of the femoral head occurred in over 50% of cases. The risk of necrosis remains with current management but the incidence is now much lower.

Twenty years ago, few surgeons would have considered operating on an older child unless the soft tissue contractures associated with dislocation had been at least partly overcome by preliminary traction. Although many continue to advise traction, either at home or in hospital, an increasing number do not, believing that shortened muscles may be lengthened at operation by tenotomy. Inevitably, financial considerations influence the decision. If traction is used it must be carefully supervised: tapes and bandaging must be regularly changed and carefully applied. It may be of simple "gallows" type or progressive abduction in flexion may be achieved if a hoop is placed over the bed. Traction in extension is particularly suitable for the older child, and modified Pugh's traction on a 45° tilted mattress is valuable as the child may lie either prone or supine and is easier to entertain.

For the child older than 2–3 years with a high dislocation, femoral shortening is often necessary to achieve reduction without femoral head compression [45, 46].

Is the Hip Reducible?

Whether or not preliminary traction has been used the child's hip should be examined under general anesthesia. Some surgeons are happy to rely solely on their clinical examination and image intensification but we recommend further evaluation by arthrography. It is essential to decide upon the shape of the femoral head and acetabulum (both of which may be largely cartilaginous). If the head reduces does it do so deeply and congruously? Are there obstacles to reduction and if so what are they? If the hip reduces what is the best position of reduction and how stable is the hip with movement?

The reducible hip: the most satisfactory reduction position should be recorded remembering that extreme positioning is not safe. This may be in 90° of flexion and 45° of abduction (the "human" position) or in modest flexion, abduction and internal rotation (typically 30° of each). It is wise to perform a tenotomy of the adductor longus. Some advise an open psoas tenotomy to further safeguard against undue head pressure. A one-and-a-half or double hip spica is applied in the safe position and changed under anesthesia 4–6 weeks later. It is wise to confirm the initial position postoperatively by MRI or CT scan. After 3 months in a hip spica an abduction brace should be used and retained until adaptive capsular shortening has occurred and the deformed cartilage of the acetabular roof has begun to ossify.

The irreducible hip: the arthrogram may show the hip cannot be reduced and clarifies the obstacles. One French school practices several weeks of traction followed always by closed reduction: where the head stands off from the acetabulum they have found that gradual penetration occurs without incarceration of the limbus. Their long-term results are very good but not yet published. Most centers recommend open reduction when the hip will not reduce under anesthesia. We prefer the anterolateral approach for these older children. The principles of this reduction are no different from those in the younger child, although femoral head deformity may be more pronounced. Femoral anteversion and valgus may be marked, and the acetabulum is shallow and anteverted. If the labrum has been inverted, it becomes more rigid, making it difficult to evert. It is sensible to carry out an intramuscular psoas tenotomy and adductor tenotomy to minimize head pressure following reduction.

In children younger than 18 months, careful reduction of the hip and capsular plication usually promote satisfactory development. In older children, a secondary bony procedure, either to realign the acetabulum or the femur, becomes increasingly advisable. Pelvic osteotomy is not recommended for children under 18 months as the bone graft used tends to crush or displace. After the age of 18 months, however, if the acetabulum is markedly dysplastic, it is wise to consider a pelvic osteotomy to make secondary operation less likely.

If, even after release of the adductors and ilio-psoas, the femoral head appears to reduce too tightly, concurrent femoral shortening should be undertaken. If extending the flexed knee provokes redislocation the hamstrings are too tight and again the femur should be shortened. It is sensible to consider coincident femoral shortening for any child over $2\frac{1}{2}$ years, for the child with a teratological dislocation, and for any child with a neuromuscular disorder such as arthrogryposis. The operation was first described in 1928 by Hey-Groves [45], but was more recently popularized by Klisic [46].

A child immobilized in a hip spica for 3 months is vulnerable to osteoporotic femoral fracture, typically a greenstick supracondylar. Gentle mobilization is important therefore after spica removal and where possible a day or two of supervised in-patient physiotherapy is helpful.

It is important to mobilize the child for a few days in hospital once a hip spica has been removed, because the osteoporotic femur may fracture. A graduated approach to splintage further reduces risks and progression from full-length hip spicas to pantaloon casts and then removable abduction braces are recommended.

While every optimism may be felt for the promptly recognized and treated neonatal unstable hip, the surgeon should be cautious of promising normal outcomes for older children. There is little doubt that the quality of the long-term result is poorer [41, 47] and each child who has been treated for hip dislocation should be reviewed at least until skeletal maturity.

Treatment in Later Childhood

The majority of children over toddler age who present with congenital hip dislocation represent the failures of earlier management. It is rare for the untreated child with congenital hip dysplasia to develop pain before adolescence. Even then, pain is likely to be experienced as discomfort or fatigue after exercise. In contrast, the child who has been treated unsuccessfully is likely to develop pain in early childhood.

Gibson and Benson [47] showed the long-term results of treatment for the older child deteriorate for a variety of reasons: femoral head and acetabular deformity become more marked, femoral anteversion increases, the acetabulum fails to develop anteriorly, and the capacity for remodeling decreases rapidly after the age of 3 years.

Where bilateral dislocation is present, the child stands with a hyperlordotic lumbar spine, which is not present in unilateral dislocation. Shortening becomes more pronounced. Palpation of the groin beneath the inguinal ligament reveals an "empty" acetabulum. The trochanter is high and proximal and may be felt deeply in the buttock, where it is carried by the increasing anteversion of the femoral head and neck.

The principles of treatment for the older child remain exactly the same as before: the hip needs to be reduced atraumatically, preventing abnormal pressure upon the reduced femoral head. To accomplish this many surgeons previously recommended preoperative skin traction but this is now rarely used. Intra-operative femoral shortening reduces the pressure upon the reduced femoral head and is almost always advisable in the child over the age of $2\frac{1}{2}$ years. Such femoral shortening may with profit be combined with derotation sufficient to counteract the excessive anteversion. It is prudent to lengthen the ilio-psoas intra-operatively to minimize further femoral head pressure.

Femoral Osteotomy

Osteotomy of the proximal femur is readily carried out through a lateral thigh incision. An L-shaped incision at its origin allows vastus lateralis to be reflected forward, just below the level of the greater trochanter; the trochanteric growth plate should not be injured. It is sensible to insert wires into the proximal femur so that, after rotation or varus, parallel alignment of the wires confirms that the desired alteration has been achieved. Image intensification should be used if possible. Ideally, the osteotomy should be performed above the level of the lesser trochanter, but this may not be possible if shortening is required. In tiny children the osteotomy is held with a small plate as a "bone suture" (Fig. 5.20). In the older child a blade plate is preferable, and from the age

of 5 or 6 years, compression at the osteotomy site obviates the need for plaster fixation.

Although femoral osteotomy may be necessary, there is a tendency to use it less often than in the past. Typically, the varus introduced at osteotomy resolves within 3 years [48] and the shortening corrects by relative overgrowth within the same period.

It is now uncommon for the child with hip dislocation who is older than 2 years to be treated non-operatively. The surgical approach favored is almost always the anterolateral, which provides the best exposure of the hip joint and its contents. In established dislocation, the superior capsule is usually firmly adherent to the side wall of the ilium above the true acetabulum and needs to be elevated and mobilized superiorly and posteriorly if the labrum is to be everted from the joint. The redundant superior capsule should be excised and a careful capsulorrhaphy performed when the head has been fully reduced.

The femoral head and acetabulum are always deformed in the long-established dislocation, but it is important to ensure that the femoral head is seated as deeply as possible in the true acetabulum. If it is impossible to evert the labrum, radial cuts should make it possible to retain it. It is unnecessary to remove the acetabular fat pad (pulvinar), but the transverse ligament should be divided. The inferior capsule may need careful release to allow the femoral head to descend fully. The posterior capsule should not be divided but in some circumstances, particularly after previous failed surgery, it cannot be avoided; great care should then be taken to divide the capsule at the acetabular margin. The procedure is most likely to be necessary where the hip has dislocated posteriorly as a consequence of excessive internal rotation at previous open reduction.

Pelvic Osteotomy

Careful preoperative analysis and intra-operative assessment should help to decide if pelvic osteotomy is necessary. The capacity of the acetabulum to remodel around the femoral head is maximal in infancy and decreases steadily after the first 3 or 4 years. If, therefore, the acetabulum contains the femoral head poorly, attempts should be made to improve the acetabular cover.

In the typical dislocation, the anterior limb of the triradiate cartilage is inadequately stimulated and the anterior acetabulum fails to develop. This produces a shallow and apparently anteverted acetabulum. If the acetabulum is flat and oval, its shape may be improved by the Pemberton [49] peri-capsular osteotomy. This is described below, but in essence a curvilinear osteotomy is made above the acetabulum and the roof is folded downward to improve acetabular congruity and cover.

If the femoral head and the acetabulum fit well but the acetabulum is too open, the Salter [50] innominate osteotomy, which rotates the whole acetabulum forward and laterally, is to be preferred. Klisic [46] made popular the simultaneous performance of open reduction, femoral shortening, and pelvic osteotomy. Some surgeons, however, prefer to reserve pelvic osteotomy for those children in whom it may be seen that the acetabulum is failing to develop adequately after reduction [51]. The stress to the child and family of multiple hip surgery in childhood and the disadvantages of repetitive plaster immobilization should not be underestimated, and where expertise and facilities allow, the surgeon should attempt both to reduce and stabilize the hip at the time of the first operation. The risk of redislocation should increase only marginally.

Wherever possible, it is best to reshape and realign the acetabulum so that articular cartilage covers the femoral head. In the child older than 4 or 5 years, acetabular and femoral head deformity may be such that this is impracticable. Under these circumstances, when the hip is subluxated and the acetabular volume reduced, a salvage procedure such as the medial displacement osteotomy of Chiari [52] or a shelf procedure may be a better solution.

Although shortening, rotational, and varus osteotomy may be necessary, both to decrease pressure upon the femoral head and to reorientate the proximal femur, it has been shown by Williamson and Benson [53] that femoral osteotomy alone in later childhood is inadequate treatment for the subluxated hip.

Because of the deteriorating results of treatment with age, many surgeons suggest that the child older than 7 years with bilateral hip dislocation should be left untreated because operation has a high chance of increasing the likelihood of adolescent hip pain. Where the dislocation is unilateral, however, most surgeons continue to advocate reduction and reconstruction in older children to preserve leg length and spinal symmetry.

The Innominate Osteotomy

Salter's osteotomy [50] is suitable for the child between the ages of 2 and 6 years with a dislocated hip and may be appropriate for the subluxating hip in the older child and adolescent. Certain criteria are necessary for the osteotomy to be undertaken. The hip should reduce concentrically and preserve a virtually normal range of movement. If open reduction is performed at the same time, hip reduction should be congruous and confirmed radiologically. It should be apparent that subluxation of the hip anterosuperiorly as it is moved from flexion into extension is prevented when the leg is internally rotated and abducted. It is precisely this

maldirectional instability that the innominate osteotomy is designed to correct.

The innominate osteotomy lengthens the leg; avoidance of this lengthening is possible by combining it with a varus rotational osteotomy [53] or by notching the upper pelvic segment in the older child [54]. Overzealous femoral internal rotation or derotational osteotomy may allow the femoral head to displace posteriorly, as the innominate osteotomy achieves improved anterolateral cover at the expense of posterior support. As already noted, in the child older than 3 years, it may be wise to shorten the femur to lessen pressure upon the reduced femoral head. Theoretically, an innominate osteotomy may increase pressure upon the femoral head, but Salter has argued that the pressure increase is trivial.

The innominate osteotomy (Figs. 5.21 and 5.22) is best performed through a transverse incision just below the iliac

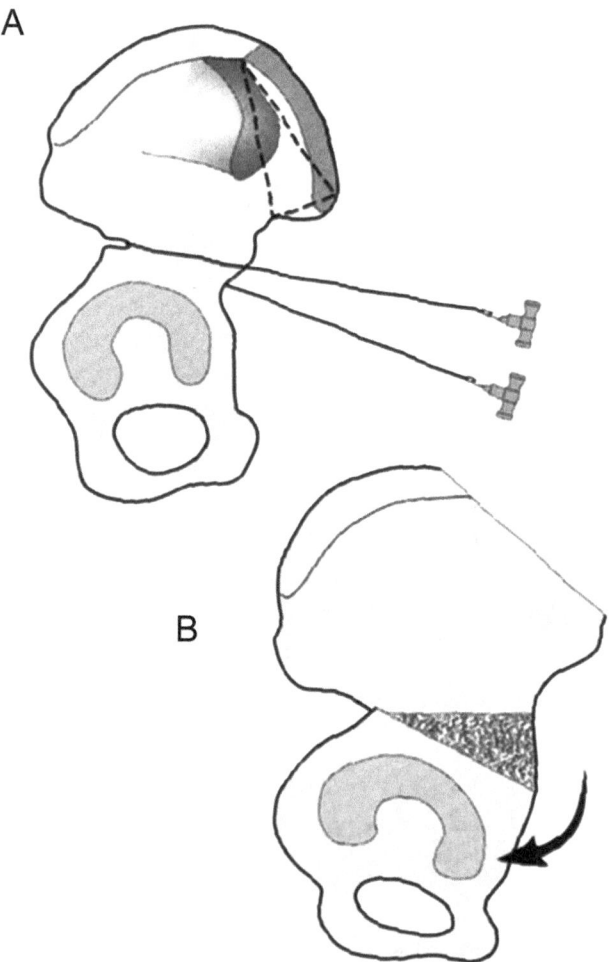

Fig. 5.21 The innominate osteotomy of Salter. (**a**) The Gigli saw transects the ilium at the level of the anterior inferior spine. (**b**) The wedge of bone harvested from the iliac crest is inserted into the osteotomy, allowing the distal pelvic fragment and acetabulum to rotate forward and laterally

Fig. 5.22 (**a**) Previously
treated DDH has left this girl
with Type II avascular necrosis,
dysplasia, and mild subluxation.
(**b**) After an arthrogram
confirmed sphericity and
congruity she was treated by
innominate osteotomy and varus
femoral osteotomy. (**c**) The
appearance 5 years later

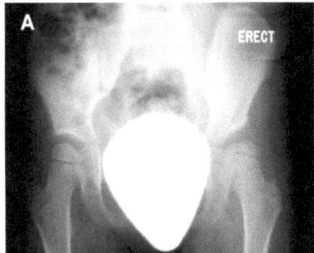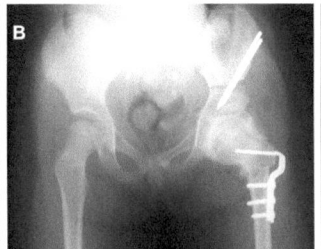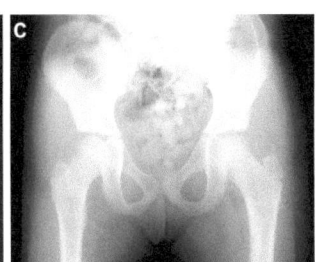

crest. The iliac apophysis is split and the split halves are elevated subperiosteally from the iliac wing, in continuity with
the gluteal muscles externally and the iliac muscles medially. Great care should be taken in exposing the sciatic notch,
and the retractors placed through this notch should be clearly
seen and felt to be subperiosteal. The psoas tendon should
be divided intramuscularly by rolling it at the level of the
pelvic brim. A curved introducer passed through the sciatic
notch allows the Gigli saw to be introduced subperiosteally
through the notch.

A transverse pelvic osteotomy is then performed at the
level of the anterior inferior iliac spine. Where the hip joint
has not been opened the thigh is placed in flexion, abduction, and external rotation. Downward leverage upon the
knee allows the distal pelvic fragment to rotate anterolaterally. Its direction may be helped by gentle downward traction
using a towel clip placed through the anterior inferior spine
or by pulling the posterior edge of the lower fragment forward with a small Lambotte hook. A wedge of bone taken
from the anterior superior iliac spine is trimmed and fash-
ioned to fit into the triangular gap so created. It is important
to keep the osteotomy closed posteriorly. Once the bone
graft is safely placed, two threaded wires should be passed
across the osteotomy and screened radiographically to ensure
that joint penetration has not occurred. The implants are cut
short, but should be left slightly proud of the closed iliac
apophysis.

The wound is closed in layers, taking care to re-appose
the iliac apophysis carefully. A one-and-a-half hip spica is
applied with the hip in 20–30° of flexion and abduction but
neutral rotation. The osteotomy unites in 6 weeks. It was
once the routine to remove these wires but they are now often
retained.

Complications that may occur with this procedure are
often the result of faulty technique [55]. The operation should
not be performed unless it is possible to reduce the hip
satisfactorily. Redislocation may occur if open reduction is
performed simultaneously [51]. The bone graft may slip or
resorb, wires may penetrate the joint or extrude, the sciatic,
femoral, or lateral femoral cutaneous nerves may be injured,
and there may be deformity of the ilium consequent upon
splitting the iliac apophysis.

Pemberton Acetabuloplasty

Where the femoral head and acetabulum do not "match," and
where arthrography has demonstrated a bilocular or "double
diameter" acetabulum in association with subluxation, it may
be wise to reshape rather than to redirect the acetabulum, in
the manner described by Pemberton [49]. Pemberton's procedure allows an incomplete iliac osteotomy to hinge through
the triradiate cartilage. This hinge alters the volume of the
acetabulum and is therefore applicable for the dysplastic oval
socket. The triradiate cartilage must be open and it is therefore most useful for children 3–11 years old. The approach
is similar to that described for an innominate osteotomy.
Careful preoperative radiographic checking is essential. A
series of curved osteotomies is passed above the hip joint,
curving medially and posteriorly to the triradiate cartilage,
usually at a distance of about 1 cm from the acetabular margin. Care must be taken to ensure that articular penetration
does not occur. A curved bone graft is taken from the anterosuperior iliac spine and inserted into the gap created as the
acetabular margin is levered down with the osteotome. When
the bone graft is tapped into place the position is usually stable so that internal fixation is unnecessary (Figs. 5.23 and
5.24).

The risk of joint penetration is real in this procedure, and
there is a slight increase in the risk of avascular necrosis from
pressure directed upon the femoral head by the levered-down
acetabular roof. The triradiate cartilage may rarely be injured
and cease to grow.

The Pemberton acetabuloplasty, just like the innominate
osteotomy, may be performed in isolation or as part of a complex open reduction in the older child, in whom it may be
combined with femoral shortening and rotation.

Other Procedures

The Dega pelvic osteotomy [56] is similar to the Pemberton,
except that the pelvic cut is not curved, but directed obliquely
downward and medially to the triradiate cartilage from an
anteroposterior axis 2 cm above the acetabular margin. It
similarly reduces acetabular size, but increases lateral rather
than anterior cover.

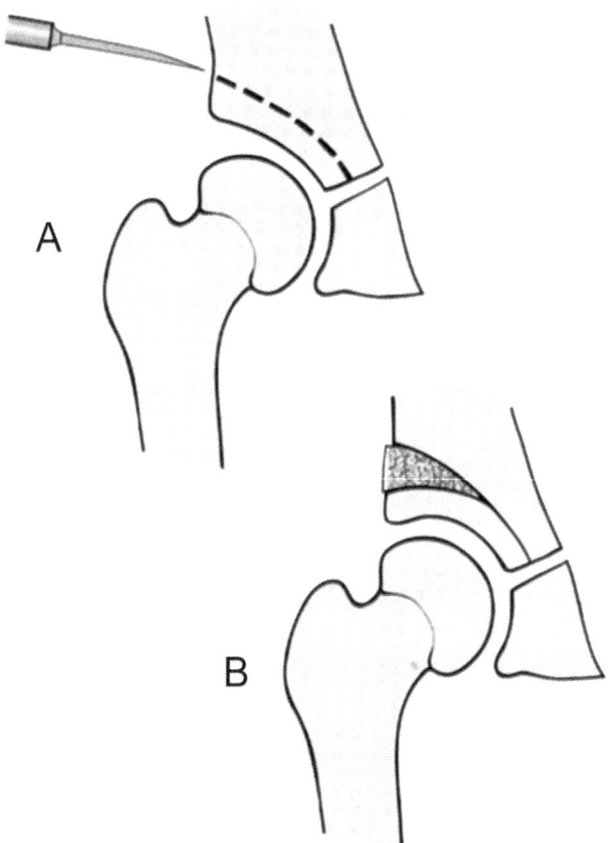

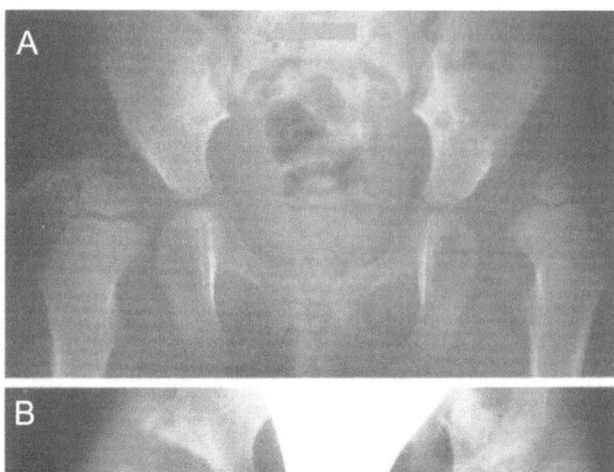

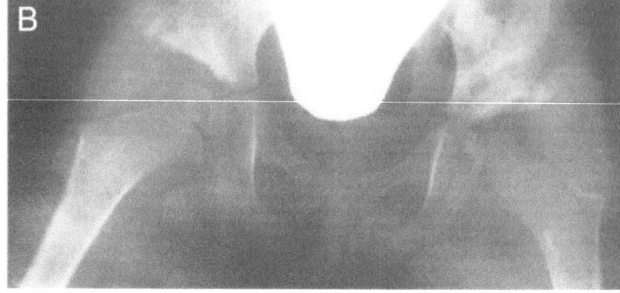

Fig. 5.24 (**a**) Two-and-a-half-year-old girl with right hip subluxation and left hip dislocation. (**b**) Following open reduction of the left hip and bilateral Pemberton osteotomy

Fig. 5.23 The pelvic osteotomy of Pemberton. (**a**) The osteotomy curves 1 cm from the acetabular margin up to the triradiate cartilage. (**b**) Hinging at the triradiate cartilage allows the acetabular roof to be levered down and stabilized with a bone graft

Macnicol [57] has described and illustrated the variety of more complex acetabular osteotomies. As skeletal maturity approaches, the Salter osteotomy in isolation may not allow sufficient rotation about the axis passing from symphysis pubis to greater sciatic notch, unless osteotomies of the superior pubic ramus and ischium are performed coincidentally. This triple innominate osteotomy, as described by Tönnis [29], allows greater rotation and displacement of the acetabulum: the innominate osteotomy element is supplemented by osteotomies of the superior pubic ramus and ischium as close as possible to the acetabulum. This allows much greater rotation of the acetabulum and improved femoral head cover. It must always be remembered that such reorientation decreases posterior cover and care is needed not to over-correct. The triple osteotomy is most useful in children aged 7–14 years whose triradiate cartilage is still open.

Residual dysplasia often merits treatment after maturity. When an adolescent or young adult develops discomfort with exercise and radiographs demonstrate marked uncovering of the femoral head, a periacetabular osteotomy should be considered. A careful history and examination may suggest the "rim syndrome" described by Klaue et al. [58]. The patient describes sudden sharp groin pain that accompanies twisting movements. There is often a feeling that the leg may "give way." Although the hip may appear to move freely at examination, pain is typically produced when the flexed hip is pressed into adduction and internal rotation. The cause is usually a torn labrum, which may be associated with a ganglionic cyst in the labrum itself or in the bony pelvis. The tear is best demonstrated by gadolinium-enhanced MRI. Increasingly hip arthroscopy is used to assess the hip since labral tears, loose bodies, and articular cartilage flaps are amenable to arthroscopic debridement. It must be remembered that unless the *cause* of the rim syndrome is addressed, further intra-articular injury is almost inevitable, with resultant osteoarthritis.

If a complex, periacetabular osteotomy is considered, careful preoperative planning is essential. A three-dimensional CT scan best allows spatially correct reconstruction of the hip joint. Significant head deformity and arthritis are contra-indications. Ganz [59] has provided clear prerequisites and technical advice for his Bernese osteotomy (Fig. 5.25). Periacetabular osteotomies are complex and risks include neurovascular injury, non-union and mal-union, and over-correction. They are less satisfactory if significant arthritis is present and are not indicated when there is poor congruity between the femoral head and acetabulum.

Fig. 5.25 The complex peri-acetabular osteotomy of Ganz. (**a**) The lines on the hemi-pelvis show the cuts necessary to rotate the acetabular fragment while preserving continuity of the posterior pelvic column. (**b**) Diagrammatic representation of the displacement highlighting that the acetabulum is not displaced laterally

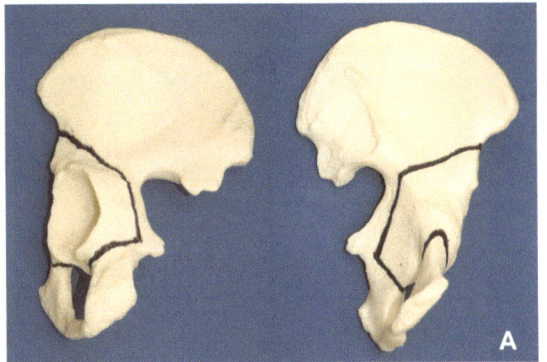
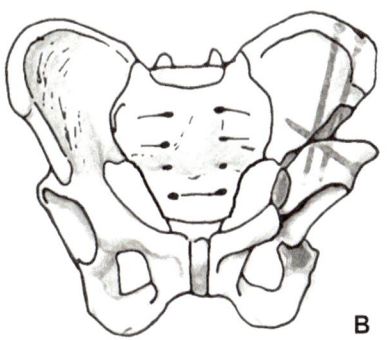

Salvage Procedures

Shelf Arthroplasty

There have been many techniques described to fashion a stabilizing bony shelf above the dysplastic hip. The Staheli technique is widely practiced [60]. Where there is mild or modest subluxation in the child whose hip is not fully containable by a dysplastic acetabulum the shelf is a low-risk procedure to stabilize the femoral head. Whenever possible, it is preferable to realign or reshape the acetabulum to cover the femoral head with true articular cartilage. If this is not possible and the child is developing fatigue discomfort the Staheli shelf arthroplasty is effective.

The superior hip capsule is exposed through a bikini incision and anterior approach. The straight and reflected heads of rectus femoris are defined. Preserving the insertion of the straight head, the reflected head is divided anteriorly and dissected backward off the hip capsule. Its posterior origin is preserved. Taking care not to injure the growth plate at the acetabular margin, a guide wire is inserted slightly cephalad above the capsular insertion. The position should be checked with an image intensifier. A curvilinear slot is made with drill holes and small osteotomes above the capsule and into this slot are inserted coraco-cancellous strips of bone taken from the outer table of the ilium. The reflected head of rectus femoris is laid on top of these bone strips and sutured back to the straight head, so applying the bone graft securely to the superior capsule. Additional cancellous graft is placed above this and the iliac apophysis repaired, holding the graft in place (Fig. 5.26). There is evidence that the graft stimulates growth of the true acetabular margin, increasing articular cartilage cover with time.

The Chiari Osteotomy

Where subluxation is fixed and the femoral head is uncovered, the Chiari medial displacement osteotomy should be considered. Although Chiari [52] first envisaged his procedure as being most applicable to the child 4 or 5 years old, it has become increasingly reserved for the older child, adolescent, and young adult with irreversible and symptomatic acetabular dysplasia. Articulation with the abnormally located false acetabulum may have to be accepted but the femoral head cover is improved to increase stability and decrease harmful shear forces. A shelf procedure affords good support if acetabular insufficiency is mild to moderate, but when the hip joint is lateralized by marked thickening of the acetabular floor, medialization of the femoral head is advisable. These greater degrees of hip deformity benefit from the salvage effect of the Chiari osteotomy, which produces an iliac bone buttress above the superior, uncovered hip capsule.

The procedure reduces loading through the femoral head both by increasing the area of contact and by medializing the fulcrum of the hip. The operation should be carried out using an orthopaedic table and with image intensifier control (Fig. 5.27). A skin-crease bikini incision affords adequate exposure and heals well [61]. The iliac osteotomy should be made just above the hip capsule. The osteotomy level must be checked radiographically as the reflected fibers of the hip capsule are often well above the elected site for osteotomy. Ideally, the osteotomy should be gently curved from front to back, to follow the contour of femoral head and capsule. The angle of the osteotomy should be almost transverse or slightly cephalad. Increasing the upward obliquity of the osteotomy imperils the sacroiliac joint and, by functionally weakening the abductor muscles, makes a persistent Trendelenburg gait more likely.

If 50% displacement at the osteotomy is planned, Benson and Jameson-Evans [62] showed that this allows only up to 2 cm of shift as the ilium is only 3 cm wide at this level. The osteotomy must not be allowed to hinge like a book posteriorly as this causes a false radiographic appearance of good femoral head cover. Anterior femoral head support can be increased by additional bone grafting although this may restrict hip flexion.

Fig. 5.26 (**a**) Diagram of the Staheli shelf arthroplasty: the graft is held on the capsule by the reflected head of rectus femoris. (**b**) A poorly covered hip treated by shelf arthroplasty

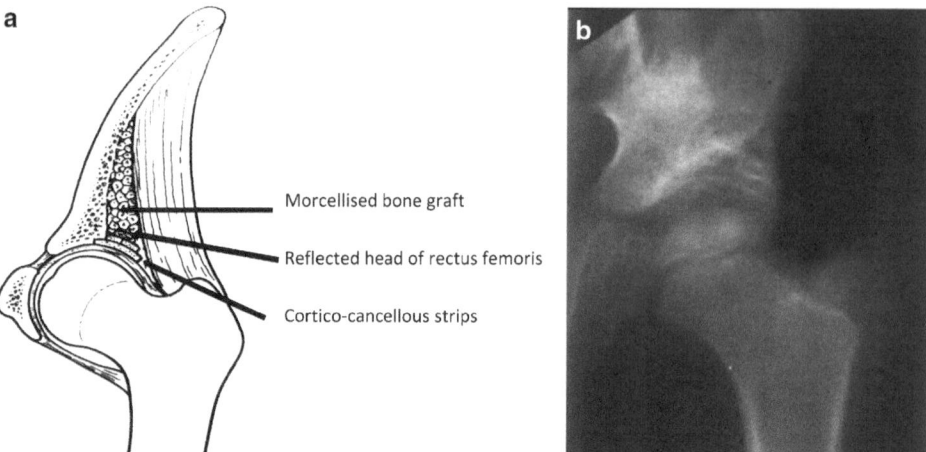

Morcellised bone graft

Reflected head of rectus femoris

Cortico-cancellous strips

Fig. 5.27 (**a**) Chiari osteotomy. Subluxation is marked; there is incongruity between head and acetabulum and a loose marginal fragment confirming instability. (**b**) After Chiari osteotomy the head is stabilized

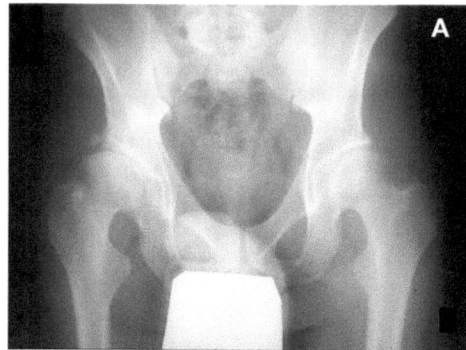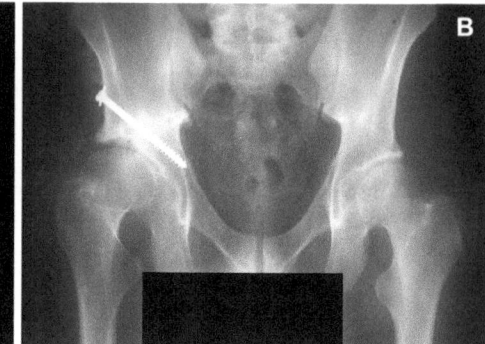

If the osteotomy is fixed with a compression screw, the leg can be moved freely during the recovery period, allowing the patient to return home using crutches a few days postoperatively. Weight bearing is progressively increased over the first 2 months and the limp usually disappears or lessens by 1 year. Because the hip is effectively stabilized, pain relief is significant and lasting. There is a concurrent halt in femoral head migration, and a gratifying degree of pelvic remodeling as Macnicol et al. have shown [63].

Early complications include too low an osteotomy, with breaching of the joint, excessive or inadequate displacement, injury to adjoining nerves and vessels, and problems with wound healing. Late complications are rare, but delayed union has been reported if internal fixation is inadequate, and pelvic ligamentous pain may retard early progress. Damage to the joint produces ankylosis, and numbness in the distribution of the lateral femoral cutaneous nerve may be remarked upon. The osteotomy is contraindicated in the presence of arthritis [64], particularly if there is significant impingement pain and stiffening. Unilateral procedures probably increase the necessity of caesarian section only slightly, bilateral osteotomies rather more. It may be appropriate to carry out a concomitant femoral realignment osteotomy, incorporating varus, valgus, rotation, or extension, depending upon the

resultant congruency of the joint. Windhager et al. [65], in their review of Chiari's own osteotomies after 20–34 years, found the overall result good in 51%, fair in 30%, and poor in 18%. They noted that results were more durable in younger patients. Remodeling of the pelvis occurs around the femoral head. If the osteotomy stabilizes the hip well revision by arthroplasty is avoided in 80% of cases 30 years postoperatively [63].

Capsuloplasty

Femoral head and acetabular deformities may become so pronounced, particularly after failed surgery, that congruous reduction cannot be achieved. If this disparity is pronounced, the Colonna [66] procedure should not be forgotten (Fig. 5.28). A circumferential acetabular capsulotomy is performed and the capsule sutured as an envelope over the femoral head. Using serial reamers, the acetabulum is enlarged to accept the femoral head enveloped in its capsular mantle. Where necessary, the femur may be shortened and rotated appropriately. The Colonna arthroplasty provides a stable articulation, but mobility is clearly less

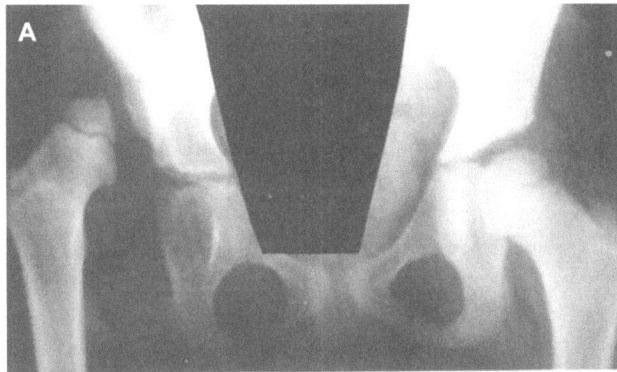

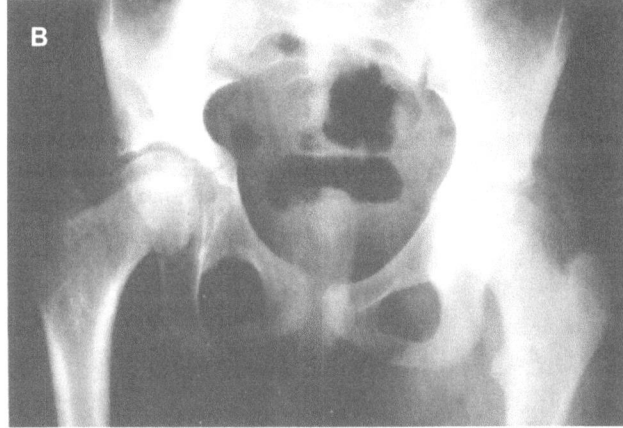

Fig. 5.28 Colonna arthroplasty. (**a**) Late dislocation and severe incongruity. (**b**) Fifteen years after the capsular arthroplasty of Colonna

satisfactory and discomfort more likely than in a more optimally reduced hip. Nonetheless, the restoration of anatomical alignment makes secondary surgery in adult life a great deal more straightforward. Pozo et al. [67] found 70% of 44 hips so treated had good function at a mean follow-up of 20 years.

Trochanteric "Overgrowth"

In children in whom acetabular development is satisfactory but limp and pain are present, the mechanics of the hip may be improved by correcting marked degrees of femoral anteversion, by shortening the femur if there is a "long leg dysplasia," and by distal transfer of the greater trochanter (Fig. 5.29) if the femoral neck is short and the abductor mechanism abnormal [68]. These relatively small surgical adjustments may give considerable improvements in function, endurance, and pain relief if they allow the coaptive relationship between the femoral head and the acetabulum to improve.

Pelvic Support Osteotomies

When the hip is dislocated in later childhood and adolescence both femoral head and acetabulum become so deformed that reduction, even if technically possible, does not provide pain relief and progressive deformity may follow. Fixed flexion, adduction, and external rotation lead to progressive apparent shortening, a deteriorating gait, and secondary back and knee discomfort.

In the adult hip arthrodesis or total joint arthroplasty is a last resort. Recent advances in hip arthroplasty, particularly surface replacement, make this a more attractive option in the young and active adult but the long-term results are still unknown. Furthermore, there is some genetic concern about metal ion release in young women. Revision arthroplasty of the fused hip is also an available but daunting option.

A Schanz sub-trochanteric osteotomy (Fig. 5.30) incorporating valgus, extension, and a little rotation may relieve pain, improve leg alignment and gait, and provide salvage for many years. It may furthermore be combined with distal femoral lengthening [69].

Fig. 5.29 (**a**) Distal transfer of the greater trochanter. Treatment of DDH has caused avascular change in the femoral head and premature growth plate closure. There is relative overgrowth of the greater trochanter. (**b**) More effective abductor power has been achieved by lateral and distal transfer of the greater trochanter, here stabilized by two screws

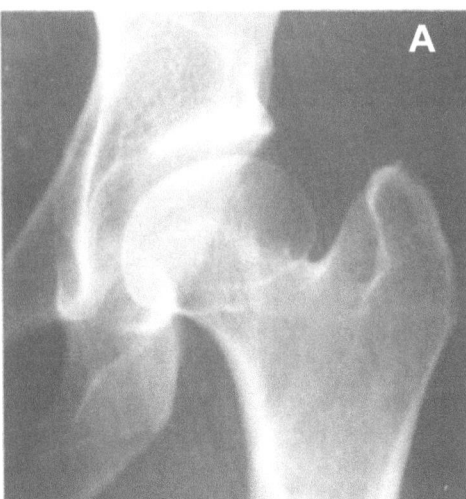

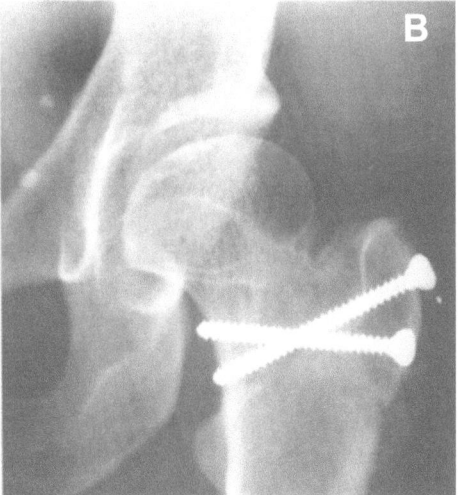

Fig. 5.30 The pelvic support osteotomy of Schanz, 30 years after sub-trochanteric valgus, extension osteotomy. Although severe arthritis has developed the major adduction and flexion deformity has not recurred

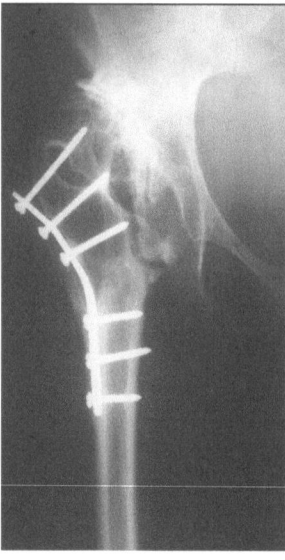

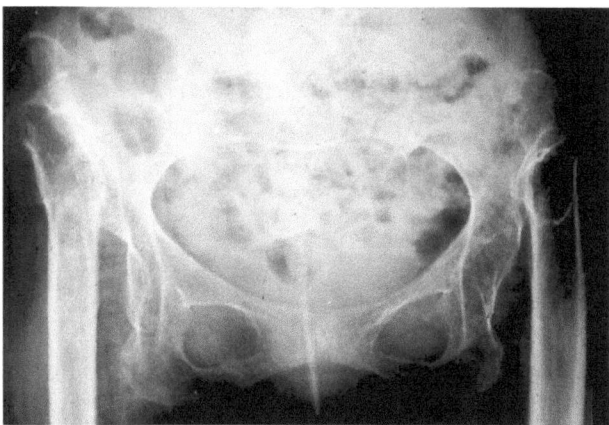

Fig. 5.31 Untreated dislocations in an 88-year-old woman. She has limped throughout her life, has modest back pain but little hip pain

Outcomes

There are few studies of untreated dysplasia. Wedge and Wasylenko [70] contacted 54 adults with 80 affected hips. Although limp was universal many did not develop pain until later adult life. Fifty-nine percent had only fair or poor grading scores. Arthritis developed earlier and was more frequent when a well-formed false acetabulum developed, especially when the hip was subluxated rather than fully dislocated. Unilateral dislocation often led to ipsilateral knee valgus and arthritis. However, the incidence of symptomatic lumbar spondylosis was not increased (Fig. 5.31).

Inevitably we have modified outcomes by treatment. Provided the hip is reducible and avascular necrosis is avoided, neonates and young infants treated promptly should develop a nearly normal hip.

Children with an irreducible hip at birth do less well. Attempts to reduce the hip neonatally may fail and lead to avascular necrosis. Teratological dislocations often present with considerable femoral head deformity so that it is not surprising to find that long-term outcomes are less satisfactory.

Malvitz and Weinstein [71] reviewed 152 young adults after they had been treated by closed reduction at an average age of 21 months. In 60% there was evidence of some proximal femoral growth disturbance; 43% of the treated hips were developing degenerative arthritis, and 36% were still subluxated.

Morcuende et al. [72] then reviewed the Iowa experience with open reduction via a medial approach. A total of 93 hips in 76 children (average age 14 months) were followed up for 4–23 years. Avascular necrotic change was observed in 43%, and 29% had residual dysplasia. The patients were too young at follow-up to assess the incidence of premature arthritis.

Angliss et al. [73] reviewed 147 children with 191 dislocated hips treated surgically for DDH at an average age of 33 years. Thirteen percent showed evidence of some avascular necrosis in the first 5 years. Mild or moderate hip arthritis developed by the mid-thirties in 40% of patients. Arthritis was more likely when the limbus was excised at operation, when residual subluxation was present, and if avascular necrosis developed. Increasing age at presentation also adversely affected the outcome.

Thomas et al. [74] recently reviewed at 45 years postoperatively those children treated by open reduction and innominate osteotomy between the ages of 18 months and 5 years. Of 51 hips with available radiographs, 22 revealed moderate or severe arthritis. Those with bilateral DDH fared worse but the age at operation seemed to make little difference.

Later treatment leads to poorer results because it is more difficult to achieve and maintain a stable reduction. The acetabulum often fails to develop sufficiently and any residual subluxation inevitably worsens with time. Unfortunately, it is not possible to predict outcome accurately for many years after treatment, because the subtle changes of growth disturbance in the proximal femur, especially premature lateral growth arrest, may not appear until adolescence. Therefore, it is imperative that all children treated for developmental dysplasia of the hip be followed by serial radiographs at least until skeletal maturity and that residual instability is recognized and treated as early as possible.

Conclusion

In dealing with displacement and developmental dysplasia of the hip, the overriding principle is to achieve a stable reduction of the femoral head. Treatment is most effective in the neonatal period. With increasing age, there is a greater reliance upon surgery. The surgeon must be constantly alert to the dangers of pressure (avascular) necrosis of the proximal femur and re-displacement. Irrevocable changes occur in the older child, particularly after failed or inadequate surgery, so that the prognosis becomes increasingly poor.

References

1. Strayer LM. The embryology of the human hip. Clin Orthop Rel Res 1971; 74:221–240.
2. Watanabe RS. Embryology of the human hip. Clin Orthop Rel Res 1974; 98:8–26.
3. Le Damany P. Variation en potordeur du cotyle humain aux divers ages. Bulletin Société des Sciences et Medicine d'Ouex 1912; 1974; 12:410.
4. Ralis ZA, McKibbin B. Changes in shape of the human hip in joint during its development and their relationship to its stability. J Bone Joint Surg 1973; 55B:780–785.
5. Portinaro NM, Murray DW, Benson MKD. Microanatomy of the acetabular cavity and its relation to growth. J Bone Joint Surg (Br) 2001; 83:377–383.
6. Trueta J. The normal vascular anatomy of the human femoral head during growth. J Bone Joint Surg 1957; 39B:358–394.
7. Chung SM. The arterial supply of the developing proximal end of the femur. J Bone Joint Surg Am 1976; 58:961–970.
8. Klisic P, Pajic D. Progress in the preventative approach to developmental dysplasia of the hip. J Paediatr Orthop 1993; Part B, 2:108–111.
9. Chan A, McCaul KA, Cundy PJ, et al. Perinatal risk factors for developmental dysplasia of the hip. Arch Dis Child Fetal Neonatal Ed 1997; 76:F94–100.
10. Carter CO, Wilkinson J. Genetic and environmental factors in the aetiology of congenital dislocation of the hip. Clinical Orthop 1960; 33:119–128.
11. Vogel I, Andersson JE, Uldbjerg N. Serum relaxin in the newborn is not a marker of neonatal hip instability J Pediatr Orthop 1998; 18(4):535–537.
12. McKibbin B. Anatomical factors in the stability of the hip in the newborn. J Bone Joint Surg 1970; 52B:148–159.
13. Barlow TG. Early diagnosis and treatment of congenital dislocation of the hip. J Bone Joint Surg 1962; 44B:242–301.
14. Macnicol MF. Results of a 25-year screening programme for neonatal hip instability. J Bone Joint Surg 1990; 72B:1057–1060.
15. Roser W. Ueber angeborene Hueftverrenkung. Langenbeck's Archiv fuer klinische Chirurgie 1879; 24:309–313.
16. Ortolani M. Un segno poco noto e sua importanza par la diagnosi di preluzzione congenitale dell'ance. Pediatria 1937; 45:129.
17. Von Rosen S. Diagnosis and treatment of congenital dislocation of the hip in the new-born. J Bone Joint Surg 1962; 44B:284–291.
18. Palmén K. Preluxation of the hip joint. Diagnosis and treatment in the newborn and the diagnosis of congenital dislocation of the hip joint in Sweden during the years 1948–60. Acta Paediatr (Suppl 129) 1961;50: 1–71.
19. Godward S, Dezateaux C. Surgery for congenital dislocation of the hip in the UK as a measure of outcome of screening. Lancet 1998; 351(9110):1149–52.
20. Graf R. Classification of hip joint dysplasia by means of sonography. Arch Orthop Trauma Surg 1984; 102:248–255.
21. Lehmann HP, Hinton R, Morello P, Santoli J. Developmental dysplasia of the hip practice guideline: technical report. Committee on Quality Improvement, and Subcommittee on Developmental Dysplasia of the Hip. Pediatrics 2000; Apr. 105(4):E57.
22. Clegg J, Bache CE, Raut W. Financial justification for routine ultrasound screening of the neonatal hip. J Bone Joint Surg 1999; 81B:852–857.
23. Morin C, Harcke HT, MacEwan GD. The infant hip: real-time US assessment of acetabular development. Radiology 1985; 157:673–677.
24. Suzuki S, Kasahara Y, Futami T, et al. Ultrasonography in congenital dislocation of the hip. Simultaneous imaging of both hips from in front. J Bone Joint Surg 1991; 73B:879–83.
25. Clarke NMP, Harcke HT, McHugh P, et al. Real-time ultrasound in the diagnosis of congenital dislocation and dysplasia of the hip. J Bone Joint Surg 1985;67B:406.
26. Engesaeter LB, Wilson DJ, Nag D, Benson MK. Ultrasound and congenital dislocation of the hip. J Bone Joint Surg 1990; 72B:197–200.
27. Dunn PM. Perinatal observations on the aetiology of congenital dislocation of the hip. Clin Orthop 1976; 119:11.
28. Bertol P, Macnicol MF, Mitchell GP. Radiographic features of neonatal congenital dislocation of the hip. J Bone Joint Surg 1982; 64B:176–179.
29. Tönnis D. Congenital Dysplasia and Dislocation of the Hip. Berlin: Springer; 1986.
30. Wiberg C. Studies on dysplastic acetabulae and congenital subluxation of the hip joint. Acta Chirurgica Scandinavica 1939; Suppl 58.
31. Severin E. Contribution to the knowledge of congenital dislocation of the hip joint. Acta Chir Scandinavica 1941; 84: Suppl 63.
32. Salter RB, Kostuik J, Dallas S. Avascular necrosis of the femoral head as a complication of treatment of congenital dislocation in young children: a clinical and experimental study. Can J Surg 1969; 12:44.
33. Kalamchi A, MacEwan GD. Avascular necrosis following treatment of congenital dislocation of the hip. J Bone Joint Surg 1980; 62A:876–888.
34. Bradley J, Weatherill M, Benson MKD. Splintage for congenital dislocation of the hip. Is it safe and reliable? J Bone Joint Surg 1987; 69B:259–263.
35. Grill F, Bensahel H, Canadell J, et al. The Pavlik harness in the treatment of congenital dislocating hip. J Pediatr Orthop 1988; 8(1):1–8.
36. Wilkinson AG, Sherlock DA, Murray GD. The efficacy of the Pavlik harness, the Craig splint and the von Rosen splint in the management of neonatal dysplasia of the hip. J Bone Joint Surg Br 2003; 85:1085–1086.
37. Nakamura J, Kamegaya M, Saisu T, et al. Treatment for developmental dysplasia of the hip using the Pavlik harness. J Bone Joint Surg 2007; 89-B:230–235.
38. Macnicol M F. Congenital dislocation of the hip. In: Bennet GC, ed. Paediatric Hip Disorders. Oxford: Blackwell; 1987: 64–113.
39. Segal LS, Schneider DJ, Berlin JM, et al. The contribution of the ossific nucleus in the structural stiffness of the capital femoral epiphysis: a porcine model for DDH. J Pediatr Orthop 1999; 19:433–437.
40. Luhmann S, Schoenecker PL, Anderson AM, Bassett G. The prognostic significance of the ossific nucleus in the treatment of congenital dysplasia of the hip J Bone Joint Surg 1998; 80-A:1719–1727.
41. Weinstein SL, Ponseti IV. Congenital dislocation of the hip: open reduction through a medial approach. J Bone Joint Surg 1979; 61A:119–124.

42. Ramsey PL, Hensiger RN, MacEwan GD. Congenital dislocation of the hip. Use of the Pavlik harness in the child during the first 6 months of life. J Bone Joint Surg Am 1976; 58:1000–1004.
43. McNally EG, Tasker A, Benson MK. MRI after operative reduction for developmental dysplasia of the hip. J Bone Joint Surg Br 1998; 79:724–726.
44. Ludloff K. The open reduction of congenital hip dislocation by an anterior incision. Am J Orthop Surg 1913; 10:438–454.
45. Hey-Groves E. The treatment of congenital dislocation of the hip. Robert Jones Birthday Volume. Oxford: Oxford University Press; 1928.
46. Klisic P. Combined procedure of open reduction and shortening of the femur in treatment of congenital dislocation of the hip in older children. Clin Orth 1976; 119:60.
47. Gibson PH, Benson MKD. Congenital dislocation of the hip. Review at maturity of 147 hips treated by excision of the limbus and derotation osteotomy. J Bone Joint Surg 1982; 64B: 169–175.
48. Sangavi SM, Szoke G, Murray DW, Benson MK. Femoral remodeling after subtrochanteric osteotomy for developmental dysplasia of the hip. J Bone Joint Surg 1996; 8B:917–923.
49. Pemberton PA. Pericapsular osteotomy of the ilium for treatment of congenital subluxation and dislocation of the hip. J Bone Joint Surg 1965; 47A:65–86.
50. Salter RB. Innominate osteotomy in the treatment of congenital dislocation and subluxation of the hip. J Bone Joint Surg 1961; 43B:518–539.
51. Macnicol MF, Bertol P. The Salter innominate osteotomy: should it be combined with concurrent open reduction? J Paediatr Orthop B 2005; 14:415–21.
52. Chiari K. Beckenosteotomie zur Pfannendachplastik. Wiener Medizinische Wochenschrift 1953; 103:707–713.
53. Williamson DM, Benson MKD. Late femoral osteotomy in congenital dislocation of the hip. J Bone Joint Surg 1988; 70B:614–618.
54. Kalamchi A. Modified salter osteotomy. J Bone Joint Surg Am 1982; 64:183–187.
55. Morscher E. Our experience with Salter's innominate osteotomy in the treatment of hip dysplasia. In: Weil UH, ed. Progress in Orthopaedic Surgery. vol 2. Berlin: Springer; 1978.
56. Dega W, Krol J, Polakowski L. Surgical treatment of congenital dislocation of the hip in children; a one step procedure. J Bone Joint Surg Am 1959; 41A(5):920–934.
57. Macnicol MF. Color Atlas and Text: Osteotomy of the Hip. London: Mosby-Wolfe; 1995.
58. Klaue K, Durnin CW, Ganz R. The acetabular rim syndrome. A clinical presentation of dysplasia of the hip. J Bone Joint Surg 1991; 73B:423–429.
59. Ganz R, Klaue K, Vinh TS, Mast JW. A new periacetabular osteotomy for the treatment of hip dysplasias. Technique and preliminary results. Clin Orthop 1988; 232:26–36.
60. Staheli LT, Chew DE. Slotted acetabular augmentation in childhood and adolescence. J Pediatr Orthop 1992; 12(5):569–80.
61. Reynolds DA. Chiari innominate osteotomy in adults: technique, indications and contraindications. J Bone Joint Surg 1986; 68B:45–54.
62. Benson MKD, Jameson-Evans DC. The pelvic osteotomy of Chiari: an anatomical study of the hazards and misleading radiological appearances. J Bone Joint Surg 1976; 58B:164–168.
63. Macnicol MF, Lo HK, Yong KF. Pelvic remodeling after the Chiari osteotomy: a long-term review. J Bone Joint Surg [Br] 2004; 86-B:648–54.
64. Högh J, Macnicol MF. The Chiari pelvic osteotomy. A long-term review of clinical and radiographic results. J Bone Joint Surg 1987; 69B:365–373.
65. Windhager R, Pongracz N, Schonecker W, Kotz R. Chiari osteotomy for congenital dislocation and subluxation of the hip. Results after 20 to 34 years follow-up. J Bone Joint Surg Br 1991; 73(6):890–5.
66. Colonna PC. Capsular arthroplasty for congenital dislocation of the hip: indications and technique. J Bone Joint Surg 1965; 47A:437.
67. Pozo JL, Cannon SR, Catterall A. The Colonna-Hey Groves arthroplasty in the late treatment of the hip. A Long-Term Rev 1987 Mar; 69(2):220–228.
68. Macnicol MF, Makris D. Distal transfer of the greater trochanter. J Bone Joint Surg 1991; 73B:838–841.
69. El-Mowafi H. Outcome of pelvic support osteotomy with the Ilizarov method in the treatment of the unstable hip joint. Acta Orthop Belg 2005; 71:686–691.
70. Wedge JH, Wasylenko MJ. The natural history of congenital disease of the hip. J Bone Joint Surg 1979; 61-B:334–338.
71. Malvitz TA, Weinstein SL. Closed reduction for congenital dysplasia of the hip. Functional and radiographic results after an average of 30 years. J Bone Joint Surg 1994; 76A:1777–1792.
72. Morcuende JA, Meyer MD, Dolan LA, Weinstein SL. Long-term outcome after open reduction through an anteromedial approach for congenital dislocation of the hip. J Bone Joint Surg 1997; 79A:810–817.
73. Angliss R, Fujii G, Pickvance E, et al. Surgical treatment of late developmental displacement of the hips: results after 33 years. J Bone Joint Surg 2005; 87-B:384–394.
74. Thomas S, Wedge J, Salter RB. Outcome at 45 years after open reduction and innominate osteotomy for late-presenting developmental dislocation of the hip. J Bone Joint Surg Am 2007; 89:2341–2350.

Chapter 6

Legg–Calvé–Perthes Disease

Andrew M. Wainwright and Anthony Catterall

Introduction

Legg–Calvé–Perthes disease is caused by infarction of the upper femoral epiphysis complicated by trabecular fracture and associated with a process of repair (Fig. 6.1) [1]. The infarct may be variable in extent and the disorder also varies in its outcome: at best the effects may be limited to a childhood limp which can resolve spontaneously. At worst, if the femoral head segmental collapses and subsequent deformity fails to remodel well, it may lead to shortening, stiffness, and premature hip arthritis.

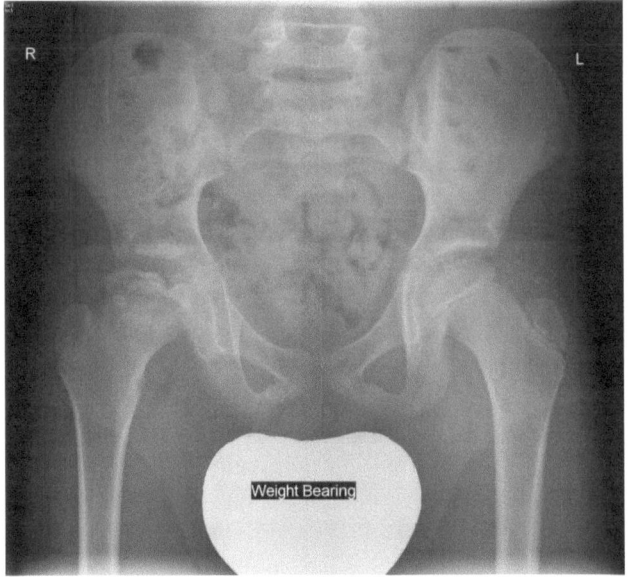

Fig. 6.1 AP view of a hip with Legg–Calvé–Perthes disease on the right side in an eight year old boy

Its Name

The condition has been known variously as coxa plana, osteochondritis deformans juvenilis, Perthes disease, Legg–Perthes disease, and Legg–Calvé–Perthes disease, to which Waldenström's name is sometimes added.

The first description of the condition is generally credited in 1909 to Henning Waldenström [2], Professor of Orthopaedics in Stockholm. He considered it to be a benign form of tuberculosis (then a common cause of hip problems). In fact, the earliest description was published in 1897 by a Czech surgeon Karel Maydl [3], Professor of Surgery in Prague [4].

The term most often used, Legg–Calvé–Perthes disease, is named after the three clinicians who independently recognized that this was a separate problem from tuberculosis of the hip in 1910:

- Arthur Legg [5] (at that time, a junior orthopaedic surgeon at Harvard Medical School, Boston)
- Jacques Calvé [6] (Director of the Institute Calvé, Berck-Plage, France)
- Georg Perthes [7] (Head of Surgery in Tübingen, Germany)

Any condition known by an eponym is intriguing and implies that the condition is not fully understood. Despite several hundred research papers, many of which are contradictory, the underlying etiology remains unknown, the course of the disease difficult to predict, and the best method of treatment not determined.

For brevity in this chapter the condition will be referred to as Perthes disease.

Epidemiology

The incidence of newly diagnosed cases is around 1 in 10,000 children per year [8, 9]. The clinical onset is usually between 4 and 7 years and rarely outside the range of 2–13 years. The

A.M. Wainwright (✉)
Nuffield Orthopaedic Centre, Oxford, UK

condition affects boys much more often than girls with a 4:1 ratio [1, 9, 10]. The condition is bilateral in 15% of patients and the disease then runs a more severe course [9, 11].

There is variation between population groups worldwide. There is a marked increased risk in white children compared with black children (10.8 compared to 0.45 per 100,000, respectively in South Africa) [12]. There is also variation regionally within counties; in the UK, the annual incidence is 5.5/100,000 in Wessex and 11.1/100,000 in Liverpool [8]. It is a condition that seems to be associated with social deprivation [9, 10].

There is no evidence that the majority of children with Perthes disease have had a preceding irritable hip. Of the few children with recurrent irritable hip only those with over 2 years delay in bone growth were found to have Perthes disease [13].

Etiology

The cause of the condition is unknown, although there are several theories about its etiology. It is generally agreed that "in a susceptible child the changes are the consequence of ischemia of variable duration, after which the process of repair produces a growth disturbance, which if uncontrolled leads to femoral head deformity with subsequent arthritis" [1].

Inherited Factors

There are some inherited conditions that are similar to Perthes disease, such as the multiple epiphyseal dysplasias. These inherited conditions which mimic Perthes disease need to be excluded when considering the evidence for inheritance in Perthes disease. Also it may be difficult to separate inherited from environmental factors in families. Despite this it is widely believed that there is no clear evidence for a strongly inherited component. This is based on studies of first-degree relatives, twin studies, and the difference in incidence between the sexes, when mimics of Perthes disease, such as the dysplasias, are excluded [14].

There are epidemiological studies that have analyzed the age of onset and associated anomalies [15, 16]. The distributions fit best with models of disease which suggest a single cause acting prenatally. This may be either genetic or environmental. When Perthes disease affects more than one family member this may be caused by environmental factors.

Thrombophilia Theory

It has been proposed that children with Perthes disease may have an underlying coagulation defect which leads to vascular thrombosis—i.e., they are thrombophilic. Reports have shown associations with hypercoagulable conditions such as protein C and protein S deficiency and resistance to activated protein C [17, 18]. Subsequent studies have failed to confirm these findings [19], although others have found a prolonged activated partial thromboplastin time [20–22]. It has been noted that children with Perthes disease with a homozygous Factor V Leiden mutation have more severe disease [23]. Other mutations have been found in the coagulation cascade [24]. The whole of this theory may support the concept of the "susceptible child."

Recurrent Infarction

Several authors have suggested that recurrent infarction is responsible for the disease, although the cause for recurrent infarction has not been established [1, 25]. Experimental work in animals [26, 27] has shown that tying a ligature around the femoral head can cause the pathological changes of ischemic necrosis but not all of those seen in Perthes disease. It is possible that the cause is a tamponade effect—this theory has been examined experimentally in dogs [28].

Growth Arrest Theory

There may be an underlying constitutional problem predisposing children to Perthes disease as it is known to be associated with delayed bone age [29]. The bone age of affected children often lags 2–3 years behind their chronological age. There are abnormalities of levels of growth factors including insulin-like growth factor binding protein 3 [30]. Other studies have shown decreased birth weight [14].

Many of these factors are also associated with social deprivation, such as small stature and delayed bone age [14, 15, 29], dietary deficiency [31], and passive smoking [32].

Course of the Disease

Waldenström described the chronological stages [33] of the disease (Table 6.1).

These stages have been modified based on the radiological appearances (the Elizabethtown classification) [34] and are now recognized as shown in Table 6.2.

Table 6.1 Waldenström's chronological stages

The evolutionary period is divided into two stages

a. *The initial stage*—the epiphysis is dense, with "decalcinated" spots, flattened, and uneven at its margins

b. *The fragmentation stage*—the epiphysis is extremely flattened and divided; it often starts with a few small pieces, progresses to many small granules, and appears atrophied

The healing period—the epiphysis becomes homogenous and there is evidence of recalcification

The growing period—normal growth and ossification of the deformed femoral head

The definite period—the permanent residual features

Table 6.2 The Elizabethtown classification

Stage I	Initial stage
Stage II	Fragmentation stage
Stage III	Healing phase
Stage IV	Definitive stage

Pathological Findings

Histologically, several changes follow sequential infarction of the femoral head [35]. A variable amount of the femoral capital epiphysis may be affected:

- *Synovial tissue* becomes inflamed and causes an effusion.
- *Articular cartilage* is mostly nourished from synovial fluid and continues to grow (even though the underlying bone has lost its source of nutrition). Cartilage becomes thicker on the medial femoral head and the acetabular floor. At its deep surface it may transform to fibrocartilage.
- *Growth plate* cartilage columns become distorted and do not undergo normal ossification. The changes occur maximally under the involved part of the epiphysis, leading to a growth disturbance and tilting of the femoral epiphysis on the neck. On the superior and lateral aspect of the femoral neck there is reactivation of the growth plate with thickened cartilage. This contributes to the formation of a coxa magna.
- *Epiphysis:* in the early phases, the trabeculae and subchondral bone plate become necrotic and fragmented due to crushing of the bony epiphysis. This starts from the anterior margin and proceeds posteriorly to a variable extent. This leads to a subchondral fracture. In the adjacent, unaffected areas of the epiphysis the appearances are normal, with some remodeling. Later in the reparative phase there is new bone deposition on the necrotic trabeculae (creeping substitution) and a callus-like cartilaginous tissue adjacent to the loose necrotic bone.

- *Metaphysis:* the central marrow contains adipose tissue; sclerotic-rimmed osteolytic lesions containing fibrocartilage occur. There is disorganized ossification and extension of the growth plate down into the metaphysis (giving the radiological appearance of metaphyseal "cysts").

In summary, two pathological processes result in the changes seen in established disease leading to a change in shape mainly in the anterior and lateral aspects of the femoral head: infarction in the epiphysis of a variable extent with trabecular fracture and a growth disturbance in cartilage and physis.

Clinical Features

Symptoms

Children present with pain in the hip or, more commonly, the knee [36]. Often the reason for orthopaedic referral is not that the child has symptoms, but that relatives or teachers have noticed a limp. In general the child feels well and has no previous medical history of joint problems.

Signs

As noted previously, the clinical onset is within a narrow age range, i.e., children of junior school age. Affected children may be of short stature and be hyperactive. The limbs may be disproportionately shorter than the trunk.

The first sign of Perthes disease is usually a limp. Waldenström reported that at first the limping may be so slight that it may not be noticeable to the eye, but heard when the child walks across the floor with shoes on [36]. In the later phases the child may develop a Trendelenburg gait because of femoral head deformity, lost abduction, trochanteric overgrowth, and/or abductor dysfunction.

Examination on the couch typically reveals fixed flexion, restricted movement, and variable leg length discrepancy. Depending upon the extent of the disease the following signs are evident:

- In *extension* there is limited abduction and internal rotation. If there is early or established femoral head deformity, the leg abducts and externally rotates as the hip flexes. An adduction contracture is a sign of severe disease with lateral impingement.

- In *flexion* there is usually no adduction or internal rotation and, with head deformity, it may not be possible to adduct to neutral.

Differential Diagnosis

Other conditions may mimic Perthes disease, affecting just one hip or both [37]:

- *Multiple epiphyseal dysplasias* must be excluded if the disease is bilateral—there are similar changes at the hip, but the changes are bilateral, symmetrical, and there may be other epiphyses involved.
- *Spondylo-epiphyseal dysplasias* produce an uninvolved but cup-shaped metaphysis. Clinical examination shows a short trunk and spinal radiographs confirm platyspondyly. Other epiphyses may be affected.
- *Hypothyroidism* leads to delayed epiphyseal maturity, a wide metaphysis and classic clinical signs.
- *Gaucher's disease* (a storage disorder) differs in that the femoral epiphysis fails to remodel and there is associated anemia, thrombocytopenia, and hepatosplenomegaly.
- *Infection*—Sub-acute septic arthritis or osteomyelitis of the femoral neck can mimic these changes; tuberculosis of the hip was the classic differential diagnosis and worldwide this condition remains prevalent.
- *Eosinophilic granuloma* often presents with a high erythrocyte sedimentation rate (ESR) and other lesions may be apparent on a skeletal survey.
- *Lymphoma* deposits in the femoral neck cause complete infarction and the change is progressive.
- *Femoral head osteonecrosis* can be associated with sickle cell disease, steroid treatment, leukemia, and immuno-suppression.
- *Hemophiliacs* may develop major femoral head infarction as a consequence of intra-articular bleeds. A positive family history and other signs of the bleeding disorder should clarify.
- *Mucopolysaccharidoses* often have delayed femoral head ossification and fragmentation.

These conditions can usually be differentiated from Perthes disease: ossification of the femoral capital epiphysis is usually delayed, the changes are often bilateral, synchronous, and symmetrical. In addition, the other systemic features of these conditions are apparent. *Bilateral Perthes disease affects each hip at a different time and with different severity.*

Radiographic Features

The radiographic features are best seen on an antero-posterior (AP) view of the pelvis and a frog lateral (Lauenstein view of the hip—i.e., in flexion, abduction, and external rotation). The changes seen depend upon the duration, stage, and severity of the disease. These changes form the basis for the classifications outlined below. One of the earliest signs is medial joint space widening. Some widening of the joint is often present in the opposite hip, compared with controls.

Classification of Severity Based on Radiographs

Radiographs yield information that allows objective assessment. For this reason there have been several classification systems that depend upon radiographic appearances alone. The classifications do offer reliable comparisons for investigators comparing the results of different treatment.

There is probably an overemphasis on radiographic findings, as these do not necessarily help to determine treatment for a particular child; this should be based more upon clinical findings.

Three systems are widely used to classify the radiological severity of Perthes disease. Each is named after its originator.

Catterall Classification

Catterall classification [37] is based on good quality AP and lateral radiographs (Fig. 6.2, Tables 6.3 and 6.4). The four groups are based on increasing proportions of femoral head involvement:

- *Group 1*—only the anterior part of the epiphysis is involved on the lateral view. No collapse of the femoral head is seen and complete absorption of the involved segment is seen without sequestrum formation. This is followed by regeneration. The AP view may show a cystic epiphysis, but there is no loss of height and metaphyseal changes are unusual.
- *Group 2*—more of the anterior epiphysis is involved and this may collapse, leaving a dense sequestrum. On the AP view a dense oval mass may be visible with viable fragments medially and laterally which maintain height. On the lateral view, a V, characteristic of this group, may separate the sequestrum posteriorly from the viable fragments.

Fig. 6.2 The Catterall classification groups I–IV, which are classified according to radiographic features of the epiphysis and metaphysis

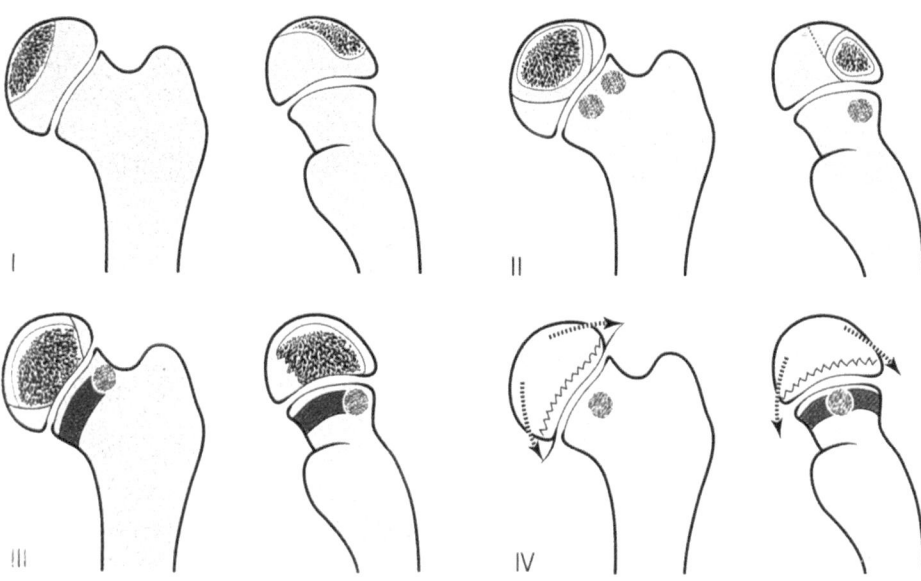

Table 6.3 Epiphyseal signs

Radiological signs	Group			
	I	II	III	IV
Sclerosis	No	Yes	Yes	Yes
Subchondral fracture line	No	Anterior half	Posterior half	Complete
Junction involved	Clear	Clear	Sclerotic	No
Uninvolved segments		Often "V"		
Viable bone at growth	Anterior margin	Anterior half	Posterior half	None
Triangular appearance to medial/lateral aspects	No	No	Occasional	Yes

Table 6.4 Metaphyseal signs

Radiological signs	Group			
	I	II	III	IV
Localized	No	Anterior	Anterior	Anterior or central
Diffuse	No	Yes	Yes	Yes
Posterior remodeling	No	No	No	Yes

- *Group 3*—only a small part of the epiphysis does not sequestrate. The AP view shows the appearance of a "head within a head," with later collapse of the central sequestrum and very small normal segments medially and laterally. The lateral segment is often small and osteoporotic and this becomes laterally displaced with collapse, producing a broadened neck. Metaphyseal changes are more generalized and associated with a broad femoral neck.
- *Group 4*—the whole epiphysis is sequestrated and total collapse of the epiphysis produces a dense line on the AP view. Early loss of height between the physis and the acetabular roof indicates flattening of the head. The epiphysis can "mushroom" anteriorly and laterally and metaphyseal changes can be extensive

Salter and Thompson Classification

Salter and Thompson described a simple two-group classification [38] based on the width of the subchondral fracture (Figs. 6.3 and 6.4), which reflects the extent of femoral head involvement:

- Group A (less than half of the head),
- Group B (more than half of the head)

The authors state that it may be applied early in the disease when the subchondral fracture is detectable. Unfortunately, the subchondral fracture line is seen radiologically in fewer than 50% of affected children.

Herring Classification

Herring et al. described a classification system [39] based upon the extent of involvement of the "lateral pillar" of the femoral head (Fig. 6.5). In the original report the lateral pillar is described as the area in the lateral 15–30% of the femoral head on a true AP film. Subsequently they have

Fig. 6.3 The Salter–Thompson classification

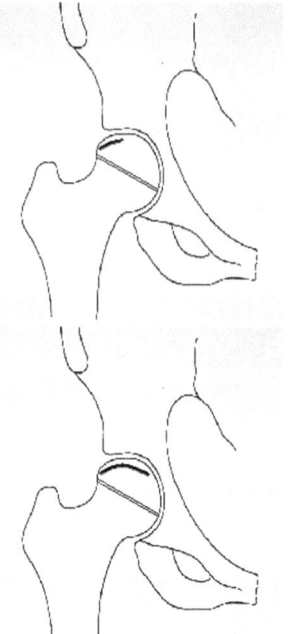

Fig. 6.5 The Herring lateral pillar classification

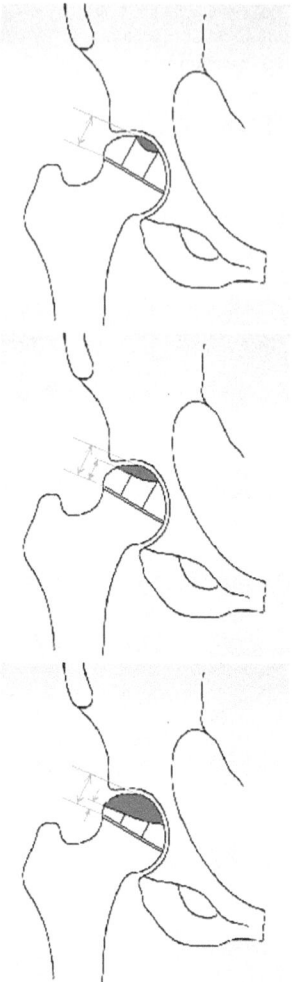

reported that the lateral pillar may be between 5–30% of the femoral head [40] so this makes the classification difficult to apply accurately.

This pillar height is compared with the unaffected hip, ignoring the amount of collapse of the central and medial pillars:

- Group A (no involvement of the lateral pillar)
- Group B (>50% of the lateral pillar height maintained)
- Group C (<50% of the lateral pillar height maintained)

A fourth group, the B/C border, has been added to this classification system by the originators. They noted that it may be difficult to differentiate between Groups B and C [40], hence the addition of this fourth, intermediate group.

Other Systems

Two more recent classification systems have been described since the description of these established systems.

Sugimoto's system assesses combined lateral and posterior pillar involvement [41]. This appears to offer a reasonable association with the amount of deformity at maturity, but needs to be confirmed by others.

Fig. 6.4 Radiographs of a subchondral fracture

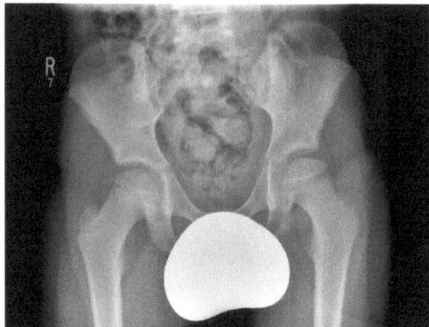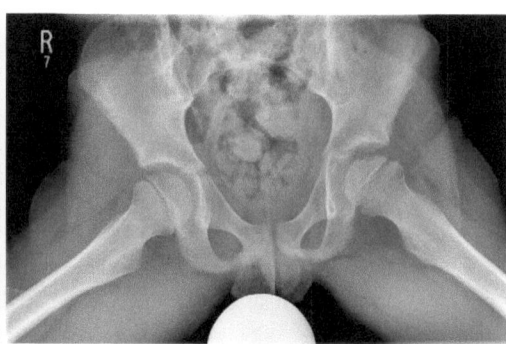

The deformity index, based upon an AP radiographic view only, has been recommended as a simple predictor of eventual radiological outcome (Fig. 6.6) [42]. While this appears to be reliable and valid in the hands of its users, only further application will determine its value. Unlike its predecessors [43, 44], it does not take into account the unseen cartilaginous part of the head seen on an arthrogram, nor does it assess different projections of the deforming femoral head. Loss of sphericity, best demonstrated arthrographically, improves prognostication by helping to differentiate between Herring Groups B and C [44].

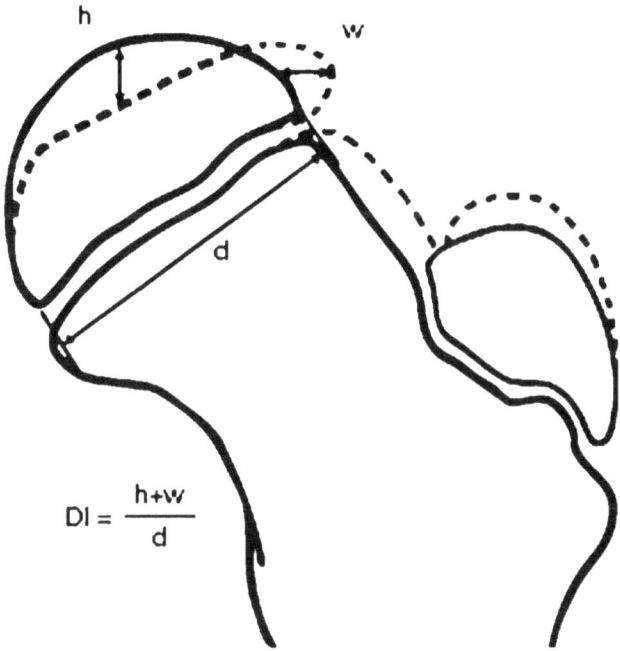

Fig. 6.6 The deformity index. Reproduced with permission and copyright © of the British Editorial Society of Bone and Joint Surgery [42]

Other Investigations and Their Value

Ultrasound scans can be useful to investigate children with hip pain, as they are safe, inexpensive, and reproducible. When combined with aspiration they help to differentiate Perthes disease from the irritable hip and septic arthritis. Capsular distension that persists for more than 6 weeks suggests Perthes disease rather than hip irritability [45]. Other diagnostic markers shown to be useful in making the diagnosis are articular cartilage thickening and quadriceps atrophy [46].

Radioisotope bone scans have a higher sensitivity and specificity than radiographs and show the onset of revascularization earlier [47]. They have been used to classify three patterns of disease [48] based on the fact that bone revascularization can occur by the recanalization of existing vessels or by neovascularization. Recanalization occurs rapidly (minutes to weeks), whereas neovascularization is prolonged (months to years). Conway reported [48] that these processes can be differentiated by scintigraphy and proposed three "tracks" that may be followed:

A. "All right track" scintigraphic pattern represents the recanalization process, a process of short duration and good prognosis.
B. "Bad track" scintigraphic pattern represents the process of neovascularization, a process of long duration and poorer prognosis.
C. "Complications" of the healing process (collapse, extrusion), particularly during the resorptive phases of bone reconstitution when the bone is weakened, can cause conversion from track A to track B.

These early tracks appear to correlate well with the radiographic-based classifications that cannot be applied until later [49]; 96% of Conway A hips later showed appearances of Herring A or B (the majority were Catterall type 2), and 82.8% of Conway B hips later showed signs of Herring C (the majority were Catterall type 3 or 4). If more severe (Herring C, Catterall 4) disease can be detected earlier with certainty, then earlier treatment may give better results in this difficult group [50].

Magnetic resonance imaging (MRI) with gadolinium enhancement has revealed Perthes disease changes in younger children which may predate the radiographic changes by up to 3 months [51]. Although MRI can give earlier information on the extent and location of involvement and healing, there is little evidence that it produces information that would alter management [52, 53]. Arthrography is as good as, or better than, MRI in determining the shape of the articular surface and lateral subluxation.

Prognosis at Maturity

There is an association between radiographic features at maturity and subsequent progression to osteoarthritis. Using concentric circular templates (Mose rings), a measure of sphericity is gauged from an AP and lateral view taken at maturity. More than 2 mm deviation between these views indicates lost sphericity and adversely affects outcome [54, 55].

Stulberg et al. assessed the sphericity and congruency of the hip at maturity [56]. From a longitudinal study over three to four decades, the prognosis for arthritis was shown to be related to the congruency between the femoral head

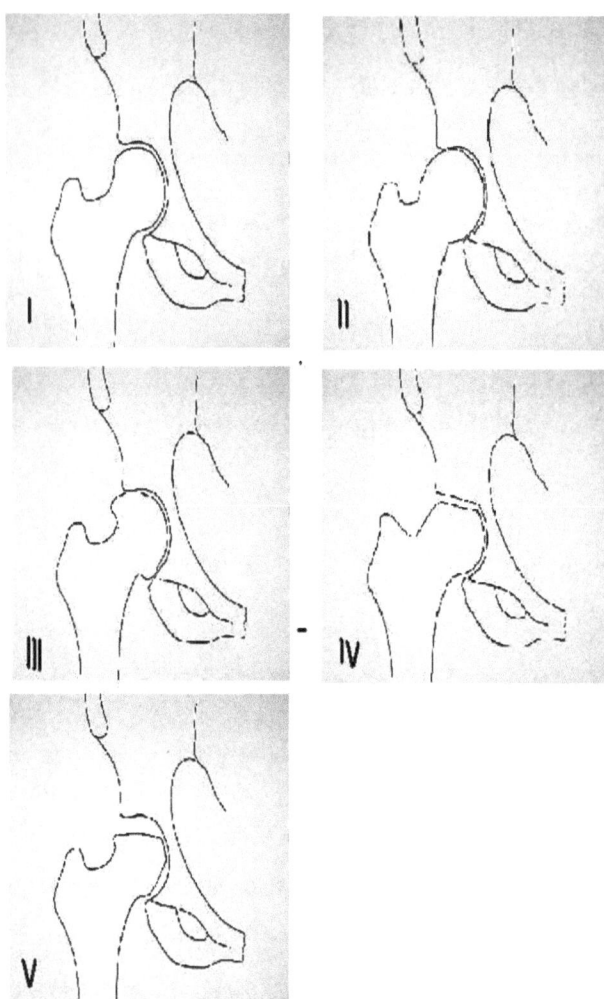

Fig. 6.7 The Stulberg classification

This system at maturity is often used as a surrogate for long-term prognosis. In the original series, the rate of arthritis at final follow-up (of an average 40 years) was 0, 16, 58, 75, and 78% for each grade (I–V), respectively. The Stulberg classes are often grouped into three types of congruency and sphericity:

1. *Spherical congruency* (class I and II hips)—in hips in this category early arthritis does not develop;
2. *Aspherical congruency* (class III hips)—mild to moderate arthritis develops in late adulthood; and
3. *Aspherical incongruency* (class IV and V hips)—severe arthritis develops before the age of 50 years in these hips

Prognosis and the "Head at Risk"

One of the challenges in Perthes disease is to determine the prognosis for an individual. A proportion of involved hips do well with no intervention but there is a group of children which does poorly with progressive deterioration in femoral head shape. Ideally the prognosis should be made early enough in the disease process to allow an intervention which will modify the natural history.

The most widely accepted prognostic factor is the patient's age at onset. This may reflect the time available for remodeling. There is a better chance of recovery when the onset is before the age of 6 years, and worse after the age of 8. This is not true for every case; although 80% of children with Perthes disease before the age of 6 have a good prognosis, half of those under 6 years with a Herring type B/C or C hip do poorly [59]. However, the older child has a higher ratio of epiphyseal bone to cartilage and consequently a greater potential for collapse of the bony epiphysis.

Girls appear to have a poorer prognosis than boys, possibly because girls reach skeletal maturity at an earlier age with less time for remodeling and also have a higher amount of head involvement (Catterall type 3 or 4).

Catterall described several clinical and radiological "head at risk" signs [60] which define factors contributing to a worse outcome (Table 6.6). Gage originally described a curved rather than straight lateral metaphysis [61] and Schlesinger has suggested that the V-shaped lytic appearance be called Catterall's sign [62].

The advantage of combining clinical with radiological assessment and looking for poor prognostic signs is that it helps to manage the individual child. A child can be managed conservatively if a good range of movement is maintained and radiographs do not show two or more of the radiological "at risk" signs. This is particularly the case in the younger child. Conversely when movement is lost early and

and acetabulum [57]. Five classes of deformity are described (Fig. 6.7 and Table 6.5).

There is considerable interobserver variability using this system. This is because some of the criteria are not clearly defined (e.g., a "flat head," and a "steep acetabulum") [58].

Table 6.5 Stulberg's classes of deformity

Class I Completely normal hip joint

Class II Spherical femoral head but with one or more of the following characteristics:
 • A larger than normal (although spherical) femoral head (coxa magna)
 • Shorter than normal femoral neck (coxa brevis)
 • Abnormally steep acetabulum

Class III Non-spherical (ovoid or mushroom shaped or umbrella shaped), but not flat, femoral head (Class II characteristics are also present)

Class IV Flat femoral head and abnormalities of the femoral head, neck, or acetabulum

Class V Flat femoral head and a normal femoral neck and acetabulum

Table 6.6 Catterall's "head at risk" signs

Clinical signs
1 An obese child
2 A decreasing range of movement
3 Adduction contracture in extension
4 Flexion with abduction

Radiological signs
1 Calcification lateral to the epiphysis
2 Diffuse metaphyseal reaction
3 Femoral head lateral subluxation
4 A horizontal growth plate
5 Gage (Catterall) sign

the sign of "flexion with abduction" appears, femoral deformity is occurring and the child may need definitive treatment. This is irrespective of age and the extent of radiological involvement.

It is generally agreed that the four major factors which determine a poor prognosis are

- greater age of the patient at onset,
- greater extent of involvement of the femoral head,
- loss of containment of the femoral head in the acetabulum in the weight-bearing position, and
- loss of motion of the hip.

Treatment Options

Several treatment options have been proposed. A large pan-European study of treatment indications in Perthes disease [63] showed that the indications varied widely between surgeons and appeared to be based more upon personal experience than on scientific data. The different potential forms of treatment are outlined below, followed by a suggested approach to management for a child who presents with Perthes disease.

Conservative Treatment

Bed Rest

Historically, treatment was aimed at preventing weight bearing until the femoral head had re-ossified. This included prolonged strict bed rest, sometimes with months in hospital (Fig. 6.8), often with the use of traction on a frame or in a spica cast. A 17-year review of this treatment in Cardiff showed that this can give good results: 88% children had a good result and only 2% a poor result [64]. Significant problems with these regimens were muscle atrophy, osteoporosis,

leg shortening, lost thoracic kyphosis, urinary calculi, social, academic, and emotional problems, and hospital costs.

Physiotherapy

Physiotherapy helps to relieve muscle spasm and regain abduction. Most children can avoid excessive physical activity, limit weight bearing with crutches, and take non-steroid anti-inflammatory drugs if their pain increases. Wherever possible the treatment should encourage children to retain hip flexibility by range of motion exercises, avoid schooling interruption, maintain social integration with their friends but minimize excessive stress through the weakened bone.

Pharmacological Treatment

It has been suggested that femoral head collapse may be reduced by medication such as bisphosphonates in the early stages of the disease. There are studies in animal models of femoral head ischemia which indicate that the use of bisphosphonates improves head sphericity [65, 66]. It will be interesting to see whether children benefit similarly in the medium to long term. Any side effects from the medication will need to be monitored closely.

Containment Treatment

Most methods of interventional treatment are based on the concept of "containment." The concept of containment assumes that the acetabulum will contain and mould the softened femoral head and result in a spherical, congruous joint, and avoid degenerative arthritis. Although containment is not clearly defined, over 80% coverage is commonly accepted to prevent extrusion of the femoral head and lateral compression. It is important that this is done at an early stage in the disease.

If containment treatment is needed, the three methods of containment that have been widely used are the weight-bearing orthosis, femoral osteotomy, and/or acetabular osteotomy.

Weight-Bearing Abduction Braces

Petrie devised an abduction brace which allowed the child to be out of hospital but caused stiff knees, very awkward ambulation, and a cumbersome cast. Devices such as the Atlanta Scottish Rite brace were designed to keep the hips abducted, while permitting mobility at the hip. Arthrography was often

Fig. 6.8 Historical treatment with bed rest

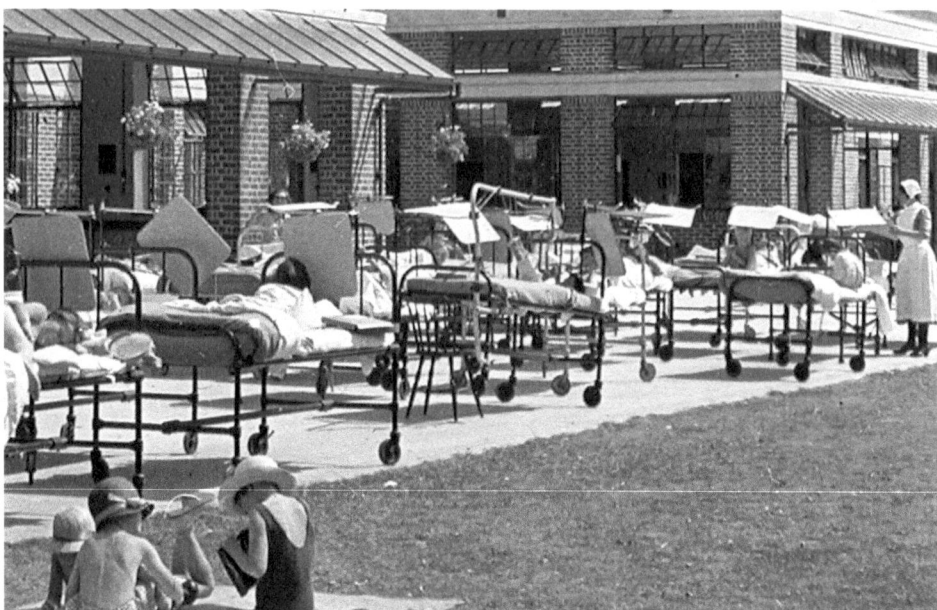

used prior to bracing to assess congruency in different positions to determine the "best-fit" position for containment, with good congruency and the avoidance of hinge abduction. Serial radiographs and clinical assessment of the range of movement were used to guide when weaning from the brace should begin. Some clinicians kept children in a brace until the lateral column re-ossified and sclerotic areas in the epiphysis had resolved.

There are problems with these abduction devices: pain and spasm may result in wide abduction of the *normal* hip and little or no abduction of the abnormal hip; then containment is not achieved. Hinge abduction may occur if the supero-lateral portion of a deformed femoral head impinges on the lateral acetabulum. This impingement damages the acetabular margin which loses its horizontal plane and slopes upward. This further increases the tendency for subluxation. In the older child bracing is difficult due to compliance and psychosocial issues. This form of treatment is not widely used in Europe [63], and in the United States several authors now advise against bracing for severely involved hips [67]. This was confirmed in the long-term follow-up by the Herring Group [68].

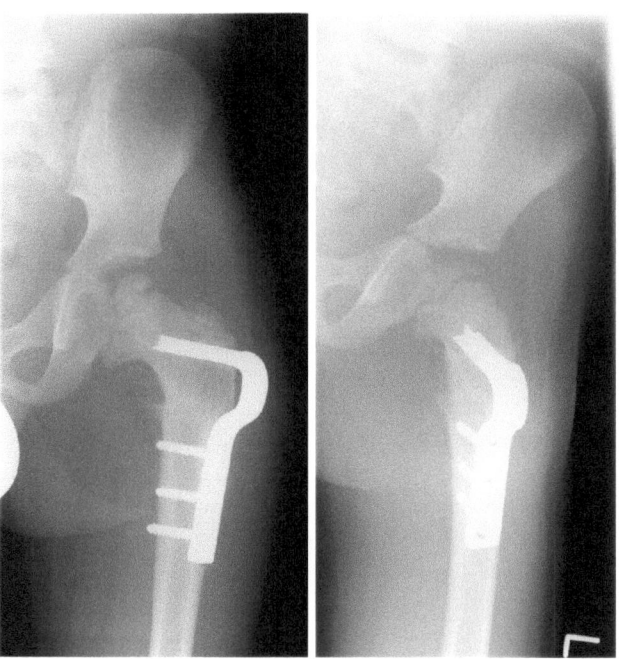

Fig. 6.9 Varus femoral osteotomy

Femoral Varus Osteotomy

Varus osteotomy of the proximal femur (Fig. 6.9) aims to center the femoral head more deeply within the acetabulum and allow weight bearing with the limb in a normal position without the encumbrance of an abduction brace. The goal is to cover the entire ossified femoral epiphysis of a "head at risk" with the ossified acetabulum [69, 70].

The prerequisites for varus derotation osteotomy include a good range of motion, hip congruency, and the ability to contain the femoral head in the acetabulum in abduction (assessed with an arthrogram). The procedure must be performed early in the initial or fragmentation stage of the disease. Many studies report good results with this operation [70–72] and it allows correction of the flexion deformity and rotational profile.

In the older child if the neck–shaft angle postoperatively is less than 115° the varus may not correct with subsequent remodeling. The greater trochanter should be kept distal to the level of the femoral head to prevent an abductor lurch. Sometime this requires distal transfer of the greater trochanter at the same operation or at a later time. Other procedures may later be required to manage limb shortening (of an already short limb), reverse the varus if it persists or remove plates and screws.

Acetabular Osteotomy

Salter described his innominate osteotomy for the subluxated hip (Fig. 6.10). He recommended that the osteotomy should be performed only in hips with a full (or almost full) range of movement, and a round (or almost round) femoral head with reasonable congruency in abduction. The child should be over 6 years old, more than 50% of the femoral head should be affected (Salter–Thompson group B) and the hip be seen to subluxate in the weight-bearing position.

Salter's osteotomy is reported to give good results, particularly in the older child with whole-head involvement [34, 73]. Potentially, it avoids further limb shortening and abductor weakness and leaves a more cosmetic scar.

The innominate osteotomy in isolation may not provide sufficient head cover or stability, particularly in the older child. Sometimes the procedure is performed in combination with a femoral osteotomy [74, 75]. This may be useful to contain a large, deformed femoral head, avoid an extreme varus neck–shaft angle, maintain leg length equality, and decrease intra-articular pressure. In the older child a triple pelvic osteotomy may be needed to rotate the acetabulum sufficiently to offer adequate head cover.

Valgus, Extension Femoral Osteotomy

This operation may be an effective salvage procedure in late-presenting cases where decreasing abduction is associated with femoral head overgrowth and mushroom deformity. When an arthrogram demonstrates femoral head deformity with unstable movement and hinge abduction in neutral but better stability in adduction and flexion, a valgus, extension upper femoral osteotomy will improve stability as the child stands and walks. It will also improve leg length and provide a more normal abductor lever arm. The rotational and sagittal correction can improve symptoms, function, and remodeling of the hip in patients with Perthes disease [76, 77] (Fig. 6.11). Care must be taken to lateralize the femoral shaft as the osteotomy is closed. Failure to do this can lead to proximal femoral deformity making potential arthroplasty more difficult. The procedure should not be undertaken before reconstitution of the femoral head nears completion.

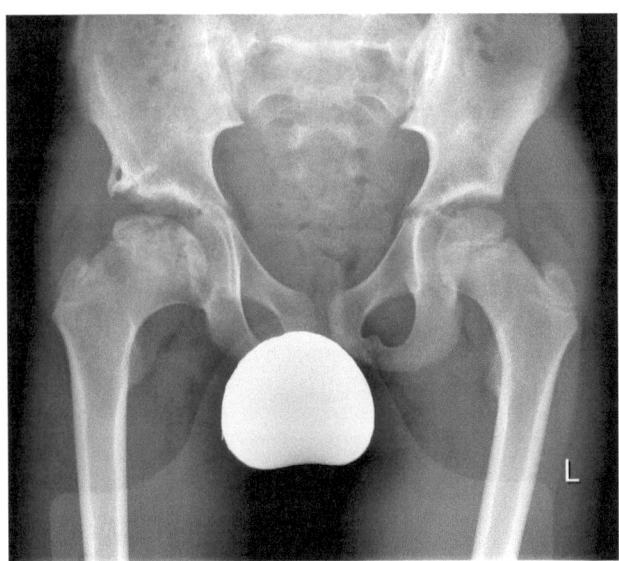

Fig. 6.11 Radiograph of shelf osteotomy

Shelf Procedures

Lateral shelf arthroplasty (Fig. 6.11) or the Chiari osteotomy may add cover to the femoral head although both rely upon capsular conversion to fibrocartilage for this improvement. The shelf arthroplasty [78, 79] is the ideal procedure for the child presenting over the age of 8 years. It increases coverage and stability of the femoral head while decreasing subluxation. If hip stability is achieved, the

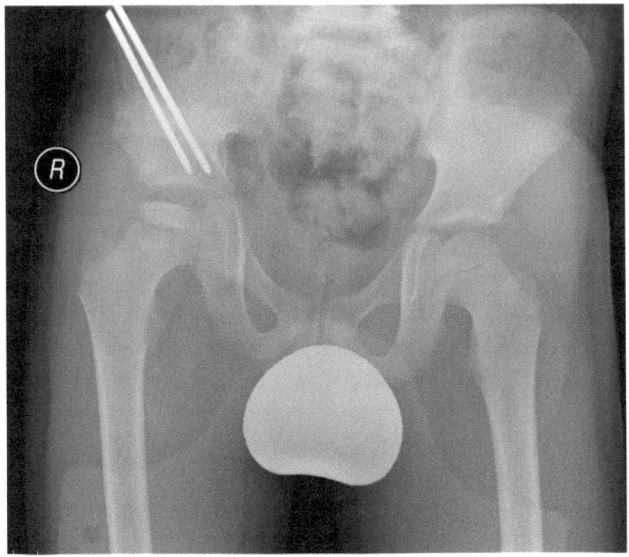

Fig. 6.10 Radiograph of Salter innominate osteotomy

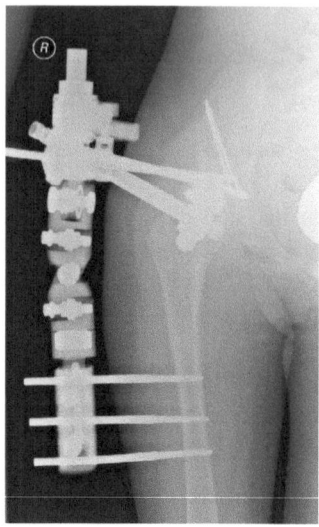

Fig. 6.12 Radiograph of distraction with external fixator

longevity of the hip improves [80]. Lateral support is helpful when there is inadequate acetabular coverage or when hinge abduction is developing. It was found to be less effective for children over the age of 11 years, especially girls [78], but offers pain relief and the maintenance of a stable, congruent hip [81]. Some suggest that shelf arthroplasty may help in the late fragmentation stage when hinging is more marked, improving moulding of the deformed femoral head.

Hip Distraction

Arthrodiastasis, distraction of the joint (Fig. 6.13), has been proposed as early treatment in the disease, before any significant collapse of the femoral head had occurred. The aim

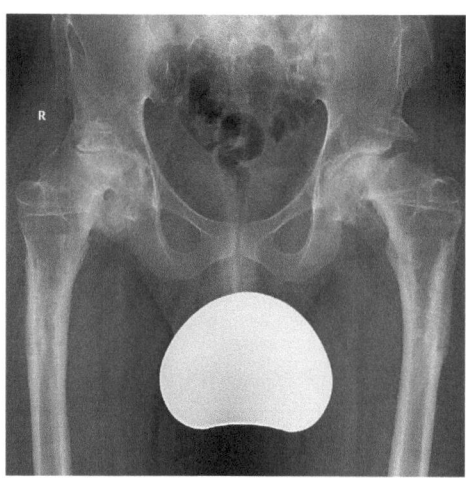

Fig. 6.13 Radiograph of a twenty year old man. He had been diagnosed with bilateral Perthes disease at age ten and had a corrective ostcotomy on both sides. Since this he experienced a reduced ROM and painful hips

is to halt further fragmentation and collapse [82]. Typically, this requires 4 months in an articulated fixator. Although the early results seemed promising, the longer term benefits have not been demonstrated (Fig. 6.12).

Other Procedures

After reossification of the femoral head there is a potential for late remodeling of the hip joint. There are circumstances when intervention is required to salvage a deformed head that is causing incongruity.

Cheilectomy

If there is femoro-acetabular impingement, excision of the extruded part of femoral head (cheilectomy) has been attempted. Ganz has shown that the hip may be dislocated with only small risk of avascular necrosis provided great care is taken to protect the posterior vessels [83, 84]. This may allow better re-shaping of the head and improve on the previously reported results of cheilectomy which often caused stiffness and pain and yielded poor long-term outcomes [85].

Arthrodesis

Surgical fusion of the hip may be indicated in young men at maturity with unilateral disease, severe functional impairment, and hip deformity.

Arthroplasty

This may be necessary after skeletal maturity if there is severe deformity and arthritis. Surface replacement may be possible and gives results equivalent to conventional replacement in Perthes disease [86].

Published Results of Treatment Regimens

It is difficult to compare previous studies. Most research has been published as case series and there are many conflicting findings following the same treatment modality. The age at onset, the stage and severity of the disease, the treatment regimens, the length of follow-up, and the outcome measures yield too many variables for easy analysis. Furthermore our measures of sphericity and head shape lack inter-observer precision. Finally, there is a long lag period of three or four decades between the onset of the disease and its degenerative effects on the hip.

There has been one proposal for a Cochrane systematic review to be published; however, the results of this review are not yet available [87].

The large prospective, multicenter study published from the Legg–Calvé Perthes Study Group in North America [68] compared the results of various interventions as determined by the treating surgeon in each center. In essence their findings by Herring type is summarized as

- *Group A hips* have an excellent prognosis and require no specific treatment.
- *Group B hips* in children whose disease started before 8 years of age have a good prognosis and require only symptomatic treatment.
- *Group B/C border hip* in children with Perthes disease starting before 8 years of age have a poorer prognosis but do not appear to benefit from surgical treatment.
- *Group B and B/C border hips* in children with Perthes disease starting after 8 years (or bone age over 6 years) have a significantly better outcome if treated with an innominate or a varus femoral osteotomy.
- *Group C hips* have an unfavorable prognosis in children regardless of age or surgical treatment (Fig. 6.13).

The other large prospective review with medium-term follow-up yielded similar findings [88]. In this series, although the lateral pillar classification was related to outcome, the strongest predictor of outcome was the percentage of femoral head involvement and age at diagnosis. The recommendation from this study was that a child aged 6 and over, with more than 50% femoral head involvement (Catterall groups 3 and 4) had a better outcome if treated with a femoral varus osteotomy.

Suggested Management of a Child with Perthes Disease

Many treatment protocols rely upon the radiographic appearances, despite the difficulties in applying classification systems early in the disease process. Although radiographs provide information that is measurable, they are not so helpful in making treatment decisions.

After making the diagnosis, management depends upon the clinical findings and the child's age at disease onset. The clinical examination gives the best assessment of the deformity of the femoral head. If there are clinical signs of deformity, the containment and congruity of the femoral head in the acetabulum in the weight-bearing position should be assessed further under anesthesia with an arthrogram.

Children who likely have a poor prognosis have clear clinical signs early in the disease, including

- poor ranges of movement
- decreased abduction in extension
- flexion into abduction
- fixed flexion deformity of over 20°
- inability to adduct or internally rotate the flexed hip to neutral
- leg length discrepancy

A suggested protocol for treatment follows based upon age and clinical findings. Under 6 years—the outlook is generally good:

- maintain range of movement, with physiotherapy and swimming
- restrict impact activities such as jumping during early phases
- crutches may be needed to help off-load the hip and relieve pain
- simple analgesia

The exception to a conservative approach is the child with whole-head involvement (Catterall group 4) when the prognosis can be improved by femoral or innominate osteotomy.

For children 6–8 years:

- as above
- monitor closely for clinical signs of a head at risk but, if clinical signs of head at risk are found, perform an examination under anesthesia and a dynamic arthrogram. This will demonstrate whether

1. the head is contained and stable. Plan monitoring and maintain hip motion and regular review for signs that would indicate the need for surgery (head at risk)
2. the head can be contained in abduction (+/–flexion). This is the indication for a femoral or pelvic osteotomy
3. the head cannot be contained but is uncovered and hinges. A lateral shelf acetabuloplasty will give support

Over 8 years as the prognosis is poorer an early examination under anesthesia and arthrogram to ascertain that

- the head is contained and stable (unusual). Any further loss of movement is an indication for definitive treatment
- the head can be contained in abduction. This is the best indication for a pelvic osteotomy or possibly a shelf procedure, before there is loss of epiphyseal height and deformity

- the head cannot be contained but is uncovered and has unstable movement with hinging. In the fragmentation or early healing stages a shelf arthroplasty is appropriate

The child at any age with late femoral head deformity:

- If the child has a painful limp with shortening and an arthrogram which shows femoral head deformity, unstable movement, and hinge abduction but stability in adduction and flexion. A valgus, extension upper femoral osteotomy, will produce stable movement, improve leg length, and produce a more normal abductor lever arm

Summary

There is still much to be learned about Legg–Calvé–Perthes disease. If the cause can be determined, then prevention or disease limitation may be possible in the future. It is apparent that a group of children need only symptomatic treatment: these tend to be younger and have a good range of movement. There is another group in which the hip progresses to a symptomatic arthropathy at an early age. One of the challenges is to improve upon the natural history by surgical intervention as soon as the clinical signs are detected.

References

1. Catterall A. Legg-Calvé-Perthes Disease. Edinburgh: Churchill Livingstone; 1982.
2. Waldenström H. Der obere tuberkulöse Cullumherd. Zeitschrift für Orthopädische Chirurgie 1909; 24: 487–512.
3. Maydl K. Coxa vara und Arthritis deformans coxae. Wiener klinische Rundschau 1897; 11:153.
4. Enersen, OD. Legg-Calvé-Perthes disease. At: http://www.whonamedit.com/synd.cfm/908.html. Accessed 7 October 2008.
5. Legg AT. An obscure affection of the hip-joint. Boston Med Surg J 1910; 162: 202–204.
6. Calvé J. Sur une forme particulière de pseudo-coxalgie greffée sur des déformations caractéristiques de l'extrémité supérieure du fémur. Revue de chirurgie 1910; 42: 54–84.
7. Perthes G. Über Arthritis deformans juvenilis. Deutsche Zeitschrift für Chirurgie 1910; 107: 111–159.
8. Barker DJP, Dixon E, Taylor JF. Perthes disease of the hip in three regions of England. J Bone Joint Surg [Br] 1978; 60-B: 478–480.
9. Kealey WDC, Moore AJ, Cook S, Cosgrove AP. Deprivation, urbanisation and Perthes disease in Northern Ireland. J Bone Joint Surg 2000; 82B: 167–171.
10. Margetts BM, Perry CA, Taylor JF, Dangerfield PH. The incidence and distribution of Legg-Calve-Perthes disease in Liverpool, 1982–1995. Ach Dis Child 2001; 84: 351–354.
11. Van de Bogaert G, de Rosa E, Moens P, et al. Bilateral Legg-Calvé-Perthes disease: different from unilateral disease? J Paediatr Orthop 1999; part B 8: 165–168.
12. Purry NA. The incidence of Perthes disease in three population groups in the Eastern cape region of South Africa. J Bone Jt Surg [Br] 1982; 64-B:286–288.
13. Keenan WNW, Clegg J. Perthes disease after "irritable hip": delayed bone age shows the hip is a "marked man." J Pediatr Orthop 1996; 16: 20–23.
14. Wynne-Davies R, Gormley J. The etiology of Perthes disease: genetic, epidemiological and growth factors in 310 Edinburgh and Glasgow patients. J Bone Joint Surg [Br] 1978; 60-B: 6–14.
15. Hall AJ, Barker DJ, Dangerfield PH, et al. Small feet and Perthes disease: a survey in Liverpool. J Bone Joint Surg [Br] 1988; 70-B: 611–13.
16. Wiig O, Terjesen T, Svenningsen S, Lie SA. The epidemiology and etiology of Perthes disease in Norway. J Bone Joint Surg [Br] 2006; 88-B: 1217—1223.
17. Glueck CJ, Glueck HI, Greenfield D, et al. Protein C and S deficiency and hypofibrinolysis: pathophysiologic causes of Legg Perthes disease. Pediatr Res 1994; 35: 383–388.
18. Glueck CJ, Brandt G, Gruppo R, et al. Resistance to activated protein C and Legg-Perthes disease. Clin Orthop 1997; 338: 139–152.
19. Hayek S, Kenet G, Lubetsky A, et al. Does thrombophilia play an aetiological role in Legg-Calvé-Perthes disease? J Bone Joint Surg [Br] 1999; 81-B: 686—690.
20. Gallistl S, Reitinger T, Linhart W, Muntean W. The role of inherited thrombotic disorders in the etiology of Legg-Calvé-Perthes disease. J Paediatr Orthop 1999; 19: 82–83.
21. Sirvent N, Fisher F, El Hayek T, et al. Absence of congenital prethrombotic disorders in children with Legg-Perthes disease. J Pediatr Orthop 2000; part B 9: 24–27.
22. Thomas DP, Morgan G, Tayton K. Perthes disease and the relevance of thrombophilia. J Bone Joint Surg 1999; 81B: 691–695.
23. Kealey WDC, Mayne EE, McDonald W, et al. The role of coagulation abnormalities in the development of Perthes disease. J Bone Joint Surg [Br] 2000; 82B, 744–746.
24. Dilley A, Hooper WC, Austin H, et al. The beta fibrinogen gene G-455-A polymorphisms a risk factor for Legg-Perthes disease. J Thromb Haemost 2003; 1: 2317–2321.
25. McKibbin B, Ráliš Z. Pathological changes in a case of Perthes disease J Bone Joint Surg [Br] 1974; 56-B (3): 438.
26. Salter RB, Bell M. The pathogenesis of deformity in Legg- Perthes disease—an experimental investigation. J Bone Joint Surg 1968; 50B: 436.
27. Kim H, Su P-H. Development of flattening and apparent fragmentation following ischemic necrosis of the capital femoral epiphysis in a piglet model. J Bone Joint Surg [Am] 2002; 84(8): 1329–1334.
28. Kemp HB. Perthes disease: an experimental and clinical study. Ann R Coll Surg Engl 1973; 52(1): 18–35.
29. Burwell RG, Dangerfield PH, Hall DJ, et al. Perthes disease. An anthropometric study revealing impaired and disproportionate growth. J Bone Joint Surg [Br] 1978; 60B: 461–477.
30. Matsumoto T, Enomoto H, Takahashi K, et al. Decreased levels of IGF binding protein 3 in serum from children with Legg Calvé Perthes disease. Acta Orthop Scand 1998; 69: 125.
31. Hall AJ, Margetts BM, Barker DJ, et al. Low blood manganese levels in Liverpool children with Perthes disease. Paediatr Perinat Epidemiol 1989; 3: 131–135.
32. Mata SG, Aicua EA, Ovejero AH, Grande MM. Legg-Calvé-Perthes disease and passive smoking. J Pediatr Orthop 2000; 20: 326–330.
33. Waldenström H. The first stages of coxa plana. J Bone Joint Surg 1938; 20: 559–566.
34. Canale ST, D'Anca AF, Cottler JM, Snedden HE. Innominate osteotomy in Legg Calvé Perthes disease J Bone Joint Surg 1972; 54-A: 25–40.

35. Catterall A, Pringle J, Byers PD. A review of the morphology of Perthes disease. J Bone Joint Surg [Br] 1982; 64B: 269–275.
36. Waldenström H. The definite form of the coxa plana. Acta Radiol 1922; 1: 384–394.
37. Catterall A. The natural history of Perthes disease. J Bone Joint Surg [Br] 1971; 53B: 37–53.
38. Salter RB, Thompson GH. Legg-Calvé-Perthes disease. The prognostic significance of the subchondral fracture and a two-group classification of the femoral head involvement. J Bone Joint Surg 1984; 66A: 479–489.
39. Herring JA, Neustadt JB, Williams JJ, et al. The lateral pillar classification of Legg-Calvé-Perthes disease. J Pediatr Orthop 1992; 12: 143–150.
40. Herring JA, Kim HT, Browne R. Legg-Calvé-Perthes Disease. Part I: classification of radiographs with use of the modified lateral pillar and Stulberg classifications. J Bone Joint Surg 2004; 86-A: 10–12.
41. Sugimoto Y, Akazawa H, Miyake Y, et al. A new scoring system for Perthes disease based on combined lateral and posterior pillar classifications. J Bone Joint Surg [Br] 2004; 86-B: 887–891.
42. Nelson D, Zenios M, Ward K, et al. The deformity index as a predictor of final radiological outcome in Perthes disease J Bone Joint Surg [Br] 2007; 89-B: 1369–1373.
43. Shigeno Y, Evans G. Revised arthrographic index of deformity for Perthes disease. J Ped Orthop 1996; 5: 44–47.
44. Ismail M, Macnicol MF. Prognosis in Perthes disease: a comparison of radiographic predictors. J Bone Joint Surg [Br] 1998; 88-B: 310–314.
45. Eggl H, Drekonja T, Kaiser B, Dorn U. Ultrasonography in the diagnosis of transient synovitis of the hip and Legg-Calvé-Perthes disease. J Pediatr Orthop 1999; part B 8: 177–180.
46. Robben SGF, Meradji M, Diepstraten AFM, Hop WCJ. US of the painful hip in childhood: The diagnostic value of cartilage thickening and muscle atrophy in the detection of Perthes disease. Radiol 1998; 208: 35–42.
47. Sutherland AD, Savage JP, Paterson DC, Foster BK. The nuclide bone-scan in the diagnosis and management of Perthes disease. J Bone Joint Surg [Br] 1980; 62B: 300–306.
48. Conway JJ. Scintigraphic classification of Legg-Calvé-Perthes disease. Semin Nucl Med 1993; 23(4): 274–295.
49. Van Campenhout A, Moens P, Fabry G. Serial bone scintigraphy in Legg-Calvé-Perthes disease: correlation with the Catterall and Herring classification. J Pediatr Orthop B 2006; 15(1): 6–10.
50. Diméglio A, Canavase F, Ali M, Kelly P. Surgical treatment of Legg-Calvé-Perthes disease; improved results for severe forms Catterall IV/Herring C. J Child Orthop 2008; 2 (Suppl 1): S27#.
51. Gent E, Antapur P, Fairhurst J, et al. Perthes disease in the very young child. J Pediatr Orthop B 2006; 15:16–22.
52. Kaniklides C, Lönnerholm T, Moberg A, et al. Legg-Calvé-Perthes disease. Comparison of conventional radiography, MR imaging, bone scintigraphy and arthrography. Acta Radiol 1995; 36: 434–439.
53. Jaramillo D, Galen TA, Winalski CS, et al. Legg-Calvé-Perthes disease. MR imaging evaluation during manual positioning of the hip—comparison with conventional arthrography. Radiol 1999; 212: 519–525.
54. Mose K. Methods of measuring in Legg-Calvé-Perthes disease with special regard to the prognosis. Clin Orthop Relat Res. 1980; 150: 103–109.
55. Mose K, Hjorth L, Ulfeldt M, et al. Legg Calvé Perthes disease. The late occurrence of coxarthrosis. Acta Orthop Scand Suppl 1977; 169: 1–39.
56. Stulberg SD, Salter RB. The natural course of Legg-Perthes disease and its relationship to degenerative arthritis of the hip. A long-term follow-up study. Orthop Trans 1977; 1: 105–106.
57. Stulberg SD, Cooperman DR, Wallensten R. The natural history of Legg-Calvé-Perthes disease. J Bone Joint Surg 1981; 63A: 1095–1108.
58. Neyt JG, Weinstein SL, Spratt K. Stulberg classification system for evaluation of Legg-Calvé-Perthes disease: Intra-rater and inter-rater reliability. J Bone Joint Surg 1999; 81: 1209–1216.
59. Rosenfeld SB, Herring JA, Chao JC. Legg-Calvé-Perthes disease: A review of cases with onset before 6 years of age. J Bone Joint Surg Am 2007; 89: 2712–2722.
60. Catterall A. Legg-Calvé-Perthes disease. Clin Orthop and Rel Res 1981; 158: 41–51.
61. Gage HC. A possible early sign of Perthes disease. Br J Radiol 1933; 6: 295–297.
62. Schlesinger I, Crider RJ. Gage's sign—revisited! J Paediatr Orthop 1988; 8: 201–202.
63. Hefti F, Clarke NMP. The management of Legg-Calvé-Perthes disease: is there a consensus? J Child Orthop 2007; 1:19–25.
64. Brotherton BJ, McKibbin B. Perthes disease treated by prolonged recumbency and femoral head containment. J Bone Joint Surg [Br] 1975; 57-B:620.
65. Little DG, McDonald M, Sharpe IT, et al. Zoledronic acid improves femoral head sphericity in a rat model of Perthes disease. J Orthop Res 2005; 23: 862–868.
66. Kim HKW, Randall TS, Bian H, et al. Ibandronate for prevention of femoral head deformity after ischemic necrosis of the capital femoral epiphysis in immature pigs. J Bone Joint Surg Am 2005; 87: 550–557.
67. Martinez AG, Weinstein SG, Dietz FR. The weight-bearing abduction brace for the treatment of Legg-Calve-Perthes disease. J Bone Joint Surg Am 1992; 74: 12–21.
68. Herring JA, Kim HT, Browne R. Legg-Calvé-Perthes Disease. Part II: Prospective Multicenter Study of the Effect of Treatment on Outcome. J Bone Joint Surg Am 2004; 86: 2121—2134
69. Somerville EW. Perthes disease of the hip. J Bone Joint Surg Br 1971; 53-B: 639–649.
70. Lloyd-Roberts G, Catterall A, Salamon P. A controlled study of the indications for and the results of femoral osteotomy in Perthes disease J Bone Joint Surg 1976; 58-B: 31–36.
71. Fulford GE, Lunn PG, Macnicol MF. A prospective study of non-operative and operative management for Perthes disease. J Pediatr Orthop 1993; 13: 281–285.
72. Coates CJ, Paterson JMH, Woods KR, et al. Femoral osteotomy in Perthes disease: results at maturity. J Bone Joint Surg [Br] 1990; 72-B:581–585.
73. Paterson DC, Leitch JM, Foster BK. Results of innominate osteotomy in the treatment of Legg-Calve-Perthes disease. Clin Orthop 1991; 266: 96–103.
74. Crutcher JP, Staheli LT. Combined osteotomy as a salvage procedure for severe Legg-Calve-Perthes disease. J Pediatr Orthop 1992; 12: 151–156.
75. Olney BW, Asher MA. Combined innominate and femoral osteotomy for the treatment of severe Legg-Calve-Perthes disease. J Pediatr Orthop 1985; 5: 645–651.
76. Bankes MJK, Catterall A, Hashemi-Nejad A. Valgus extension osteotomy for 'hinge abduction' in Perthes disease: results at maturity and factors influencing the radiological outcome. J Bone Joint Surg [Br] 2000; 82-B:548–554.
77. Yoo WJ, Choi IH, Chung CY, et al. Valgus femoral osteotomy for hinge abduction in Perthes disease. Decision-making and outcomes. J Bone Joint Surg [Br] 2004; 86; 726–730.
78. Daly K, Bruce C, Catterall A. Lateral shelf acetabuloplasty in Perthes disease: a review at the end of growth. J Bone Joint Surg [Br] 1999; 81-B: 380–384.

79. Willett K, Hudson A, Catterall A. Lateral shelf acetabuloplasty: an operation for older children with Perthes disease. J Pediatr Orthop Surg 1992; 12:563–568.

80. Kruse RW, Guille JT, Bowen JR. Shelf arthroplasty in patients who have had Legg-Calvé Perthes disease: a study of long-term results. J Bone Joint Surg [Am] 1991; 73-A:1338–1347.

81. Freeman R, Kandil Y, Wainwright A, et al. The outcome of patients with hinge abduction in severe Perthes disease treated by shelf acetabuloplasty. J Children Orthop 2007; 1 (Suppl 1): S35.

82. Maxwell SL, Lappin KJ, Kealey WD, et al. Arthrodiastasis in Perthes disease. Preliminary results. J Bone Joint Surg [Br] 2004; 86(2):244–250.

83. Ganz R, Gill TJ, Gautier E, et al. Surgical dislocation of the adult hip a technique with full access to the femoral head and acetabulum without the risk of avascular necrosis. J Bone Joint Surg Br 2001; 83: 1119–1124.

84. Lavigne M, Parvizi J, Beck M, et al. Anterior femoroacetabular impingement: part I. Techniques of joint preserving surgery. Clin Orthop Relat Res 2004; 418:61–66.

85. Rowe SM, Jung ST, Cheon SY, et al. Outcome of Cheilectomy in Legg-Calve-Perthes disease; Minimum 25-year follow-up. J Pediatr Orthop 2006; 26: 204–210.

86. Boyd HS, Ulrich SD, Seyler TM, et al. Resurfacing for Perthes disease: an alternative to standard hip arthroplasty. Clin Orthop Relat Res 2007; 465: 80–85.

87. Maxwell L, Kealey D. Surgical management of Perthes disease (Protocol). Cochrane Database of Systematic Reviews 2002; 2: CD003829.

88. Wiig O, Terjesen T, Svenningsen S. Prognostic factors and outcomes of treatment in Perthes disease: a prospective study of 368 patients with five-year follow-up. J Bone Joint Surg [Br] 2008; 90-B: 1364–1371.

Chapter 7

Slipped Capital Femoral Epiphysis

Malcolm F. Macnicol and Michael K. D. Benson

Introduction

Posterior slipping of the upper (capital) femoral epiphysis (SUFE) is the most common cause of hip disability in early adolescence, until the growth plate closes. A number of factors contribute to a relative weakening of the growth plate and its surrounding fibrocartilaginous perichondrial ring, culminating in a shearing displacement through the zone of hypertrophic cartilage. The resultant symptoms and loss of function may be trivial or profound. Treatment is directed at preventing progressive slippage, minimizing deformity, and avoiding the major complications of avascular necrosis (AVN) and chondrolysis. Incidence: The incidence of SUFE is 2–3 per 100,000 children and adolescents [1] and is dependent upon race, gender, and geographical region. Minor slips which stabilize are often missed and the incidence also seems to be rising as a result of increasing obesity in youngsters [2]. The male predominance is now less marked, a ratio of 2:1 being recorded [3]. Boys usually present between the ages of 14 and 16 years whereas girls are afflicted between 11 and 13 years; after menarche girls are almost immune to the condition. The left hip is affected in 60% of cases initially but in 20–25% of cases the contralateral epiphysis may slip at a later date [4]. Subtle changes of pre-slipping in the opposite hip are evident in a further 40%. Rarely, both epiphyses may displace simultaneously but usually there is a delay of 6–18 months [5–7] between the sides, sometimes as long as 4–5 years. Younger boys are particularly at risk of a contralateral slip. Stasikelis et al. [8] found the Oxford pelvic bone age score [9] to be predictive: all their male patients under 11 years and 7 months developed a contralateral slip whereas only 9 of 22 did so between the ages of

11 years 8 months and 14 years 11 months. No cases presented secondarily over the age of 15 years, in accordance with the finding that closure of the triradiate cartilage is protective [10].

Racial variations are recognized, SUFE being relatively rare in southern Asia, Japan, China, and Africa but 4–5 times as common in Polynesians and 2.2 times in African-Americans compared to whites [1]. Obesity and variable radiographic surveillance may account for some of the differences in prevalence but neither Loder et al. [11] nor Kordelle et al. [12] have been able to establish acetabular morphological changes as contributory. Bilaterality is twice as common in African-Americans (34%) than in whites, Hispanics, and Asians. Hansson et al. [13] noted increased rates of SUFE during summer and autumn and in rural versus urban populations living above the 40° northern latitude, perhaps implicating physical activity as a precipitant. According to Rennie [14] the disorder appears to be autosomal dominant with variable penetrance, causing a 7% risk of a second family member being affected.

Etiology

The interplay of factors that contributes to SUFE is intriguing, mechanical stress, repetitive trauma, anatomical factors, endocrinopathies, and immunological abnormalities being considered separately and together as etiologically important.

Biomechanical Factors

Chung et al. [15] showed that the perichondrial fibrocartilaginous ring surrounding the growth plate contributes significantly to the ability of the epiphysis to withstand shear

M.F. Macnicol (✉)
University of Edinburgh, Edinburgh, UK; Royal Hospital for Sick Children, Edinburgh, UK; Murrayfield Hospital, Edinburgh, UK; Royal Infirmary; Edinburgh, UK

forces. It is firmly bound to neighboring subperiosteal meta-physeal bone and is the strongest during infancy. The ring decreases in volume and strength progressively and coincidentally the physeal plate widens during the growth spurt in early adolescence. At this stage the mammillary processes at the epiphyseal–metaphyseal junction offer more intrinsic resistance to shearing forces than the perichondral ring.

Shear stress across the growth plate is minimized by a horizontal physis and anteverted femoral neck. Gelberman et al. [16] found SUFE to correlate with neck retroversion and it is highly unusual to encounter the condition in a patient with femoral anteversion. Whereas anteversion averages 10.6° in adolescents of normal physique the figure also decreases to 0.4° in the obese [17]. Mirkopoulos et al. [18] found that patients with a slip had a more vertical proximal femoral physis, the effective decrease in neck–shaft angle also contributing to increased shear forces. Rarely, the epiphysis may slip into a valgus position although it is not known if this occurs when the growth plate is more horizontal. Because 5–6 times of body weight is applied to the femoral head during running and jumping it is also established that body weight and repetitive trauma contribute to the risk of SUFE.

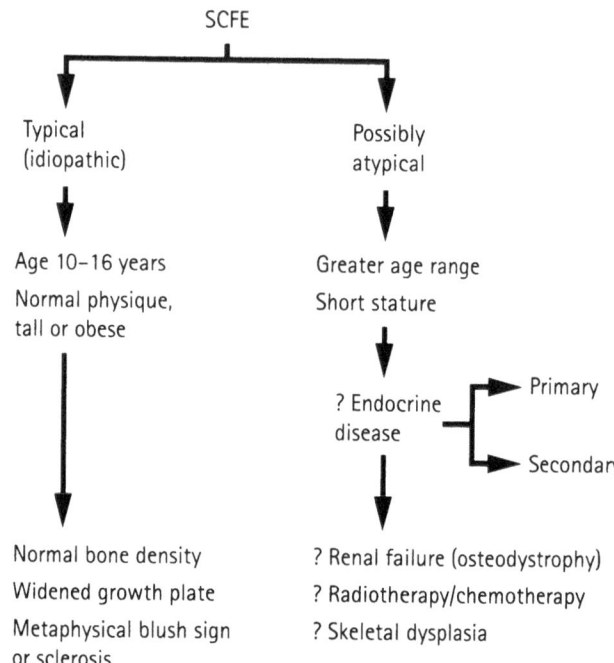

Fig. 7.1 Clinical differences between typical and atypical cases of slipped epiphysis

Endocrine Factors

Short stature, extremes of physique, and hypogonadism may predispose to SUFE, especially at an earlier stage in childhood when bilateral slips may develop. Appreciation of this atypical slip is important (Fig. 7.1) and these children should be referred for review by a paediatrician. Blethen and Rundle [19] found that growth hormone (GH) treatment for established GH deficiency, Turner's syndrome, or chronic renal failure enhances the risk of SUFE. Estrogen is known to increase the strength of the growth plate by causing it to narrow so that girls after menarche are protected from SUFE. When children with pan-hypothyroidism are treated with growth hormone, there is a significant risk of slip, particularly if sex hormones are not given concurrently. A deficiency of sex hormones will delay epiphyseal closure, thus increasing the time span when slipping may occur. This hormonal imbalance may also result in obesity, adding to the adverse mechanical factors.

Other endocrinopathies have been implicated, including hypothyroidism, primary and secondary hyperparathyroidism (where epiphyseal slips may also occur at the wrist), hypogonadism, and an association with craniopharyngioma and optic glioma. Previous irradiation therapy may also increase the risk of SUFE in a dose-related manner [20].

Immunological Factors

Eisenstein and Rothschild [21] reported an association between SUFE and increased serum immunoglobulins, particularly IgA. Patients with chondrolysis showed a greater increase in IgM. It was proposed that epiphyseal slipping was either a localized manifestation of a generalized inflammatory disorder or, more probably, that the slip exposes a tissue proteoglycan that acts as an antigenic stimulus for immunoglobulin and complement (C3) production.

Synovial fluid assays in SUFE sometimes reveal elevated immune complexes compared to normal joints, at a time when serum levels are normal. Cell death and the local inflammatory response could therefore increase the risk of further slippage and chondrolysis. As yet, the evidence for these associations is unconvincing.

Pathophysiology

The growth plate structural changes in SUFE have been assessed mainly by core biopsies. Apart from hyperparathyroidism, when the displacement may occur in the metaphysis, the slip develops through the zone of hypertrophic cartilage where the enlarging chondrocytes lie in irregular clusters [22] within a matrix which is weakened by a lack of collagen fibrils. Abnormal accumulation and distribution of glycoproteins and proteoglycans may inhibit the process of chondrocyte apoptosis [23, 24].

In the pre-slip stage the synovium is edematous and hyperemic while the growth plate appears widened [25]. Softening and decalcification of the metaphysis produce juxta-epiphyseal osteopenia radiographically. In the second stage of true displacement the slip progresses incrementally, although a sudden shearing force may lead to the so-called acute-on-chronic slip. In reality, displacement results from pathological movement not of the epiphysis but of the femoral neck which adducts, externally rotates, and shifts proximally like the fractured neck of femur in the elderly.

The capital epiphysis remains within the acetabulum, constrained by the ligamentum teres, the labrum, and surface tension. Griffiths [26] confirmed that the epiphysis comes to lie posterior to the femoral neck but that an anterior radiographic projection of the hip gives a misleading appearance of medial displacement. It is therefore helpful to rotate the femur during surgery to fix the epiphysis as this identifies the precise position of the epiphysis and screw tip under image intensifier. In rare cases the slip is acute, catastrophic, and unstable [27], so that imaging of a true lateral of the hip proves almost impossible.

The periosteum is torn through anteriorly as the slip progresses while posteroinferiorly, where it is lifted up from the neck of the femur, the callus forms. In the chronic slip with a history of over 3 weeks re-modeling of the callus stabilizes the displaced epiphysis, as with any fracture. The posterior retinacular vessels are stripped up with the periosteum and eventually shorten. Manipulation may therefore stretch the arterial supply and produce epiphyseal ischemia. The uncovered, anterior portion of the residual proximal femoral growth plate appears bluish-grey with islands of bone and cartilage. Impingement may later develop anteriorly between this metaphyseal "bump" and the acetabular rim although re-modeling in lesser slips eventually reduces this.

The synovial membrane and periosteum remain hyperemic and edematous throughout the slipping phase. Eventually, the inflammatory process subsides and the growth plate closes prematurely, on average 19 months after the onset of symptoms in the untreated case.

Clinical Features

Pain in the groin or knee, limp, and restricted hip movements characterize SUFE. Despite a limp, which may be painless, and an externally rotated leg (Fig. 7.2), diagnosis may be delayed by weeks or months. The knee may be the only symptomatic site [28] and radiographs are mistakenly confined to that joint. It is therefore essential to examine and possibly image the hips in any child or adolescence with a limp

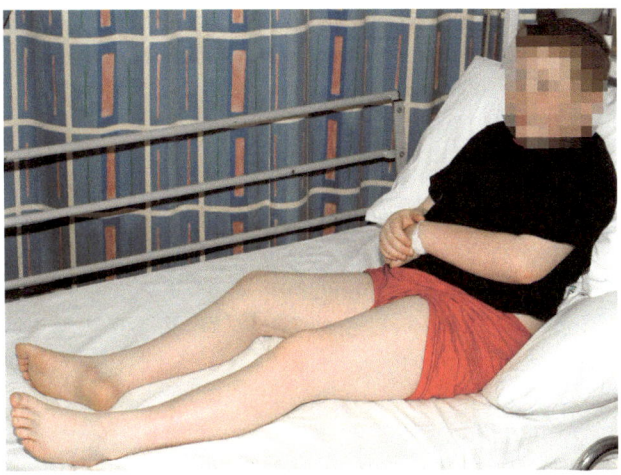

Fig. 7.2 External rotation and shortening of the right leg as a result of slipped epiphysis

and knee pain, particularly if knee examination is normal. An antalgic or Trendelenburg gait should also be tested for.

Classification

The condition is graded by the length of history, the extent of the slip, and by the disability in regard to weight bearing. Loder et al. [27] proposed that an unstable acute slip prevents the patient from weight bearing due to pain, even when crutches are being used. Active straight leg raising is also impossible with an unstable SUFE.

The involved limb lies in external rotation and adduction when displacement is severe. With a mild slip internal rotation and adduction of the flexed hip are painful and possibly limited. In more marked slipping abduction, flexion and internal rotation are decreased. As the examiner flexes the affected hip the thigh rolls typically into external rotation, producing the "figure 4" position. Flexion may be more limited than extension. Movement is more restricted in the acute slip, probably because the hemarthrosis or tense effusion causes pronounced muscle spasm. Shortening of the leg is rarely more than 2 cm, a combination of real and apparent loss of length.

Acute Slip

The history is less than 2–3 weeks by definition and the symptoms are usually marked. Approximately 20% of cases present acutely and AVN may complicate the condition in up to 50% of cases. A type I (Salter–Harris) fracture is a different entity, occurring in a normal patient with no prodromal symptoms who has been injured by a severe traumatic event. In both conditions reactive bone changes are yet to be seen on radiographs or scans.

Chronic Slip

The history is more than 3 weeks' duration with no defined trauma or sudden pain. Limp may be painless and unnoticed by the patient or family. Radiographs reveal posterior tilting of one or both capital epiphyses with associated metaphyseal re-modeling.

Acute-on-Chronic Slip

Although the patient has been symptomatic for more than 3 weeks, a sudden increase in pain and disability suggests a rapid further displacement of the epiphysis. This presentation accounts for about half of all treated cases.

It is not entirely clear why some epiphyses slip minimally and then stabilize, and why others displace progressively or in one, catastrophic shift. Knight et al. [29] found that of the 30% who present with a chronic slip, 50% have displaced less than 30°. Acute episodes of slipping superimposed upon chronic mild displacement result in periods of hip irritability and variable deformity.

Measuring the Slip

Although radiographic alterations are evident on the anteroposterior radiographs in SUFE the classic lateral projection method was proposed by Southwick [30] (Fig. 7.3) when describing his corrective proximal femoral osteotomy. If pain and spasm allow, a frog lateral view is attempted. Forcible positioning is both uncomfortable and risky so it may be wiser to obtain a "cross-table" lateral.

Radiographic imaging of the slip at operation is difficult and may be misleading. When the leg is externally rotated the epiphysis appears to be tilted medially; when the hip is internally rotated the tilt appears to be posterolateral. To demonstrate the displacement best the hip should be flexed 20–30°, the knee flexed to 90° and the thigh supported in 30° of external rotation. This reduces the parallax effect [26, 31] which can also be reduced by screening the hip while rotating the leg until the epiphysis is best visualized.

The degree of posterior slip is defined as follows:

Mild – the head–shaftangle is less than 30° (Fig. 7.3)
Moderate – the angle is 30–60°
Severe – the angle is more than 60°

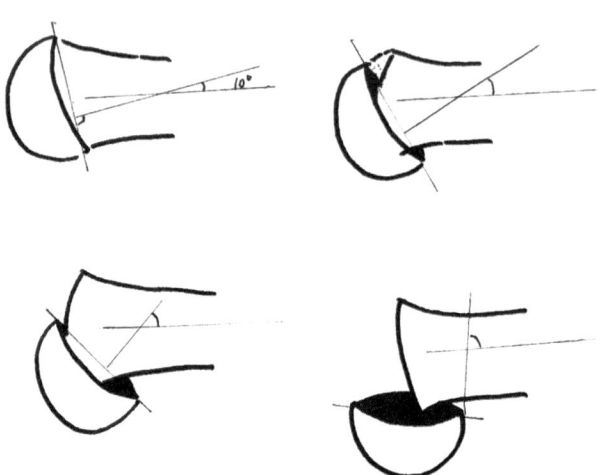

Fig. 7.3 The lateral projection of the affected hip shows neck retroversion and the extent of epiphyseal displacement in degrees

The tilt is compared to the contralateral hip which is often retroverted or may also be affected by a mild slip. Southwick also noted that the anteroposterior (AP) view offered a measure of the axis of the femoral neck versus the base of the capital epiphysis, considering the normal angle to be 145°.

Wilson [32] quantified displacement on the lateral view using the ratio of slip distance to the diameter of the femoral neck proximally. A mild slip is less than 33%, a moderate is 33–50%, and severe is more than 50% displacement. Complete displacement (100%) is a 90° Southwick angle.

Figure 7.4 shows some of the changes seen on an AP radiograph of a slip:

1 Klein's line [33] intersects the lateral segment of the epiphysis but this intersection is reduced or absent on the abnormal side (Trethowan's sign).
2 A break in Shenton's arc develops progressively.
3 Scham's sign [34] describes the absence of the normal overlap between the proximal, medial metaphysis, and the acetabular wall (pubic component).
4 Steel's metaphyseal blanch sign [35] develops as the posteriorly slipping epiphysis overlaps the proximal femoral neck.
5 Concurrently, the height of the epiphysis reduces as it tilts.
6 Relative osteopenia occurs in the femur and hemipelvis on the abnormal side as weight bearing is reduced.

It is particularly important to look for these subtle signs and to augment this with a frog lateral view. Computed tomography (CT) scans or magnetic resonance (MR) imaging depict the anatomy accurately and are therefore of value, principally in the established or healed case when corrective osteotomy is being planned.

Fig. 7.4 The anteroposterior radiographic projection shows a number of signs. See text for the six alterations

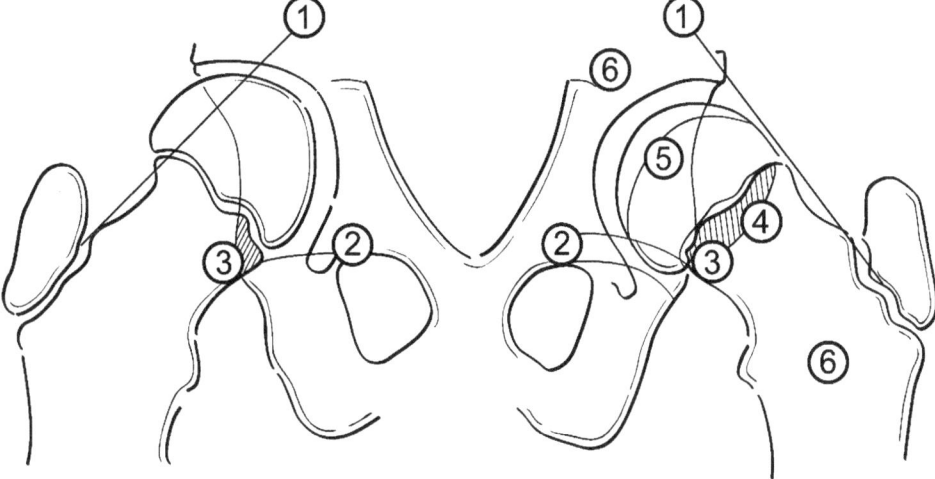

Alternative Imaging (Early)

Imaging of the hips by radiography can be augmented by ultrasound [36] which demonstrates the effusion and possibly the shift of the epiphysis on the metaphysis. Similarly, MR scanning may be appropriate in the acute situation, allowing some definition of the abnormal anatomy and possible changes in the "pre-slipping" phase, although the value of this over radiographs has been disputed [37]. Images are degraded by the presence of metallic implants in the proximal femur postoperatively.

Alternative Imaging (Late)

Bone scanning with technetium (Tc-99m) was assessed prior to treatment by Rhoad et al. [38]. Since ischemia was identified in 6 of the 10 unstable but none of the stable hips the scan was a useful predictor of outcome prior to surgical treatment. None of the unstable hips with normal isotope uptake subsequently developed AVN. Owing to restrictions in the acute availability of this investigation in many health care systems, bone scanning cannot yet be considered a standard investigation in the urgent management of SUFE.

Bone scans are more commonly used to assess the presence of AVN or chondrolysis postoperatively, particularly in the severe slips or after corrective osteotomy at the femoral neck. These two complications invariably lead to stiffness and discomfort but whereas AVN leads to reduced epiphyseal isotope uptake, chondrolysis produces increased uptake in the acetabulum as well as the epiphysis.

CT scans are of value postoperatively, first to assess the position of the screw if there is concern about implant position or joint penetration, and second to improve later realignment surgery (Fig. 7.5). Axial CT scans allow detailed

measurement of the slip angle between the axis of the femoral neck and the tangent across the base of the epiphysis [39]. Bone stock and femoral dimensions can also be gauged with 3D CT scanning (Fig. 7.6).

Surgical Treatment

The objectives of orthopaedic management are as follows:

1 Early diagnosis and definition of the slip
2 Avoidance of forced manipulation (Fig. 7.7)
3 Stable fixation of the slipped epiphysis
4 Consideration of the risks of contralateral slippage
5 Monitoring for AVN or chondrolysis
6 Timed contralateral distal femoral epiphysis for leg length discrepancy
7 Later corrective osteotomy if appropriate.

In Situ Fixation

Conservative treatment with a hip spica cast is no longer appropriate and carried a high rate of complications. Percutaneous fixation (Fig. 7.8) is effective for mild to moderate chronic and acute-on-chronic slips, using a single cannulated, full-threaded screw placed as centrally in the epiphysis as possible [40]. For greater degrees of slip the guide wire and subsequent screw need to be placed through a more anterior site in the femoral neck. Even if the line of the insertion is marked out on the skin of the proximal thigh using anterior and lateral projections on the image intensifier it is often necessary to expose the femur more formally.

Fig. 7.5 CT scans reveal the posterior epiphyseal slip and three artifacts from previous pinning

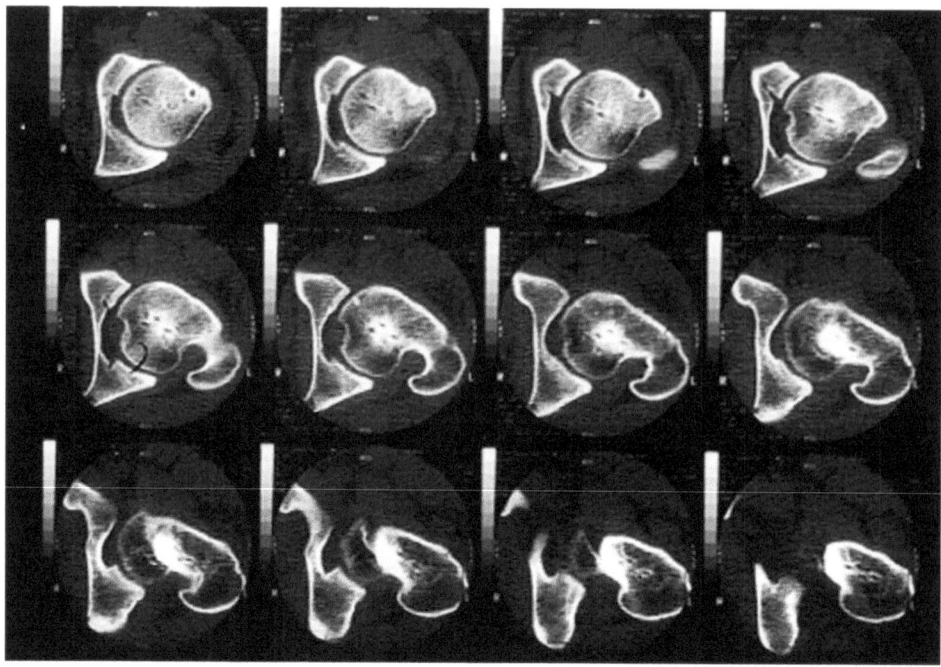

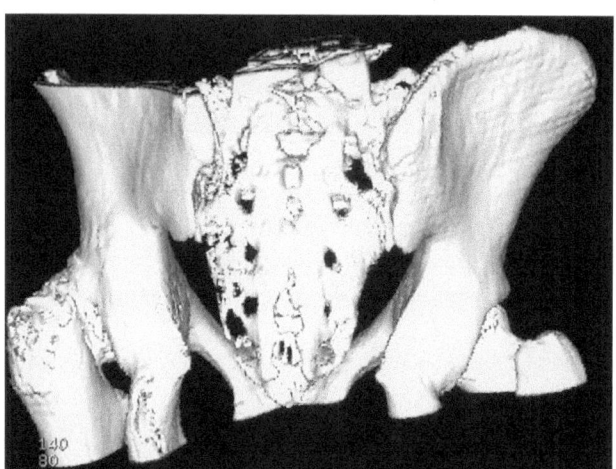

Fig. 7.6 Imaging with 3D CT shows posterior shift of the epiphysis and external rotation of the femur

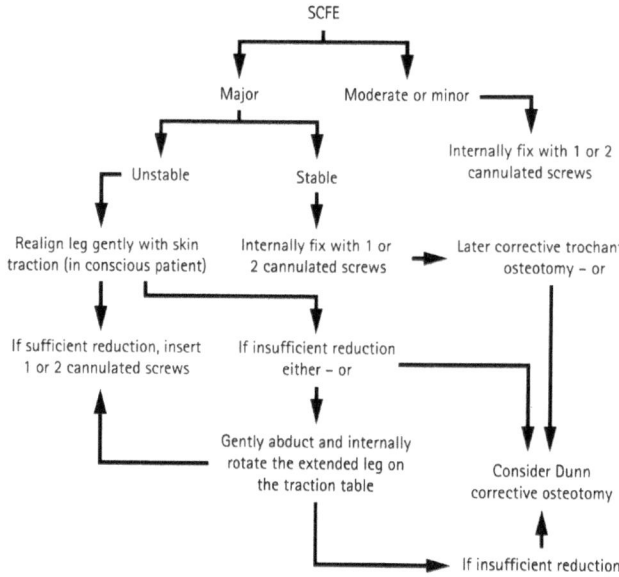

Fig. 7.7 Flow diagram to outline the surgical approach for slipped epiphysis

The epiphysis must be clearly visualized throughout the procedure to ensure that the guide wire or screw do not penetrate the joint. Greenhough et al. [41] reported a high complication rate with multiple pins but a single cannulated screw applied with compression and five threads in the epiphysis [42] should offer good stability. An arthrogram has been recommended after pinning [43] or cannulated screw insertion [44], while the patient is still anesthetized, although this does not rule out joint penetration completely [45]. The hip should also be assessed through a full range of movement to check for crepitus or obstruction and definitive AP and lateral radiographs obtained at the end of the procedure.

With slips of greater than 30° the medullary aperture begins to close (Fig. 7.9) and an anterior neck insertion is inevitable (Figs. 7.10 and 7.11). This helps to avoid the crucial lateral epiphyseal vessels which enter the epiphysis at its posteroinferior quadrant [46] and anastomose with vessels from the ligamentum teres and other retinacular vessels.

Fig. 7.8 The stages in percutaneous pinning

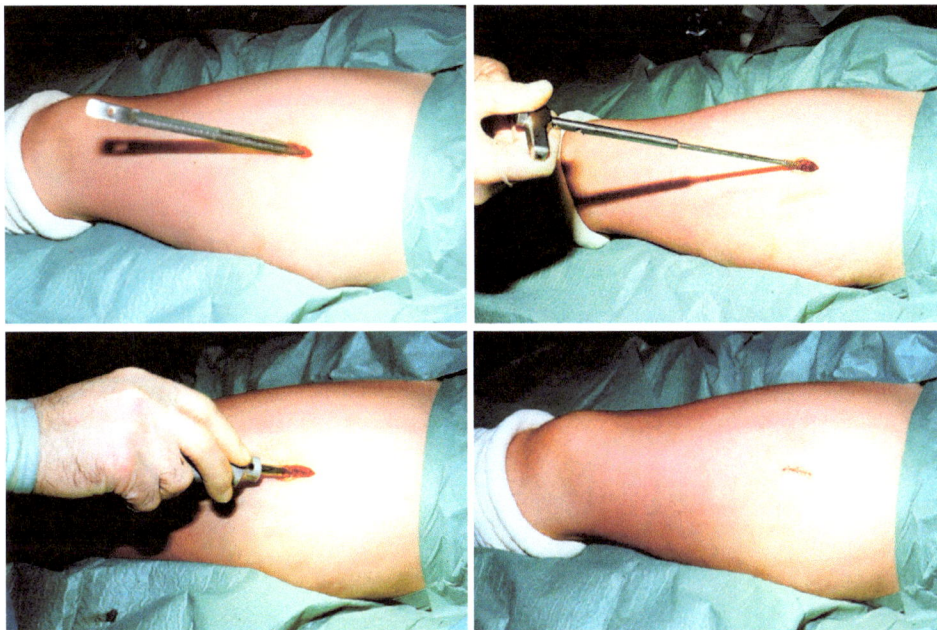

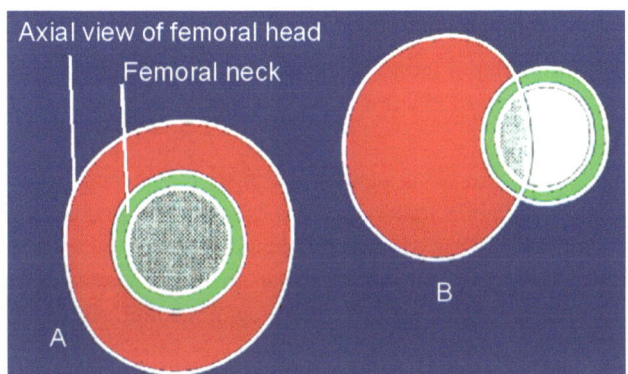

Fig. 7.9 The aperture shared by the femoral neck and epiphysis (**a**) gradually closes off as the slip increases (**b**)

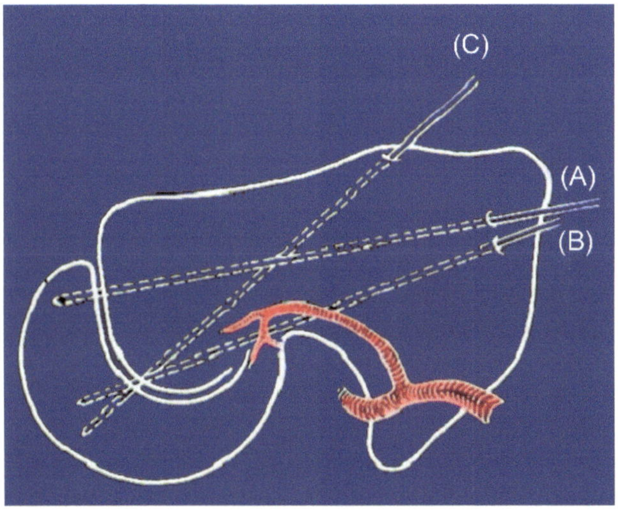

The Unstable Slip

Management of the major acute slip is controversial and beset with concerns. The risk of stretching the posterior retinacular vessels is considerable when the leg is manipulated under general anesthesia to reduce the slip. Gently rolling the extended leg internally with the thigh supported and slightly abducted may lessen the slip angle, making in situ fixation possible [47]. In the heavier child double guide wire fixation may be indicated to achieve epiphyseal stability, while maintaining internal rotation and some abduction of the hip. This permits double screw fixation [48] thus increasing implant strength by 33% [49], although complications may be increased. De Sanctis et al. [50] found that single cannulation screw fixation was effective for both stable and

Fig. 7.10 The trajectory of the guide wire is important. A conventional insertion may either result in a poor fixation in the anterior epiphysis (**a**) or, if directed more posteriorly, may breach the posterior cortex of the neck and thus injure the vital retinacular vessels (**b**). A more anterior starting point with the guidewire will allow the neck to be traversed within the neck and the center of the epiphysis to be reached (**c**)

unstable slip if the implant was properly positioned in the epiphysis.

Timing the surgery may be important in the management of the unstable hip. Kalogriantis et al. [51] have suggested treatment within 24 h if possible, when the risk of stretching the retinacular vessels with gentle manipulation may be less (Fig. 7.7). AVN complicated those hips treated between 24 and 72 h. In view of the isotope bone scan results of Rhoad

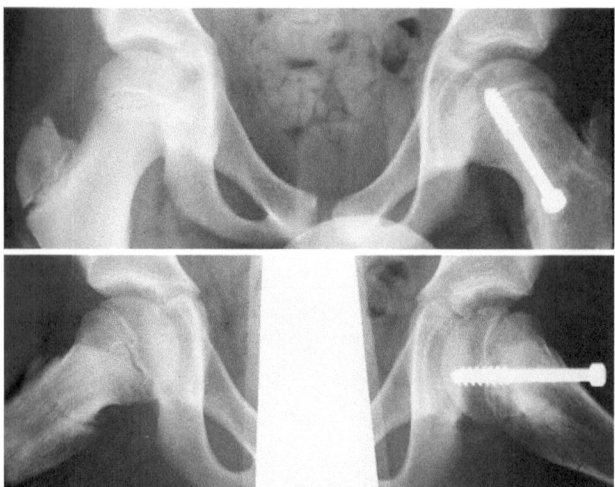

Fig. 7.11 Radiographs to show cannulated screw fixation of a moderate slip

et al. [38] it still remains a concern as to whether there is any truly safe period to operate upon the acute, severe slip [52].

The etiology of this chondrolysis is unclear although pin penetration and the obsolete use of a spica cast produce high rates. It may complicate subcapital, basal neck (cuneiform) [53, 54], and even later corrective trochanteric osteotomy. An increased risk in African-American and Hawaiian children has been reported [55].

The joint space narrows due to softening and thinning of articular cartilage on both sides of the joint. A villous synovitis develops with the eventual formation of adhesions. As cartilage is lost the subchondral bone is exposed, leading to pain and progressive osteoarthritis.

Treatment comprises physiotherapy to maintain as much hip movement as possible. If symptoms are severe, weight bearing is reduced for a variable period and non-steroidal anti-inflammatory drugs may be appropriate. Infection should be ruled out by joint aspiration and a CT scan will visualize whether the screw or pin has penetrated the joint. Arthrodesis or hip resurfacing arthroplasty is a later option, but realignment, sometimes useful in cases of segmental AVN, is not effective. Standard bone grafting and vascularized fibular grafts are ineffectual.

Later Proximal Femoral Osteotomies

In cases where the growth plate has closed following in situ fixation, with an established slip angle of 30–60°, a later corrective intertrochanteric osteotomy is indicated. For lesser slips re-modeling may improve alignment in the younger

patient, but this phenomenon ceases with skeletal maturity. Osteoplasty by removal of the prominent neck bump anteriorly [56] may be indicated when there is evidence of femoro-acetabular impingement.

Urgent Subcapital Osteotomy

There is a limited place for these procedures, provided that the surgeon is experienced in this demanding technique. When the epiphysis proves to be irreducibly displaced through 70–90°, the Dunn procedure [57, 58] allows the slip to be fully corrected. It is imperative to obtain full surgical access through an anterolateral or anterior approach. The plane of dissection is between the abductors and tensor fasciae latae, with or without greater trochanteric osteotomy, exposing the femoral neck superiorly and anteriorly (Fig. 7.12). The operation may be undertaken with the patient lying supine [59] or lying on the unaffected side with the image intensifier positioned appropriately.

The posterior retinacular vessels of the femoral neck must not be damaged and this is ensured by

1 leaving the soft tissues over the posterior neck undissected
2 shortening the femoral neck 1–2 cm to allow gradual repositioning of the epiphysis without tensioning the vessels
3 gentle positioning of the thigh in abduction and slight internal rotation while inserting a central, cannulated screw with compression

The curved line of the femoral neck and the saucer-shaped inferior epiphyseal surface (Figs. 7.13 and 7.14) should fit together snugly and the hip carefully screened to assess stability of fixation and possible pin penetration. Postoperative mobilization depends upon the security of fixation and whether a greater trochanteric osteotomy has been used. If hip movements comparable to the normal side are regained rapidly over the first few days the likelihood of AVN is low. Partial weight bearing can be permitted with crutches within the first week postoperatively, with full weight bearing by 6 weeks.

AVN is reported in 20–25% of patients [60] (Fig. 7.15), with varying rates of chondrolysis in different series [59]. Shortening of the affected leg is approximately 1.5 cm and since the growth plate has been ablated the discrepancy may increase unless contralateral prophylactic fixation of the proximal epiphysis has been deemed advisable. If this is not the case, particularly with the younger patient, a distal femoral epiphysiodesis should be undertaken at the appropriate time [61].

Fig. 7.12 Stages in the Dunn osteotomy

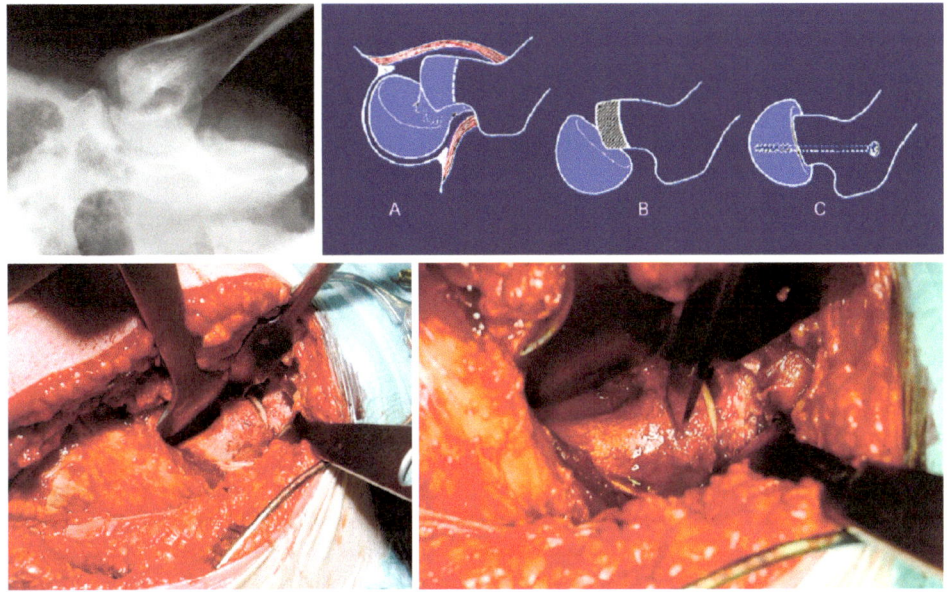

Fig. 7.13 The femoral neck must be shortened so that repositioning the epiphysis does not stretch or damage the posterior retinacular vessels

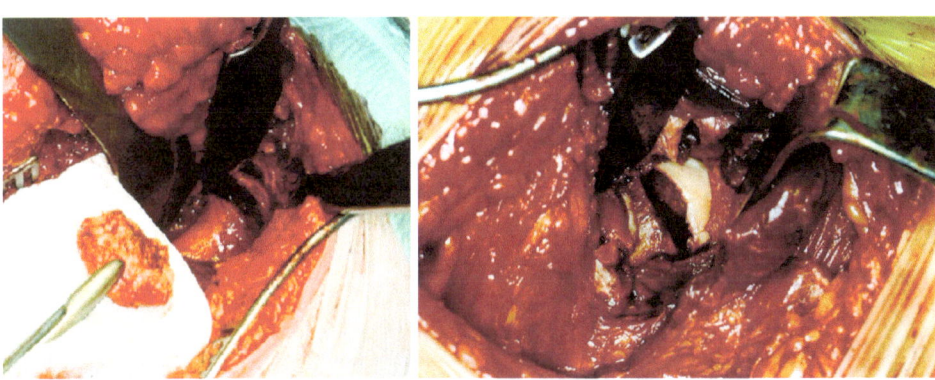

The Fish osteotomy [62, 63] is a similar procedure undertaken less acutely. Provided that the growth plate is still open, best confirmed by axial CT scanning, correction is possible by removing callus and an appropriate wedge of proximal metaphyseal bone. The anterolateral approach is used and the growth plate defined with a needle. The AVN and chondrolysis rates remain as complications.

Contralateral Prophylactic Fixation

Bilateral epiphyseal slips occur in 95% of patients with chronic renal osteodystrophy [64] and in 61% of endocrinopathies [65]. These slips are usually severe and therefore merit bilateral fixation unlike the often asymptomatic minor slips seen in athletic individuals [66] which may still predispose to later osteoarthritis due to femoro-acetabular impingement (Fig. 7.16)

The risk of severe contralateral slip is greater in younger children who have already suffered from an unstable slip, so there is a case for bilateral fixation, particularly if social circumstances cause concern. Jerre et al. [4] reported a contralateral slip rate of 20–25% and since only one in ten of these will be unstable, the risk of developing an unstable contralateral slip is in the order of 1–2%. Nevertheless, the risks of a later, major contralateral slip is such that careful monitoring every 3–6 months is warranted [67].

The complications from contralateral fixation are low [68], particularly as operative techniques have improved. It is therefore prudent to fix the contralateral hip in prepubertal children, particularly if the triradiate cartilage is open or when the Oxford pelvic bone age score, as modified by Stasikelis et al. [69], confirms that the patient is relatively immature. Vigilant follow-up in the orthopaedic outpatient clinic is mandatory until the proximal femoral growth plates fuse. It is a calamity if a patient with a poor result from one unstable slip sustains a contralateral unstable slip with subsequent complications.

Fig. 7.14 Dunn procedure
a) the right hip treated by Dunn
procedure with b) right hip of the
same patient three years later
after metal removal c) acute slip
of the left hip in 13 year old boy
d) after Dunn procedure without
trochanteric osteotomy

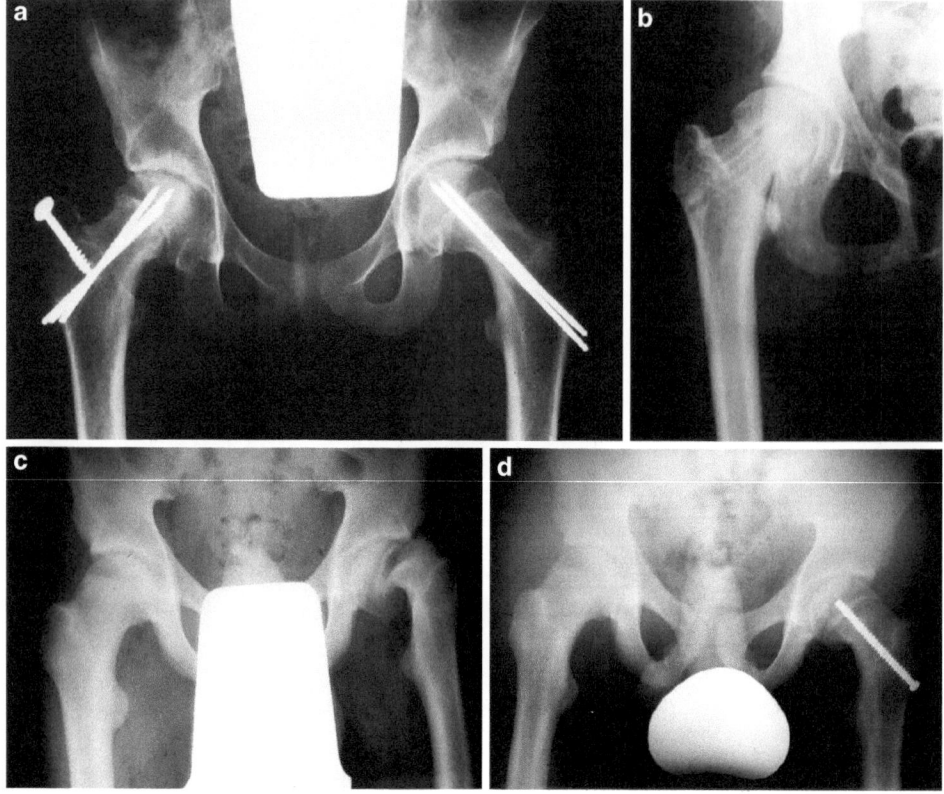

Fig. 7.15 The radiographic
appearances 20 years after a right
Dunn osteotomy complicated by
segmental avascular necrosis and
subsequent osteoarthritis

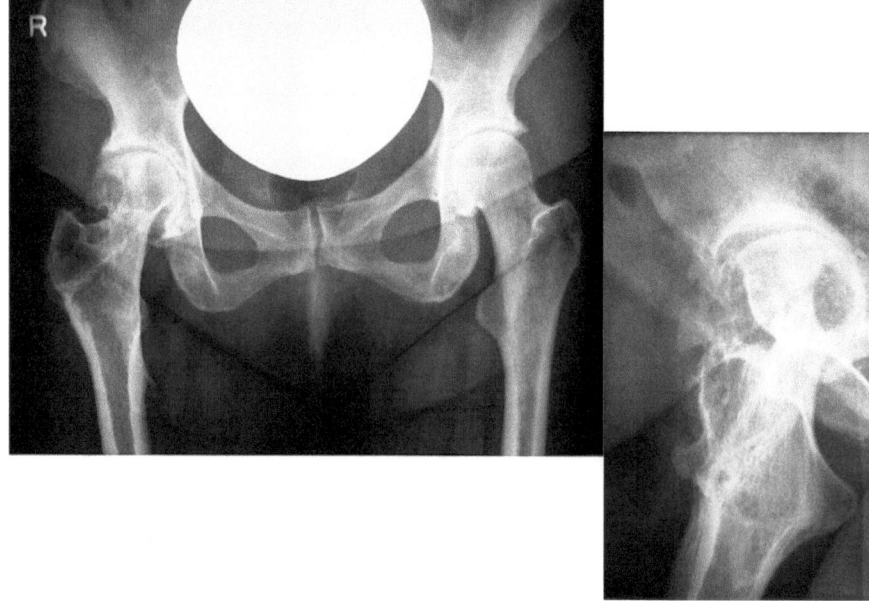

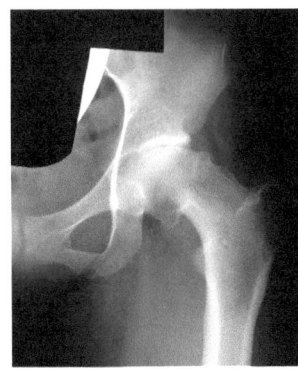

Fig. 7.16 Pistol grip deformity of the left hip in a 20 year old girl, who had an acute-on-chronic slip on the left side at age 14 years

Complications

Operative

Difficulties in imaging the true lateral view of the hip, both preoperatively and during the surgical procedure, may result in the pins or cannulated screw being inserted inaccurately leading to later loss of reduction, implant breakage or penetration into the joint. The guide wire may fracture if it bends during positioning of the leg to maintain slip reduction thus snaring against the cannulated reamer. The surgeon should therefore be prepared to enlarge the wound if these technical difficulties arise. Migration of pins may occur and clustering their tips may produce segmental necrosis [46]. A fracture may develop at the stress riser where the implant has been inserted. Lastly, the standard surgical complications of nerve and vessel injury, infection, and hypertrophic scar may occur.

Avascular Necrosis

As previously discussed the most common cause of AVN is manipulative reduction of the slipped epiphysis (Fig. 7.17) although it can occur rarely in the untreated, unstable hip. The rate of AVN increases if the partial or complete reduction has been for a mild slip (12.5%), a moderate slip (70%), or a severe slip (75%) [70].

Postoperative stiffness is the first sign that necrosis may be present, cell death producing a continuing reactive effusion and muscle spasm. The radiographic changes are evident by 6–12 months (Fig. 7.17) [71], although minor changes and loss of femoral head sphericity may not appear until a few years later, with the inevitable hastening of osteoarthritis. MR and isotope bone scanning confirm AVN,

which may be partial (segmental) or total, at an early stage postoperatively.

Chondrolysis

This complication has been discussed in relation to the unstable slip. An autoimmune reaction has been proposed [21], resulting in a lack of synovial fluid production. There is no clear-cut association with intra-articular pin penetration [41, 72].

Later Surgical Procedures

Corrective Femoral Osteotomy

Southwick described his triplane valgus, extension, and internal rotation distal segment correction in 1967 [30]. With the removal of carefully executed bone wedges at the level of the lesser trochanter (Fig. 7.18) following preoperative planning, the principal components of the deformity can be corrected. Fixation with fixed angle blade plates and screws (Fig. 7.19) avoids the need for postoperative immobilization and achieves excellent or good results in 87% of patients at 18 years.

Imhauser [73, 74] and Griffiths [26] corrected the extension and external rotational deformities, satisfactory results being reported for moderate and severe SUFE [75]. These intertrochanteric osteotomies are distal to the site of deformity and correction is limited but usually sufficient to improve gait. AVN is not a risk although loss of fixation (with re-operation needed), delayed union, fracture, and occasionally chondrolysis have been reported. Later osteoarthritis still develops in many cases. In patients where the growth plate was open Southwick found that closure of the physis was probably hastened by the realignment which increased axial compression when weight bearing.

Implant Removal

As many of these patients will require a later hip arthroplasty, removal of blade plates and screws is advisable once the growth plate and osteotomy have united. Apart from requiring a second anesthetic the removal of implants is often difficult, so an asymptomatic single cannulated screw should be left in situ.

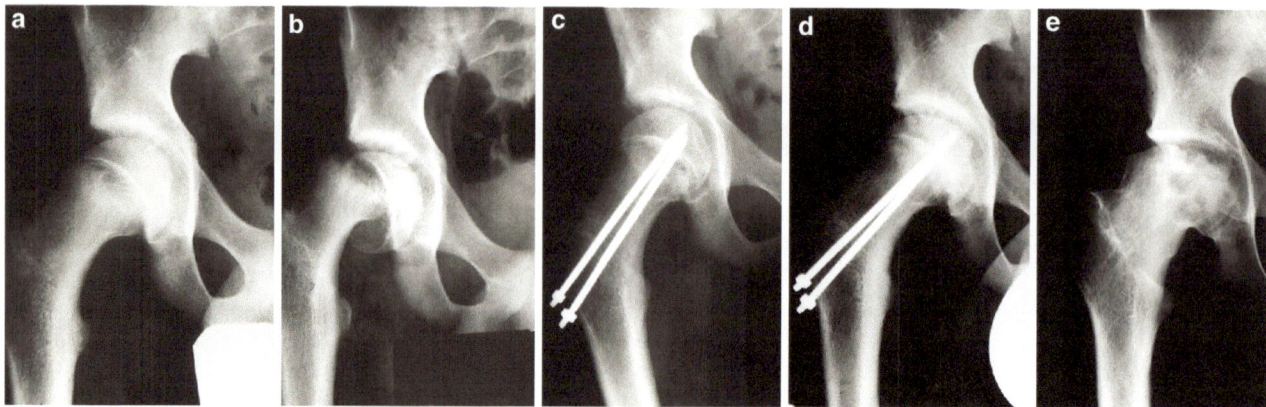

Fig. 7.17 A minor slip of the right upper femoral epiphysis was not appreciated although many of the pathological signs detailed in Fig. 7.4 are present (**a**). The epiphysis slipped significantly a few days later (**b**) and was reduced anatomically by manipulation under anesthesia (**c**). Avascular necrosis and loss of joint space became progressively more obvious (**d**, **e**)

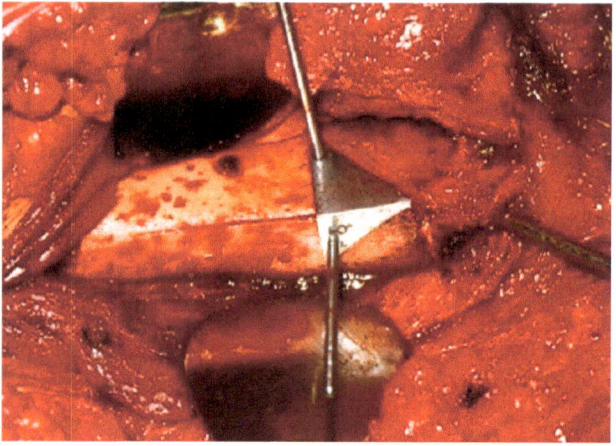

Fig. 7.18 Metal templates allow the excision of precisely measured bone wedges as part of a Southwick, triplane osteotomy

Conclusion

Failure to diagnose the slipped capital femoral epiphysis remains the main concern in this condition. As a cause of limp in childhood, it accounts for only 0.5% of the total number of hip conditions that are encountered. It is this relative rarity that makes slipped epiphysis difficult to diagnose, coupled with its insidious onset in some children and adolescents, and the fact that pain is commonly referred to the ipsilateral knee. In any child who is abnormally short, or in whom the medical history is complex, and particularly in the later stages of childhood and in adolescence, the possibility of slipped upper femoral epiphysis must be entertained.

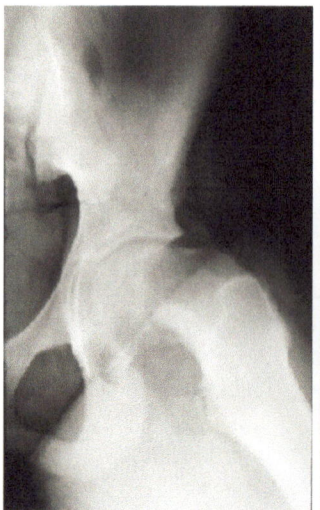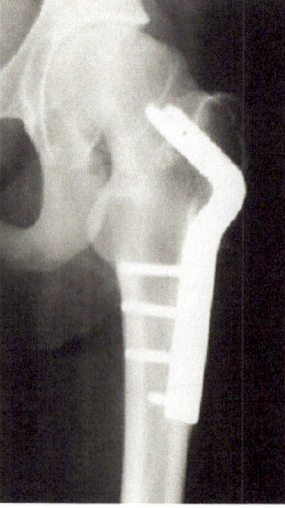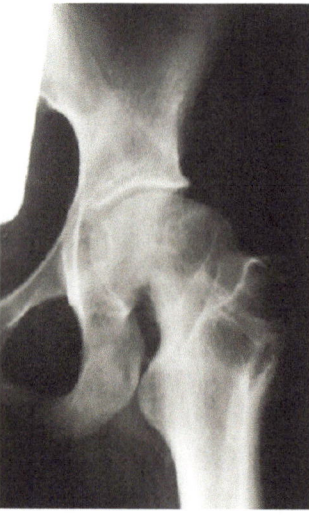

Fig. 7.19 A valgus, derotation (biplanar) proximal femoral osteotomy corrects leg alignment although some head–neck deformity has to be accepted

References

1 Loder RT. The demographics of slipped capital femoral epiphysis. An international multicentre study. Clin Orthop 1996; 322:8–27.

2 Kelsey JL, Acheson RM, Keggi KJ. The body build of patients with slipped capital epiphysis. Am J Dis Child 1972; 124:276–81.

3 Hansson LI, Hagglund G, Ordeberg G. Slipped capital femoral epiphysis in Southern Sweden 1910–1982. Acta Orthop Scand Suppl 1987; 226:1–67.

4 Jerre R, Billing L, Hansson G, et al. The contralateral hip in patients treated for unilateral slipped upper femoral epiphysis: long term follow up of 61 hips. J Bone Joint Surg [Br] 1994; 76B:563–7

5 Sorensen KH. Slipped upper femoral epiphysis. Clinical study on etiology. Acta Orthop Scand 1968; 39:499–517.

6 Hagglund G, Hansson LI, Ordeberg G. Bilaterality in slipped upper femoral epiphysis. J Bone Joint Surg [Br] 1988; 70B:179–81.

7 Loder RT, Aronson DD, Greenfield ML. The epidemiology of bilateral slipped capital femoral epiphysis: a study of children in Michigan. J Bone Joint Surg [Am] 1993; 75A:1141–9.

8 Stasikelis P, Sullivan C, Phillips W, et al. Slipped capital femoral epiphysis: prediction of contralateral involvement. J Bone Joint Surg [Am] 1996; 78A:1149–55.

9 Acheson R. The Oxford method of assessing skeletal maturity. Clin Orthop 1957; 10:19–26.

10 Puylaert D, Dimeglio A, Bentahar T. Staging puberty in slipped capital femoral epiphysis: importance of the triradiate cartilage. J Pediatr Orthop 2004; 24:144–7.

11 Loder RT, Mehbod AA, Meyer C, et al. Acetabular depth and race in young adults, a potential explanation of the differences in the prevalence of slipped capital femoral epiphysis between different racial groups. J Pediatr Orthop 2003; 23:699–702.

12 Kordelle J, Richolt JA, Millis MB, et al. Development of the acetabulum in patients with slipped capital femoral epiphysis: a three-dimensional analysis based on computed tomography. J Pediatr Orthop 2001; 21:174–8.

13 Hansson LI, Hagglund G, Ordeberg G. Epidemiology of slipped capital epiphysis in Southern Sweden. Clin Orthop 1984; 191: 82–94.

14 Rennie AM. The inheritance of slipped upper femoral epiphysis. J Bone Joint Surg [Br] 1982; 64B:180–4.

15 Chung SMK, Batterman SC, Brighton CT. Shear strength of the human capital epiphyseal plate. J Bone Joint Surg [Am] 1976; 58A:99–103.

16 Gelberman RH, Cohen MS, Shaw BA, et al. The association of femoral retroversion with slipped capital femoral epiphysis. J Bone Joint Surg [Am] 1986; 68A:1000–7.

17 Galbraith RT, Gelberman RH, Hajek PG, et al. Obesity and decreased femoral anteversion in adolescence. J Orthop Res 1987; 5:523–8.

18 Mirkopulos N, Weiner DS, Askew M. The evolving slope of the proximal femoral growth plate relationship to slipped capital femoral epiphysis. J Pediatr Orthop 1988; 8:268–73.

19 Blethen SL, Rundle AC. Slipped capital femoral epiphysis in children treated with growth hormone: a summary of the national cooperative growth study experience. Horm Res 1996; 46:113–6.

20 Loder RT, Hensinger RN, Alburger PD, et al. Slipped capital femoral epiphysis associated with radiation therapy. J Pediatr Orthop 1998; 18:630–6.

21 Eisenstein A, Rothschild S. Biochemical abnormalities in patients with slipped capital femoral epiphysis and chondrolysis. J Bone Joint Surg [Am] 1976; 58A:459–67.

22 Mickelson MR, Ponseti IV, Cooper RR, et al. The ultrastructure of the growth plate in slipped capital femoral epiphysis. J Bone Joint Surg [Am] 1977; 59A:1076–81.

23 Kerr JFR, Wyllie AH, Currie AR. Apoptosis—basic biological phenomenon with wide-ranging implications in tissue kinetics. Brit J Cancer 1972; 26:234–42.

24 Roach HI, Aigner T, Kouri JB. Chondroptosis: a variant of apoptotic cell death in chondrocytes? Apoptosis 2004; 9:265–79.

25 Howorth B. Slipping of the capital femoral epiphysis: pathology. Clin Orthop 1966; 48:33–9.

26 Griffiths MJ. Slipping of the upper femoral epiphysis. Ann Roy Coll Surg 1976; 58:34–42.

27 Loder RT, Richards BS, Shapiro PS, et al. Acute slipped capital femoral epiphysis: the importance of physeal stability. J Bone Joint Surg [Am] 1993; 75A:1134–40.

28 Matava MJ, Patton RM, Luhmann S, et al. Knee pain as the initial symptom of slipped capital femoral epiphysis: an analysis of initial presentation and treatment. J Pediatr Orthop 1999; 19:455–60.

29 Knight DJ, Dreghorn C, Main SG. Slipped capital femoral epiphysis in Glasgow. J Pediatr Orthop 1987; 7:283–7.

30 Southwick WO. Osteotomy through the lesser trochanter for slipped capital femoral epiphysis. J Bone Joint Surg [Am] 1967; 49A:807–34.

31 Billing I, Severin E. Slipping epiphysis of the hip; a roentgenological and clinical study based on a new roentgen technique. Acta Radiol 1959; 51:1–76.

32 Wilson PD. The treatment of slipping of the upper femoral epiphysis with minimal displacement. J Bone Joint Surg [Am] 1938; 20A:379–99.

33 Klein A, Joplin RJ, Reidy JA, et al. Roentgenographic features of slipped capital epiphysis. Am J Roentgenol 1951; 66:361–74.

34 Scham SM. The triangular sign in the early diagnosis of slipped capital femoral epiphysis. Clin Orthop 1974; 103:16–7.

35 Steel HH. The metaphyseal blanch sign of slipped capital femoral epiphysis. J Bone Joint Surg [Am] 1986; 68A:920–2.

36 Kallio PE, Mah ET, Paterson DC, et al. Ultrasound in slipped capital femoral epiphysis. Diagnosis and assessment of severity. J Bone Joint Surg [Br] 1991; 738:884–9.

37 Tins BJ, Cassar-Pullicino VN. Slipped upper femoral epiphysis. In: Davis AM, Johnson K eds. Imaging of the hip and bony pelvis. Techniques and applications. Springer, Berlin 2005; pp 173–94.

38 Rhoad RC, Davidson RS, Heyman S, et al. Pre-treatment bone scan in SCFE: a predictor of ischemia and avascular necrosis. J Pediatr Orthop 1999; 19:164–8.

39 Cohen MS, Gelberman RH, Griffin PP, et al. Slipped capital femoral epiphysis: assessment of epiphyseal displacement and angulation. J Pediatr Orthop 1986; 6:259–64.

40 Morrissy RT. Slipped capital femoral epiphysis: technique of percutaneous in situ fixation. J Pediatr Orthop 1990; 10:347–50.

41 Greenhough CG, Bromage JD, Jackson AM. Pinning of the slipped upper epiphysis—a trouble-free procedure? J Pediatr Orthop 1985; 5:657–60.

42 Carney BT, Birnbaum P, Minter C. Slip progression after in situ single screw fixation for stable slipped capital femoral epiphysis. J Pediatr Orthop 2003; 23:584–9.

43 Bennet GC, Koreska J, Rang M. Pin placement in slipped capital femoral epiphysis. J Pediatr Orthop 1984; 4:574–8.

44 Lehman WB, Minche D, Grant A, et al. The problem of evaluating in situ pinning of slipped capital femoral epiphysis. An experimental model and review of 63 consecutive cases. J Pediatr Orthop 1984; 4:297–303.

45 Shaw JA. Preventing unrecognised pin penetration into the hip joint. Orth Rev 1984; 13:142–52.

46 Brodetti A. The blood supply of the femoral neck and head in relation to the damaging effects of nails and screws. J Bone Joint Surg [Br] 1960; 428:794–801.

47 Aronsson DD, Loder RT. Treatment of the unstable (acute) slipped capital femoral epiphysis. Clin Orthop 1996; 322:99–110.

48 Macnicol MF, Macindoe N. Management of severe slippage of the capital femoral epiphysis. Curr Orth 1996; 10:180–4.

49 Karol LA, Doane RM, Cornicelli SF, et al. Single versus double screw fixation for treatment of slipped capital femoral epiphysis: a biochemical analysis. J Pediatr Orthop 1992; 12:741–6.

50 De Sanctis N, DiGennaro G, Pempinello C, et al. Is gentle manipulative reduction and percutaneous fixation with a single screw the best management of acute and acute on chronic slipped capital epiphysis. A report of 70 patients. J Pediatr Orthop B 1996; 5:90–5.

51 Kalogriantis S, Khoon Tan C, Kemp GJ, et al. Does unstable slipped capital femoral epiphysis require urgent stabilisation? J Pediatr Orthop B 2007; 16:6–9.

52 Weinstein S. Natural history and treatment outcomes of childhood hip disorders. Clin Orthop 1997; 344:227–34.

53 Kramer WG, Craig WA, Noel S. Compensating osteotomy at the base of the femoral neck for slipped capital femoral epiphysis. J Bone Joint Surg [Am] 1976; 58A:796–800.

54 Barmada R, Bruch RF, Gimbel JS, Ray RD. Base of the neck extracapsular osteotomy for correction of deformity in slipped capital femoral epiphysis. Clin Orthop 1978; 132:98–101.

55 Carney BT, Weinstein SL, Noble J. Long-term follow-up of slipped capital femoral epiphysis. J Bone Joint Surg [Am] 1991; 73A:667–74.

56 Heyman S, Herndon C, Strong J. Slipped femoral epiphysis with severe displacement: a conservative operative technique. J Bone Joint Surg [Am] 1957; 39A:293–303.

57 Dunn DM. The treatment of adolescent slipping of the upper femoral epiphysis. J Bone Joint Surg [Br] 1964; 46B:621–9.

58 Dunn DM, Angel JC. Replacement of the femoral head by open operation in severe adolescent slipping of the upper femoral epiphysis. J Bone Joint Surg [Br] 1978; 60B:394–403.

59 Macnicol MF, ed. Color Atlas and Text of Osteotomy of the Hip. London: Mosby-Wolfe; 1996:139–44.

60 Szypryt EP, Clement DA, Colton CL. Open reduction or epiphysiodesis for slipped upper femoral epiphysis. J Bone Joint Surg [Br] 1987; 64B:737–42.

61 Macnicol MF, Gupta M. Epiphysioidesis using a cannulated tube saw. J Bone Joint Surg [Br] 1997; 97B:307–9.

62 Fish J. Cuneiform osteotomy of the femoral neck in the treatment of slipped capital femoral epiphysis. J Bone Joint Surg [Am] 1984; 66A:1153–68.

63 Fish J. Cuneiform osteotomy of the femoral neck in the treatment of slipped capital femoral epiphysis. J Bone Joint Surg [Am] 1994; 76A:46–59.

64 Loder RT, Hensinger RN. Slipped capital femoral epiphysis associated with renal failure osteodystrophy. J Pediatr Orthop 1997; 17:205–11.

65 Loder RT, Wittenberg B, DeSilva G. Slipped capital femoral epiphysis associated with endocrine disorder. J Pediatr Orthop 1995; 15:349–56.

66 Murray RO, Duncan C. Athletic activity in adolescence as an aetiological factor in degenerative hip disease. J Bone Joint Surg [Br] 1971; 53B:406–19.

67 Maclean JGB, Reddy SK. The contralateral slip. An avoidable complication and indication for prophylactic pinning in slipped upper femoral epiphysis. J Bone Joint Surg [Br] 2006; 88B:1497–501.

68 Seller K, Raab P, Wild A, et al. Risk benefit analysis of prophylactic pinning in slipped capital femoral epiphysis. J Pediatr Orthop 2001; 10:192–6.

69 Robb JE, Annan IH, Macnicol MF. Guidewire damage during cannulated screw fixation for slipped capital femoral epiphysis. J Pediatr Orthop B 2003; 12:219–22.

70 Tokmakova KP, Stanton RP, Mason DE. Factors influencing the development of osteonecrosis in patients treated for slipped capital femoral epiphysis. J Bone Joint Surg [Am] 2003; 85A:798–801.

71 Krahn TH, Canale ST, Beaty JH, et al. Long term follow up of patients with avascular necrosis after treatment of slipped capital femoral epiphysis. J Pediatr Orthop 1993; 13:154–8.

72 Vrettos B, Hoffman EB. Chondrolysis in slipped upper femoral epiphysis: long-term study of the etiology and natural history. J Bone Joint Surg [Br] 1993; 75B:456–61.

73 Imhauser G. Zur Pathogenese und Therapie der jugendlichen Huftkopflosung. Orthop 1957; 88:3–41.

74 Imhauser G. Spaetergebnisse der sog Imhauser Osteotomie bei der Epiphysen loesung. Z Orthop 1977; 115:716–25.

75 Parsch K, Zehender H, Buehl T, Walker S. Intertrochanteric corrective osteotomy for moderate and severe chronic slipped capital femoral epiphysis. J Pediatr Orthop B 1999; 8:223–30.

Chapter 8

The Knee

David M. Hunt and Malcolm F. Macnicol

Introduction

The child's knee is vulnerable to mechanical problems, although the relative frequency of complaints varies with age. For example, instability of the knee in a child is more likely to result from a patellofemoral problem than from a torn meniscus. Isolated congenital abnormalities are often of minor degree, whereas more severe problems are usually found in association with lower limb dysplasias and syndromes. The stiff, congenital knee dislocation that is seen in Larsen's syndrome is an example. Because the growth plates above and below the knee make such a major contribution to longitudinal growth, trauma and infection at these sites in early life can have disastrous consequences, causing leg length discrepancy and deformity. Primary tumors found in the region of the knee, both benign and malignant, are specific for age (see Chapter 14).

Referred pain from the hip and lumbar spine can sometimes be confusing: in such conditions as slipped capital femoral epiphysis, the first radiograph in the patient's file is invariably one of the knee. Further difficulty and confusion become apparent when a psychological cause for knee pain or bizarre gait is suspected. It is a mistake to focus so much on the knee as to forget the child and the parents. Great caution and diplomacy should be exercised in this area.

The classic presentation of knee malfunction includes pain (particularly in the older child), clicking and/or giving way, effusion, and locking which is most likely to be the pseudo-locking of patellar instability or tibiofemoral subluxation than meniscal (discoid lateral meniscus or an unstable tear). Yet in many cases the younger child will have no complaint to make; it is parental concern about deformity, whether resolving and benign or structural and progressive, which promotes orthopaedic review. As detailed

in Chapter 2, gait, knee alignment, patellar tracking, and increases or decreases in the four arcs of movement (flexion/extension, coronal laxity, rotation, and anteroposterior glide) should be recorded and compared to the opposite knee. Testing should quantify mild, moderate, and major effusions [1], areas of diagnostic tenderness, and maltracking of the patella both passively and under load with the patient sitting at the edge of the examining couch.

Knee Deformity

Genu Recurvatum

Familial joint laxity is a common cause of symmetrical physiological genu recurvatum, usually seen in girls. Such laxity may predispose the child to ligament sprains and may be associated with patellar instability. When unilateral or severe, recurvatum is more likely to be pathological. One must distinguish between congruous hyperextension, anterior subluxation of the tibia, and complete anterior dislocation of the tibia on the femur.

Congenital Dislocation of the Knee

Congenital dislocation of the knee is rare [2], about 1% of the frequency of developmental dysplasia of the hip (DDH), which is detected in 1–2 per 1000 live births. It is clinically obvious and therefore unlikely to be missed although varying degrees of knee hyperextension may be erroneously included. Curtis and Fisher [3] represented the increasing severity of the deformity (Fig. 8.1a), the joint appearing "back to front" with an obvious transverse anterior skin crease (Fig. 8.1b) and the femoral condyles prominent posteriorly because the tibia is displaced. The hamstring tendons subluxate anteriorly, potentiating the deformity.

D.M. Hunt (✉)
Department of Orthopaedics, St. Mary's Hospital, London, UK

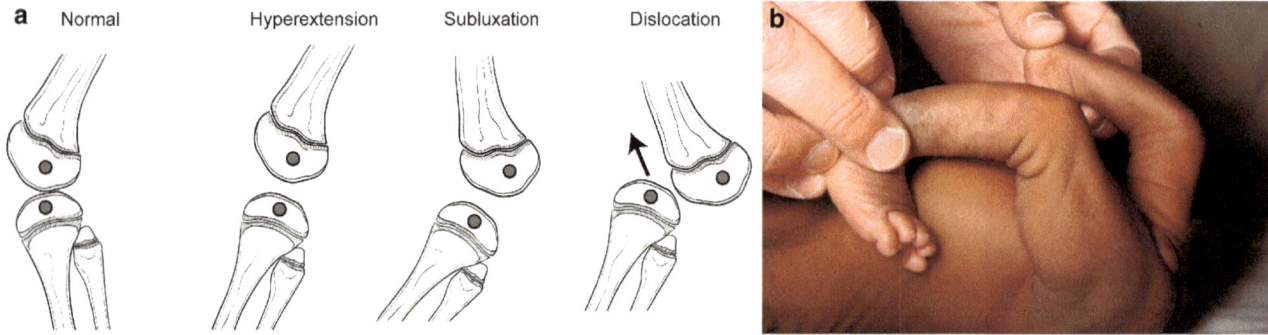

Fig. 8.1 (**a**) Congenital dislocation of the knee is a continuum of deformity although a grading of severity has been proposed [3]. (**b**) The knee is clearly abnormal with a transverse anterior skin crease

Hyperextension with slight subluxation is probably an intrauterine moulding deformity, analogous to neonatal hip instability. In normal infants the knee often reduces with a clunk as it is flexed, the hamstrings and iliotibial band shifting to the flexor side of the knee axis. If the knee can be flexed to 30–40°, splintage with increasingly flexed anterior casts and physiotherapy produces a satisfactory result. Splintage can be discontinued at 6–8 weeks, the knee returning to a normal shape, with minimal residual hyperextension and slight loss of flexion.

More severe knee dislocation is recalcitrant to conservative measures. Other abnormalities are usually present including a dysplastic patella tethered proximally by a shortened, fibrotic quadriceps tendon, and obliteration of the suprapatellar pouch. Ultrasound scanning can be helpful in identifying the patella (Fig. 8.2) [4]. Abnormalities or absence of the cruciate ligaments are present [5] and associated anomalies include DDH, clubfoot, calcaneovalgus, dislocation of the elbow, and syndromes such as arthrogryposis.

Skeletal traction is contraindicated so a sequential release is undertaken, involving the fascia lata and vastus lateralis, a V–Y lengthening of the distal quadriceps and any tethering adhesions. The surgery is best undertaken by 6 months of age so that secondary changes are avoided. Delay may lead to a progressive, sloping deformity where the posterior tibia abuts against the distal, anterior femur, a deformity that makes stable open reduction difficult. Failure to elongate the lateral tethers leads to a valgus deformity, again difficult to correct.

An extremely rare form of congenital snapping knee has been described [6,7]. The tibia subluxates anteriorly in extension and reduces with a pronounced clunk at 30° of flexion. The condition is often part of a syndrome (Larsen's, Catel-Manzke, or congenital short tibia) and the dysmorphic nature of the joints becomes obvious as the child grows. Division and possibly re-routing of the iliotibial band together with suturing of the biceps tendon to the vastus lateralis control the subluxation.

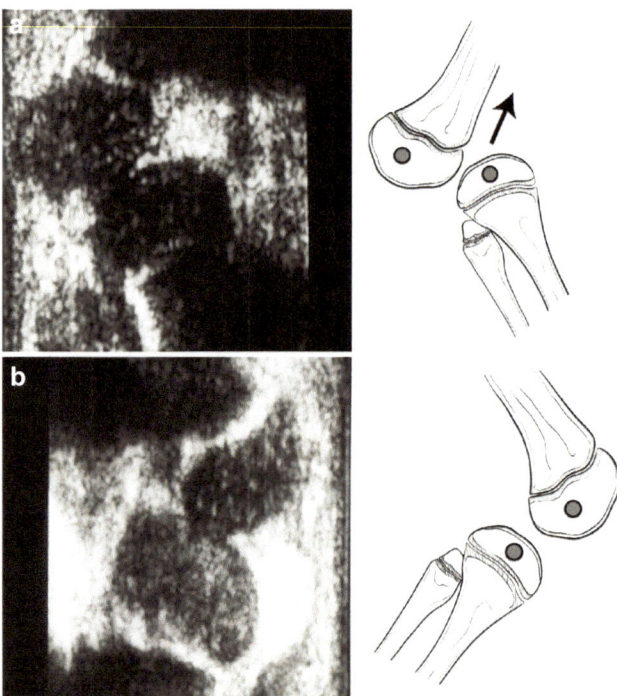

Fig. 8.2 Ultrasound of congenital dislocation of the knee. (**a**) At birth. (**b**) Reduced

Neurological Hyperextension

Secondary Genu Recurvatum

The hyperextended knee is a common feature of several neurological conditions. The usual mechanism is muscle imbalance, in which a strong or spastic quadriceps group overcomes the action of weak hamstrings. Very occasionally, the hamstring deficit may be due to excessive and inappropriate release in patients with cerebral palsy.

In poliomyelitis, hamstring paralysis in the presence of active quadriceps can produce stretching of the posterior soft tissues of the knee, and eventually a gross recurvatum that is extremely difficult to control without a caliper. Posterior soft tissue reefing procedures are not successful, and probably the best surgical option at maturity is the anterior patellar bone block, fixing the patella to the upper tibia so that it acts as a "doorstop" in extension.

In the totally flail knee, it is well to remember that slight hyperextension enables the patient to lock out and therefore stabilize the knee when walking.

A second cause of neurological recurvatum arises when the knee is forced into hyperextension by an equinus foot; this is seen in cerebral palsy and sometimes after head injury. Early lengthening of the tendo-Achilles will prevent progression of knee deformity and improve gait.

Post-traumatic Tibial Recurvatum

Injury to the anterior half of the proximal tibial growth plate and the apophysis of the tibial tuberosity may produce a progressive recurvatum of the knee if there is sufficient skeletal growth remaining (Fig. 8.3a) [8]. The Salter–Harris type V fracture, with or without a splitting of the physis, results from compression if the knee is hyperextended and may be associated with cruciate ligaments tears.

Moroni et al. [9] described the role of proximal tibial osteotomy at skeletal maturity. If the injury is recognized earlier than this, an epiphysiodesis or posterior stapling will prevent the inexorable increase in angulation and a contralateral proximal tibial epiphysiodesis should be considered to prevent leg length discrepancy.

The osteotomy should be supratubercular (Fig. 8.3b), as close to the deformity as possible. An anterior opening wedge using bank bone is effective, without osteotomy of the fibula. A posterior closing wedge osteotomy [10] may be more risky and further shortens the tibia. Choi et al. [11] have described the successful use of the Taylor spatial frame to produce graded correction of the proximal tibial slope. The osteotomy should start below the tibial tuberosity if patellar positioning is acceptable although in most cases the lack of anterior tibial growth produces a relative patella alta.

Tibial recurvatum also develops in certain skeletal dysplasias. Associated ligament laxity may prevent successful correction and the subchondral plate is characteristically softened and unreliable. Iatrogenic recurvatum is now rare but used to complicate prolonged traction with the knee in extension (frame knee), cast immobilization, proximal tibial traction wire or pin fixation, and tibial tuberosity transfer before skeletal maturity.

Flexion Deformity

During the first few days of life, a mild physiological flexion deformity of the knee is commonplace and rapidly resolves. More obvious and permanent fixed flexion may be seen at birth in arthrogryposis and spina bifida, whereas in cerebral palsy, myopathic and infective conditions, and juvenile idiopathic arthritis the deformity appears later. Serial plaster splints or slabs applied during the first few weeks of life can be effective, but attention needs to be paid to the skin, especially in children who have impaired sensation. The chief shortcoming of serial splintage is that, although the knee may indeed straighten, the correction is often spurious, with the knee hinging open at the back and the tibia impacting against the femoral condyles and failing to glide forward in a normal and congruous fashion. To overcome this problem, reverse dynamic slings [12] have been used in hemophilia and are certainly applicable in the older child.

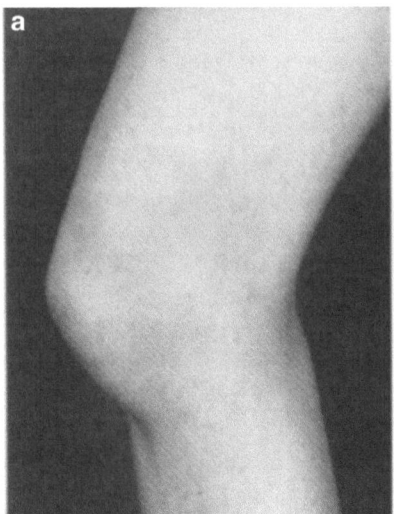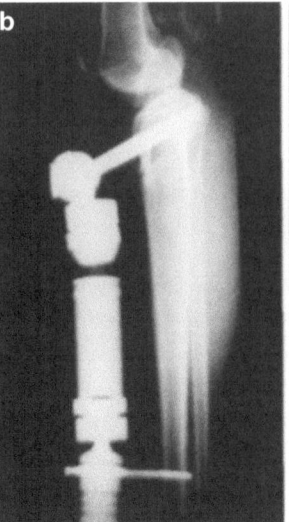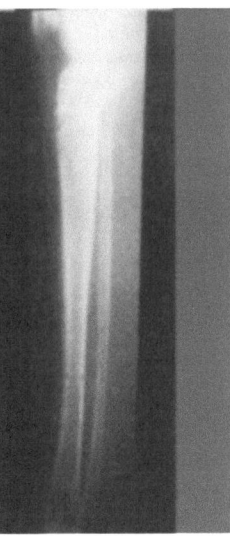

Fig. 8.3 (**a**) Recurvatum after proximal tibial growth plate injury: Note the prominence of the posterior femoral condyles (**b**) Pre- and postoperative lateral radiographs after correction of genu recurvatum using a distraction frame

Fig. 8.4 Supracondylar extension osteotomy of the femur for fixed flexion deformity. Recurrence of the knee flexion deformity with growth and later reversal of some of the correction

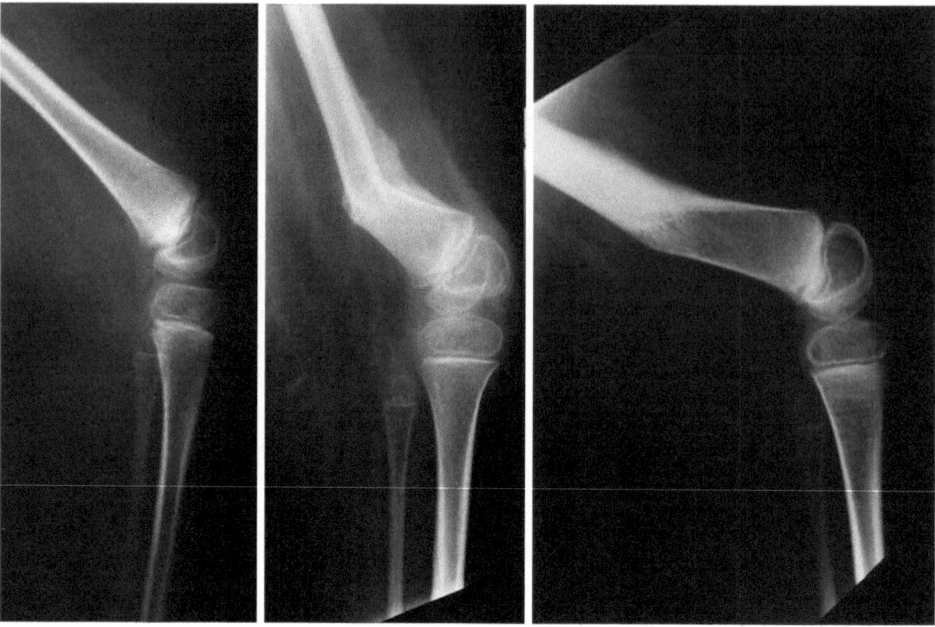

The surgical correction of paediatric deformity includes an extensive soft tissue release since the effects of supracondylar extension osteotomy alone will reverse with further skeletal growth (Fig. 8.4). The posterior exposure is achieved by medial and lateral longitudinal incisions or a transverse lazy "S" incision provided that skin is allowed to heal postoperatively before stretching casts are applied. The hamstring tendons and posterior cruciate ligament are divided after careful identification of the popliteal vessels and the common peroneal and posterior tibial nerves. The posterior capsule should be released fully after opening the joint space posteriorly.

Nerves and vessels must be protected from the deleterious efforts of rapid extension of the knee, the same principle applying to correction of severe valgus. In younger patients serial casts work well but they lose their effectiveness after puberty. Arthrogrypotic deformity corrects reasonably well with soft tissue release and possibly osteotomy [13, 14] (see Chapter 20) or by circular frame distraction [15].

Valgus Deformity

Physiological valgus of the knee ceases to be a functional or cosmetic problem in most children by the age of 6 years, the tibiofemoral angle spontaneously decreasing [16]. An intermalleolar distance of greater than 5 cm when standing may merit review in mid-childhood but there is no evidence that osteoarthritis will develop prematurely in the valgus knee.

It is invidious to state that a definite intermalleolar distance at the age of 12 years should be surgically corrected but concern about function is legitimate if the distance exceeds 15 cm, allied to a valgus angulation of 15°. Medial ligament pain, limp, and the onset of patellar subluxation reinforce the decision to operate, although physiotherapy, weight reduction when appropriate and medial shoe wedges may prove effective.

When valgus appears to be increasing medial stapling [17, 18] or epiphysiodesis [19, 20] are effective. A standing radiograph film will demonstrate any obliquity of the knee joint and confirm whether staples should be placed above rather than below the knee. Strong implants are required and experience has shown that a 10-cm intermalleolar gap will close in approximately 1 year. Obviously, there must be sufficient potential growth to effect the correction and the staples must be removed as soon as physiological alignment is achieved. Failure to time staple removal accurately will convert a knock-knee to a bow leg deformity, causing immense dissatisfaction. Staples should be inserted extraperiosteally, as should any form of plate and screw anchorage. Even with correctly timed removal the effects of the stapling may persist causing over-correction [21] (Fig. 8.5), so careful clinical and radiographic monitoring is essential until skeletal maturity.

Distal femoral osteotomy is the only option at the end of growth [22, 23]. Valgus deformity may be secondary to loss of abduction due to stiffness in the ipsilateral hip or may present as a complex deformity in skeletal dysplasia, requiring an abduction (valgus) osteotomy of the proximal femur as well as corrective osteotomies above and below the knee (Fig. 8.6).

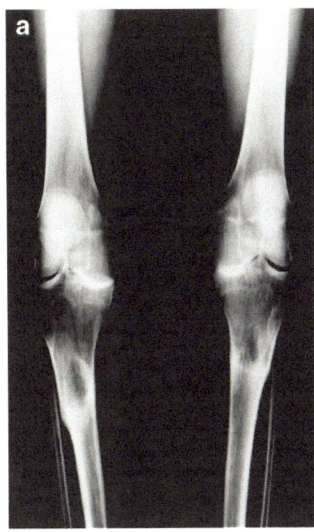

Fig. 8.5 Surgical over-correction of genu valgum in adolescence led to genu varum and later osteoarthritis in adult life

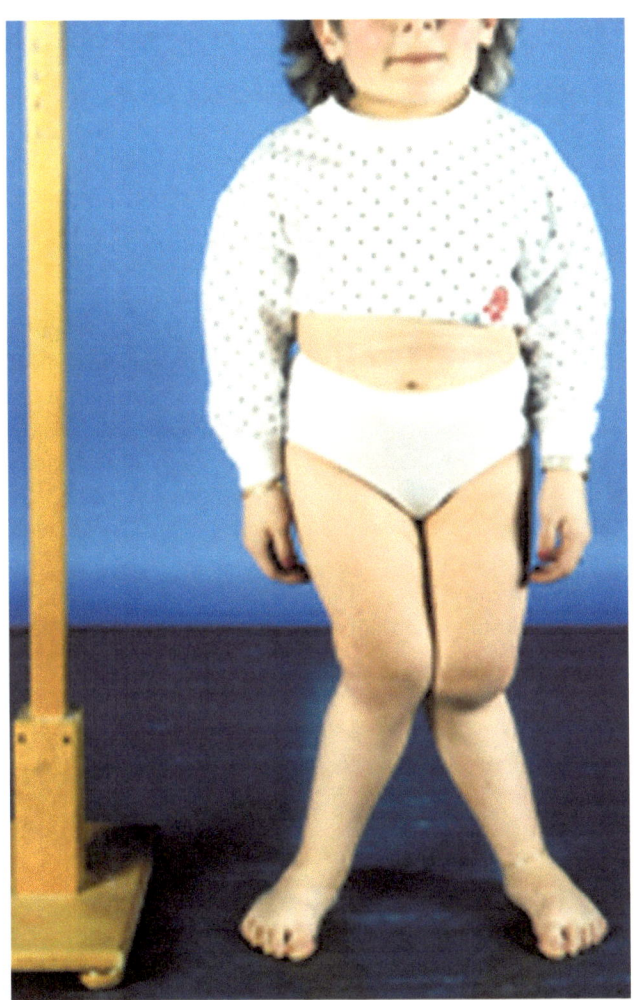

Fig. 8.6 Complex deformity with hip adduction and genu valgum requiring multi-level osteotomies

Post-fracture Genu Valgum

Unilateral and initially progressive genu valgum may follow a proximal, metaphyseal tibial fracture [24], particularly if there is tibial comminution and associated fibular fracturing (Fig. 8.7). Many theories have been advanced to explain the asymmetrical physeal growth, including inadequate primary reduction or splintage, differential vascular stimulation of the growth plate, unusual loading through the proximal tibia, interposition of soft tissues in the fracture site medially (pes anserinus, periosteum, tibial collateral ligament), and tethering by the shortened (united) fibula. It is wise to await the spontaneous correction of the deformity although this is not always assured.

Genu Varum

Babies are usually born with bow legs which persist through the toddler stage. The appearance may be accentuated by internal tibial torsion and these "late correctors" may be a cause of great anxiety for parents. Resolution or progression of the deformity can be monitored photographically and the diagnosis of a possibly pathological deformity is made by asking five questions:

1. Is the child short or disproportioned as may occur in skeletal dysplasia or endocrine disorders?
2. Is the deformity unilateral or asymmetrical, perhaps following trauma or infection?
3. Is there a family history of a syndrome such as familial hypophosphatemic rickets?
4. Is the deformity excessive for the child's age? (progressive varus after the age of 3 years)
5. Is the angulation within the physiological pattern for age (Fig. 8.8)?

Tibia vara or Blount's disease [25] was first recognized by Erlacher in 1922 [26], before an extensive review of the condition by Blount. Repetitive, compressive injury of the proximal tibial growth plate medially leads to progressive varus. There is later overgrowth of the lateral tibial physis and of the distal, medial femoral epiphysis.

Langenskiold [27] classified infantile tibia vara into grades of severity that worsened with increasing age (Fig. 8.9). Stages I and II can be expected to resolve fully but surgical realignment by osteotomy becomes increasingly likely thereafter. The radiographic tibiofemoral [15] and metaphyseal–diaphyseal [28] (Fig. 8.10) angles are monitored, the latter being pathological when it exceeds 15°.

Fig. 8.7 Post-proximal tibial metaphyseal fracture valgus correcting spontaneously with growth

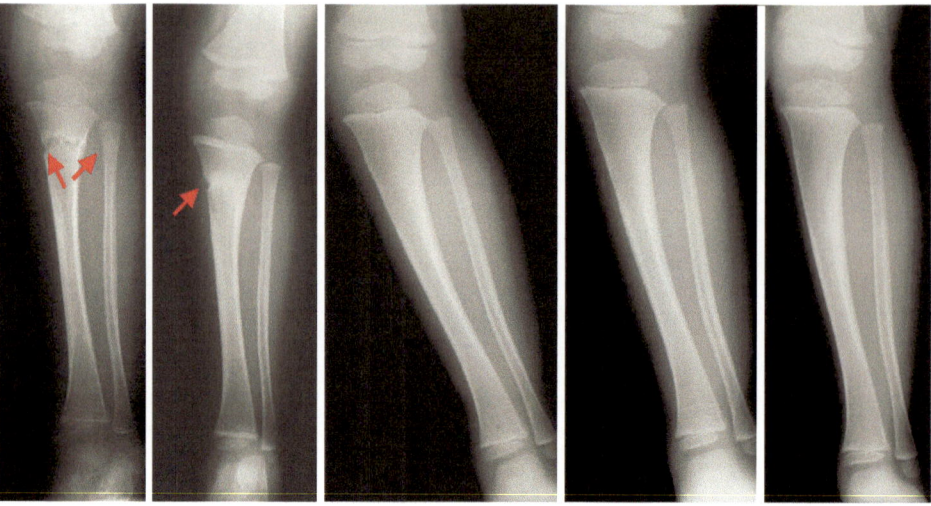

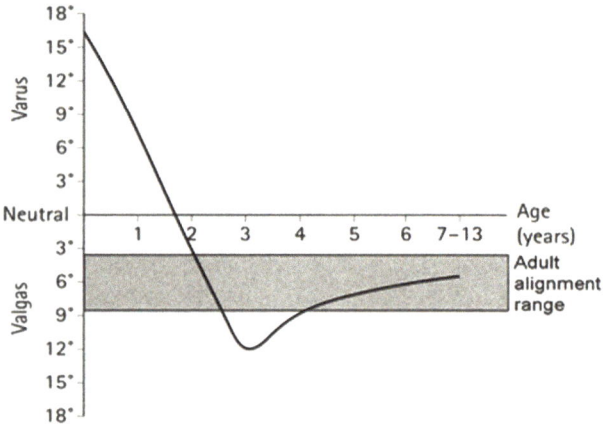

Fig. 8.8 Graph showing normal progression from varus to valgus with age

The etiology of Blount's disease includes increased body weight, level of activity, and angular deformity. The postero-medial corner of the proximal tibial growth plate fails under load and in severe cases the femur may develop a lateral bow. The incidence is estimated at 0.05 per 1000 live births

with variations between populations dependent upon age of walking [29], body mass, and the stage at which surgical correction is undertaken. Satisfactory correction from a single tibial osteotomy is more certain if undertaken by the age of 4 years [30] although the Scandinavian experience is of a more benign condition that can be surgically treated effectively up to the age of 8 years [31]. The internal rotation deformity should also be corrected. Recurrence is likely if a bone bar is missed.

The bone bar or tether can be mapped by magnetic resonance (MR) scanning (see Chapter 41) and should be excised in patients under 10 years of age at the time of osteotomy. After this age corrective osteotomy can be combined with a lateral or complete epiphysiodesis, and in unilateral Blount's disease a contralateral proximal tibial epiphysiodesis will prevent a leg length discrepancy. In severe or late, neglected cases elevation of the medial tibial plateau [32, 33] is achieved with an elevating osteotomy (Fig. 8.11) or using a distraction frame.

Adolescent Blount's disease is usually unilateral and less severe than the infantile form. Pain may precede the deformity and shortening of up to 2 cm develops. Internal tibial

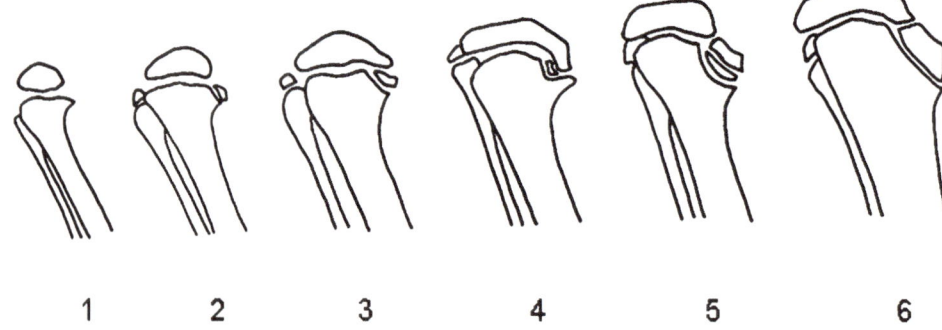

Fig. 8.9 Grades of severity in Blount's disease [26]

1   2   3   4   5   6

Fig. 8.10 The metaphyseal–diaphyseal angle of Levine and Drennan [27] (**a**) Clinical photograph. (**b**) Radiological metaphyseal–diaphyseal angle

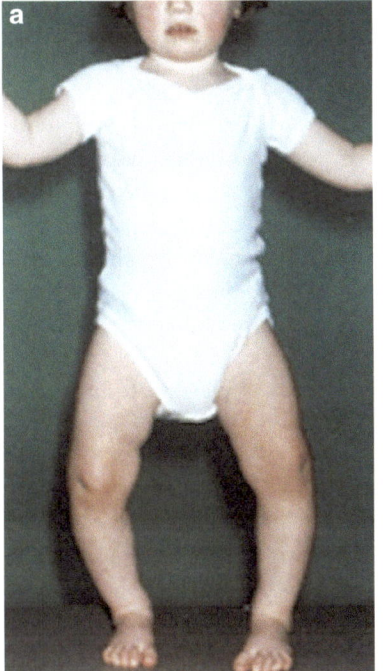
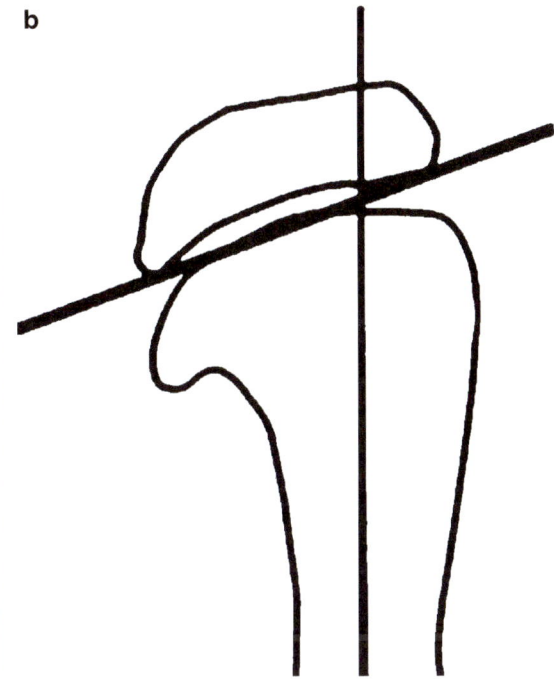

Fig. 8.11 (**a**) MRI showing the unossified medial tibial condyle. (**b**) Pre- and postoperative radiographs of elevation of the medial tibial plateau which is occasionally required in the neglected or recurrent case

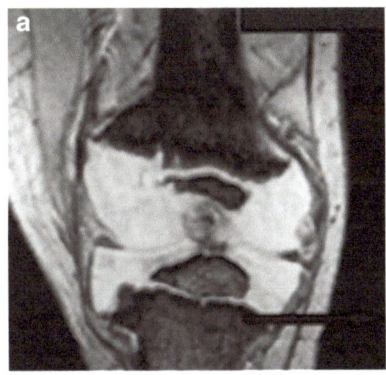
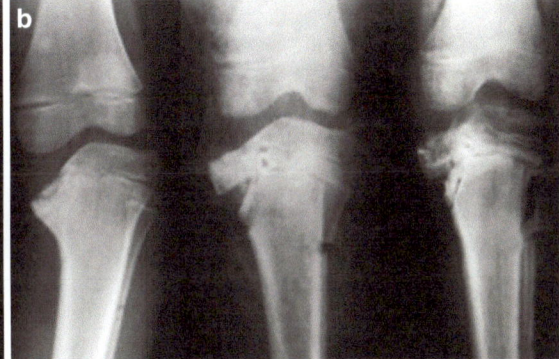

torsion is less obvious and the shape of the tibial epiphysis is relatively normal with no beaking of the medial tibial metaphysis. The proximal tibial and lateral, distal femoral growth plates are widened.

Corrective osteotomy with lateral proximal tibial epiphysiodesis is a reliable means of improving alignment. Leg length discrepancy is prevented by appropriately timed epiphysiodesis above and below the opposite, normal knee joint. Distraction osteogenesis offers an alternative approach [34] with further refinements described by Coogan et al. [35].

A variety of osteotomies have been described (Fig. 8.12):

- Transverse opening or closing wedge [36]
- Inverted arcuate [37]
- Dome or arcuate [38]
- Oblique coronal [39]
- Serrated W–M [40]
- Oblique sagittal [41]
- Spike [42]

Traditionally the dome osteotomy has been popular and is relatively easy to perform [43]. Correction of coronal, sagittal, and axial (rotational) deformities is not possible with the transverse, spike, oblique, and serrated osteotomies. Conventional fixation with Steinmann pins, screws, or plates requires precision, so external fixation may be preferred, allowing alignment to be adjusted postoperatively.

Complications of proximal tibial osteotomy [44] include common peroneal and other nerve deficits, compartment syndrome, laceration of the anterior tibial artery, inaccurate correction, failure of fixation with recurrent deformity, pin site and wound infections, and limb length inequality. The correction of the internal rotation of Blount's disease may

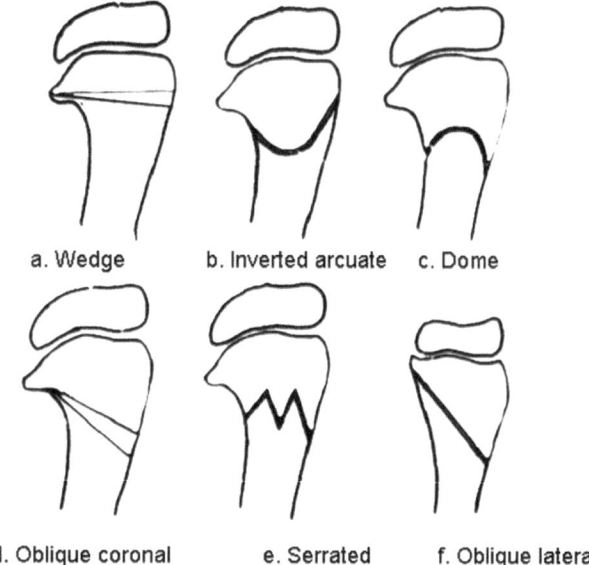

a. Wedge   b. Inverted arcuate   c. Dome

d. Oblique coronal   e. Serrated   f. Oblique lateral

Fig. 8.12 Proximal tibial corrective osteotomies described in the literature

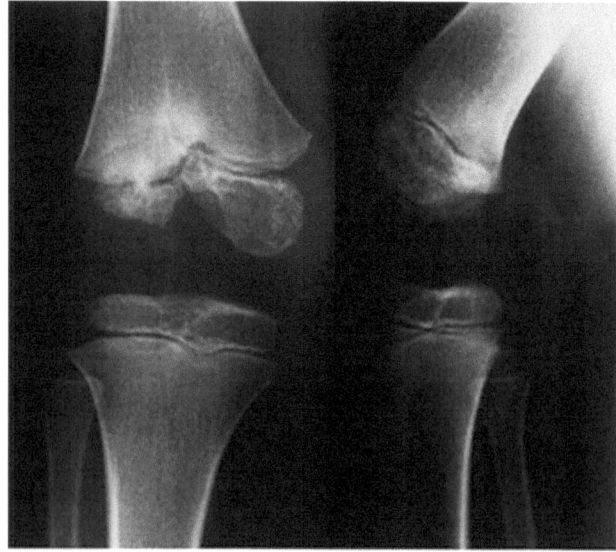

Fig. 8.13 Post-infective knee deformity following meningococcal septicemia

imperil arterial supply at the level of the proximal tibial diaphysis.

Coronal deformity may follow infection (Fig. 8.13) or trauma, nutritional and renal rickets, or skeletal dysplasia, including focal fibrocartilaginous dysplasia which affects the tibia or, very rarely, the femur [45]. Leg lengthening may also increase or produce angulation at the knee.

Anterior Knee Pain

Many of the diagnoses associated with anterior knee pain produce similar symptoms which accounts for the confusion about this condition. Aglietti, Buzzi, and Insall [46] have stressed that there is no single symptom or sign that is in itself diagnostic of patellar pain. There is, however, a pattern of symptoms which are specific for patellar pain and the patella is the usual cause of true "anterior knee pain." The importance of taking a thorough and careful history regarding, for example, the onset and the site of the pain and aggravating factors cannot be over-emphasized. The aim is to make a specific diagnosis in each case and not to lump these patients together as "just anterior knee pain" and untreatable. The onset of symptoms may follow an acute event such as a direct blow on the knee or a twisting injury with minor subluxation of the patella, both resulting in chondral damage and subsequent pain. Often the onset is slow, as a result of over-use such as excessive running. Careful examination will indicate the site of the pain and whether or the lesion is in bone, cartilage, or soft tissue.

It is then helpful to consider the causes of anterior knee pain under the headings "Distinct diagnoses" and "Obscure diagnoses" (see Table 8.1)[47]. The first group is made up of mainly focal pathological lesions, for which logical treatment can be applied and outcome predicted. The second is a spectrum of conditions ranging from anterior knee pain of unknown cause through chondromalacia to dynamic problems of maltracking, subluxation, and excessive lateral pressure. It includes pain referred either from the spine or the hip which must be considered when the examination of the knee is normal.

Table 8.1 Causes of anterior knee pain

Distinct diagnoses	Obscure diagnoses
Overuse	
Osgood–Schlatter's condition	Idiopathic knee pain
Sinding–Larsen–Johansson syndrome	Chondromalacia patellae
Bipartite patella	Maltracking and malalignment
Stress fracture, tendinitis	Shift/tilt and instability
Trauma	Excessive lateral pressure syndrome
Osteochondritis dissecans	Neurogenic pain
Bone bruising	Regional pain syndrome
Meniscal and ligament tears	Referred pain
Syndromes and dysplasias	Psychogenic
Tumors	
Plicae and bursae	
Iatrogenic	
Infrapatellar contracture, e.g., post-ACL reconstruction or patellar realignment	
Scar neuroma	

Distinct Causes of Anterior Knee Pain

Osgood–Schlatter's Condition

This is a condition affecting the young athlete. Pain is situated very precisely over the tibial tuberosity so diagnosis is rarely a problem as patients point exactly to where the pain is. It has been estimated to occur in 21% of athletic children but only in 4% of non-athletes [48]. Boys are more commonly affected between the ages of 13 and 14. In girls the onset is earlier (10–11 years). The cause is repetitive microtrauma at the insertion of the patella tendon into the tibial tuberosity apophysis which, being softer and thus weaker than the normal attachment of tendon to bone (Fig. 8.14), stretches or microfractures the tuberosity, giving rise to the pain. The bone is growing faster than soft tissue and therefore in this condition, tightness of the quadriceps and hamstrings is a feature. The tuberosity will increase in size, resulting in a large bump over the front of the tibia. This can develop into a separate ossicle which may cause persistent pain after skeletal growth ceases, interfering with kneeling and requiring surgical removal at maturity. The most important feature of the pain is that it rapidly settles with rest and never occurs at night. The condition resolves spontaneously when soft tissue growth catches up, usually in 1–2 years. There is really no differential diagnosis but sometimes there is alarm about a possible tumor. A radiograph is a definitive but unnecessary investigation. Ultrasound scanning can relieve anxiety about malignancy.

Treatment consists of reassurance and a policy of allowing activity but letting the child stop when the pain starts. The problem is that these children are often athletically gifted and are under pressure to perform. The importance of a good warm-up and stretching program has recently been appreciated and is very helpful in overcoming muscle tightness, thus reducing symptoms.

Appreciation of the value of a stretching program has rendered the use of casts or bracing obsolete. The application of

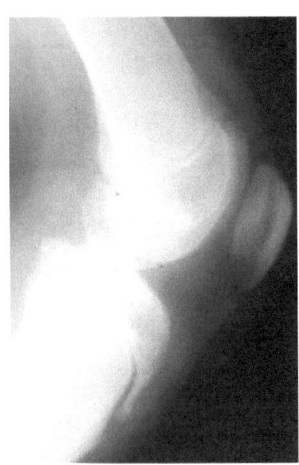

Fig. 8.14 A lateral radiograph of Osgood–Schlatter's condition

an anti-inflammatory, non-steroid gel may relieve local tenderness but is little more than a placebo. Occasionally, an acute flexion injury will avulse part of the tibial tuberosity which must not be confused with Osgood–Schlatter's condition (see Chapter 32).

Sinding–Larsen–Johansson

This occurs in the same age group of children but the point of tenderness and pathology are located at the lower pole of the patella. The lateral radiograph of the patella may be normal or there may be speckled calcification or a small ossicle at the lower pole. It occurs in the same age group and patient population as Osgood–Sclatter's condition and treatment is the same. Acute pain and tenderness following a sudden flexion injury should raise the possibility of a sleeve fracture of the patella when ultrasound is more revealing than a plain radiograph [49] (Fig. 8.15). Both Osgood–Schlatter's and Sinding–Larsen–Johansson conditions are more likely with patella alta.

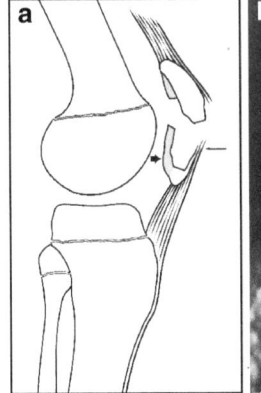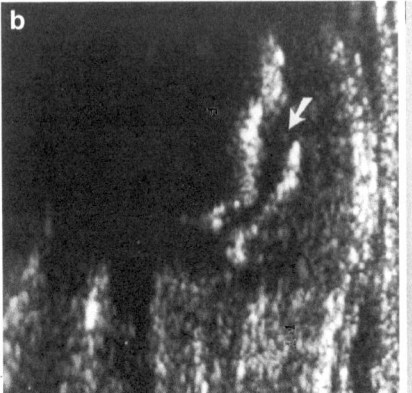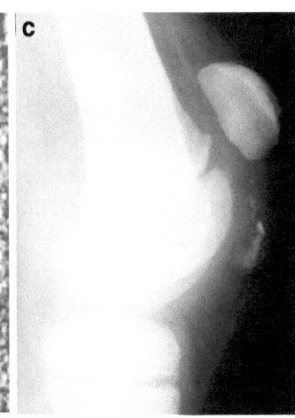

Fig. 8.15 (**a**) Line drawing of a patellar sleeve fracture. (**b**) Ultrasound showing the periosteal sleeve. (**c**) Later radiograph of a missed case showing new bone formation in the sleeve, giving the appearance of a double patella

Bipartite Patella

The patella ossifies from multiple centers. Any of these may persist, failing to fuse. Occasionally they can be painful, probably a form of traction apophysitis in the immature skeleton. By far the most common is the supero-lateral center and traction is from the vastus lateralis. The pain is made worse by squatting. Treatment is as for other traction conditions such as Osgood–Schlatter's disease, employing an effective thigh muscle stretching program until symptoms settle. Very occasionally, a sudden flexion injury can cause avulsion of the fragment in which case reattachment is required to preserve the integrity of the extensor mechanism.

Sleeve Fracture of the Patella

This is a diagnosis which is often missed. It presents as an acutely painful knee after a fall or landing heavily, forcing the knee into flexion. The swelling may be minimal and the only finding is a variable degree of patellar alta and tenderness at the lower pole. Active knee extension is restricted or impossible. The avulsed periosteal sleeve, usually from the lower pole of the patella, is not visible radiographically. Ultrasound is very helpful but an awareness of the possibility of this injury is the most important factor (Fig. 8.15). Open reduction and reattachment of the sleeve is necessary to avoid an extensor lag and the embarrassment of a large bony lump appearing at the lower end of the patella [49].

Stress Fractures of the Patella

Stress fractures of the lower pole of the patella occur in spastic children with flexed knee gait and are a cause of pain and further deterioration in walking [50]. These fractures cannot heal unless steps are taking to correct the fixed flexion deformities of the knees.

Osteochondritis Dissecans

Osteochondritis dissecans is one of the causes of anterior knee pain. The symptoms are initially non-specific and related to activity, not necessarily to the site of the lesion. Rarely, the lesion is on the patella or in the trochlear groove, in which case the pain will be truly anterior.

Males are affected twice as commonly as females. Two distinct types are recognized: the juvenile type which starts before the growth plates fuse, commonly before the age of 12 years, and the adult type starting after the growth plates have fused.

The cause of the lesion is not known. Repetitive trauma is unlikely as the condition is often bilateral and symmetrical. It usually occurs on the lateral side of the medial femoral condyle which is not a site subjected to trauma except perhaps in those with excessive recurvatum which allows the tibial spine to impinge against the femoral condyle more easily (Fig. 8.16).

Transient ischemia of the affected part is another possibility, resulting in an ossification defect which fails to heal [51]. The lesion starts in the subchondral bone and may lead to separation and fragmentation, causing the overlying articular cartilage to split and the fragment to hinge and eventually displace.

The child often walks with an antalgic gait, resisting full extension. In addition to a sensation of catching or of giving way and, later, locking, there may be an effusion and Wilson's sign can be helpful if positive: the knee is flexed to 90°, the tibia is internally rotated and the knee extended. A positive sign is pain felt at the 30° mark when the medial tibial spine impinges against the medial femoral condyle at the classic site. It is relieved by external rotation of the tibia and reproduced again on internal rotation. Often with careful examination, a tender spot at the site of the lesion can be found.

The first investigation should be the four standard radiographic views of the knee, of which the notch or tunnel view is usually the most helpful. A technetium bone scan will assess the presence or absence of hyperemia at the site of the lesion and this has been linked to the likelihood of healing [52].

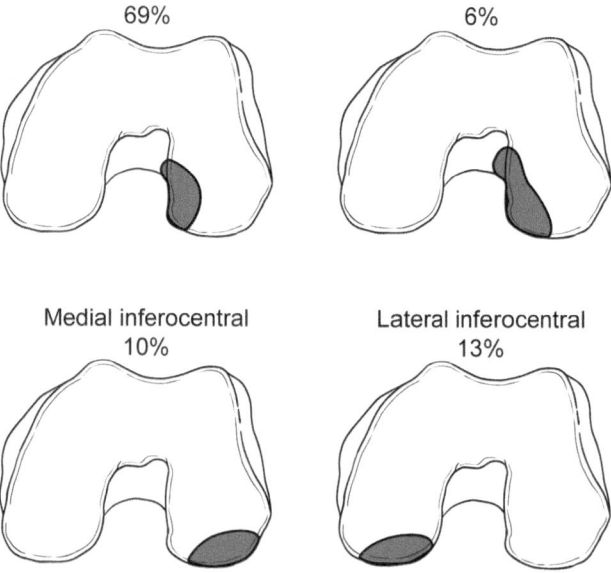

Fig. 8.16 The incidence of osteochondritis dissecans in different positions in the knee [56]

Table 8.2 MRI signs of osteochondritis dissecans (De Smet 1997)

1. A line of high signal intensity > 5 mm long deep to the OCD lesion (T2)
2. An area of homogeneous signal >5 mm in diameter deep to the lesion (T2)
3. A focal defect > 5 mm in the articular surface (T1)
4. A line of high signal crossing the subchondral plate into the lesion (T2)

The biggest advance in the management of this condition has been magnetic resonance imaging (MRI) which has largely replaced isotope bone scanning, especially when combined with arthrography in the form of gadolinium enhancement. De Smet [53] identified four MRI signs, observing that the volume of the area of high signal behind the lesion was the most valuable for predicting outcome (Table 8.2).

The high signal line on T2 and the articular cartilage breach on T1 are the most relevant for predicting healing. The advantage of MRI is that surgical intervention in the form of arthroscopy may be avoided and repeat scans can be used to monitor progress (Fig. 8.17).

The aim of treatment is to promote healing. In the juvenile type, where the growth plates are open, the chances of spontaneous healing are high. Treatment is non-operative with a program of rest followed by graduated activity. This extends for a minimum of 3 months. The initial treatment is rest from all activity using crutches and a brace. Protected weight bearing is allowed. After 6 weeks, if the knee is pain-free and not swollen, the brace is discontinued but protected weight bearing is continued for a further 6 weeks. Physiotherapy can start with a supervised, progressive program of mobilizing exercises and low-impact quadriceps and hamstring strengthening. The child should do this for at least 3 months before adding running, jumping, or side-stepping movements. An MRI showing healing is helpful at this stage.

Arthroscopy is indicated in the older child, or the occasional younger one when symptoms persist for more than 6 months, particularly if there are episodes of locking, sharp pain, and an effusion. Characteristically, there is progression and separation of the lesion with a breach in the articular cartilage.

The lesion is inspected and probed. If stable, drilling with a Kirschner wire often stimulates healing. This can be done retrograde under image intensifier control from a point on the femoral condyle just distal to the growth plate. The arthroscopic guides used for the placement of tunnels in cruciate ligament reconstruction are helpful for accurately drilling into the lesion from the deep surface. Alternatively, transarticular drilling, either open or arthroscopically, is acceptable. If the lesion is unstable but not displaced, it can be held with bone pegs taken from the proximal tibia, with biodegradable pins or using variable thread headless screws (Fig. 8.18).

Debate surrounds the management of the bone fragment when it is almost totally detached or has become loose in the joint. Nearly all affected patients are skeletally mature. Small fragments, less than 1.5 cm in diameter, are probably best removed and the base curetted. Drilling or microfracture with chondral picks stimulates the influx of pluripotential cells into the defect to produce fibrocartilage [54].

Lesions greater than 1.5 cm should be replaced if possible. The base of the defect should again be curetted, drilled, or microfractured (Fig. 8.19). The fragment may need to be trimmed to fit the defect and then fixed as for the stable lesion. The end result must leave a smooth, congruous, or even slightly depressed surface. If an accurate fit is not possible the fragment should be discarded. Treatment of these defects by chondrocyte transplantation is an area where this newer technique may be successful [55].

Rehabilitation must be taken slowly after any of these procedures, with protected weight bearing for at least 9 months.

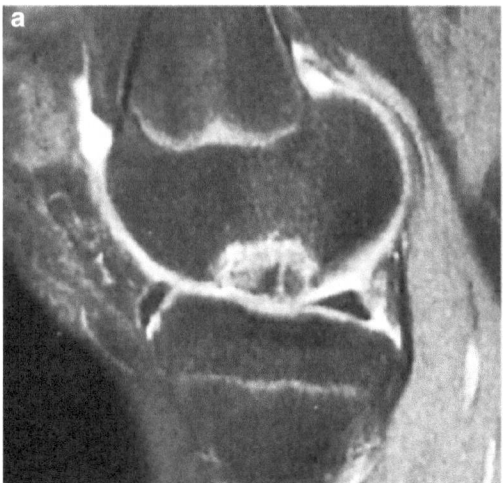
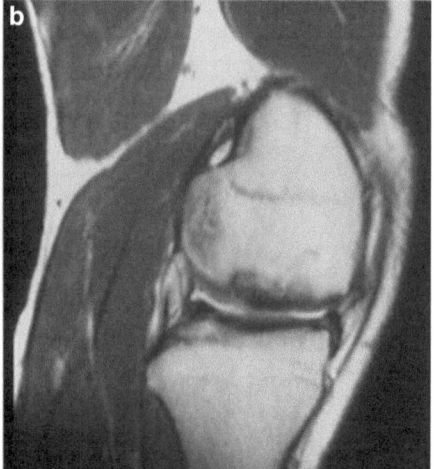

Fig. 8.17 (**a**) T2-weighted MRI showing osteochondritis dissecans of the medial femoral condyle with a line of high signal deep to the lesion. (**b**) T1-weighted MRI of an osteochondritis dissecans lesion in the lateral femoral condyle showing a breach in the articular cartilage

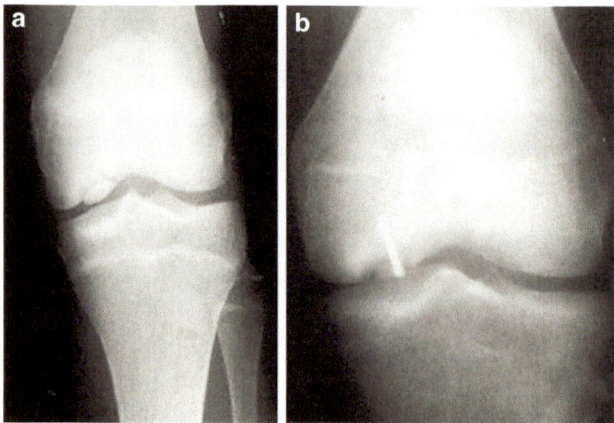

Fig. 8.18 (**a**) An osteochondritis dissecans lesion in the extended classical position in the medial femoral condyle. (**b**) Fixation with a variable thread screw

In summary, the natural history of osteochondritis dissecans depends upon the age of the child at the onset of symptoms. The juvenile type, before skeletal maturity, heals with minimal risk of developing osteoarthritis at 30 years if it is in the classical position. In any other position, osteoarthritis is likely particularly if it involves a weight-bearing surface. Lesions of the lateral femoral condyle appear to do worst but these comprise only 15% of all cases [56]. The adult type does less well and the fragment may not heal, predisposing to osteoarthritis [57]. It is a reasonable estimate to say that the onset of osteoarthritis is accelerated by 10 years.

Bone Bruises

The entity of the bone bruise or contusion was largely theoretical until the advent of MRI which shows bruising very clearly. Following a direct blow or a high-velocity fall, often in association with anterior cruciate and medial collateral ligament injury, the lateral femoral condyle impacts on the posterior tibial plateau as the knee twists. Similarly, acute varus angulation can produce a lateral ligament tear and medial bruising. They are self limiting and no treatment is required apart from protection from similar injuries until the symptoms of pain and possibly swelling have settled.

Reassurance, backed up by a positive MRI, is enough to convince the child and parents of the need to modify activity, usually for about 6 weeks.

Plicae and Bursae

Popliteal Cysts

Popliteal cysts are twice as common in boys and usually present before the child has reached the age of 10 years as an asymptomatic fluctuant swelling just to the medial side of the popliteal fossa. If there is doubt about the cystic nature of the lesion, trans-illumination will settle the issue. This technique is a great deal, less expensive than ultrasound or MRI scanning which is unnecessary. If there is concern about enlargement or a possible diagnosis of villonodular synovitis or chondromatosis, an ultrasound is all that is required. The most common cause is a semi-membranosus bursa which is better felt in extension than in flexion; the knee is otherwise normal. Dinham [58] drew attention to the very high recurrence rate after surgical removal, and the natural tendency of these cysts to disappear spontaneously. Operation without a very good reason is unjustified and reassurance is all that is required.

Plicae

Much has been made of the importance of plicae in knee surgery. The common sites of plicae are well known (Fig. 8.20) and they are very rarely of significance in children. They can cause pain over the medial femoral condyle on squatting especially when thickened in some skeletal dysplasias or inflammatory conditions. They do not cause "snapping" of the knee which in children is due to a discoid meniscus or rarely to the semi-membranosus during flexion.

Ganglion Cysts

Ganglia occur at many sites in the knee. They are found in the substance of the anterior or posterior cruciate ligaments

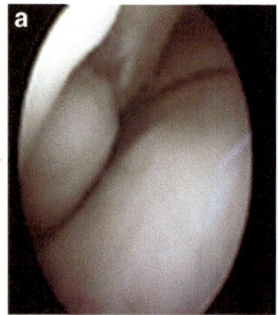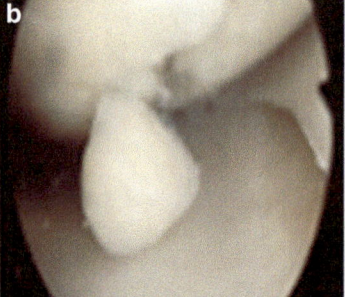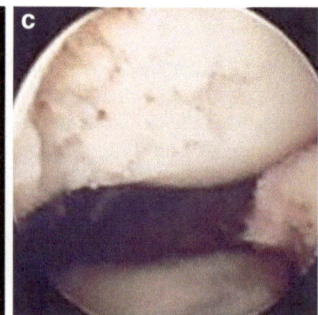

Fig. 8.19 (**a–c**) An osteochondral fragment detached and with an irregular fit; it was removed and the defect treated by microfracturing

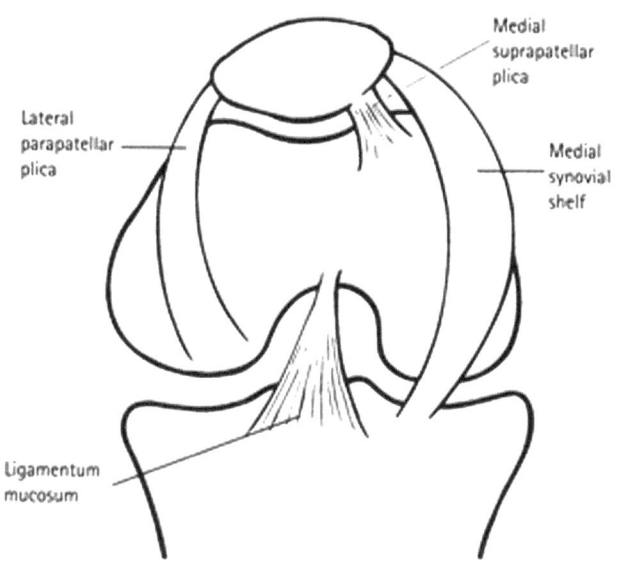

Fig. 8.20 The sites of synovial plicae

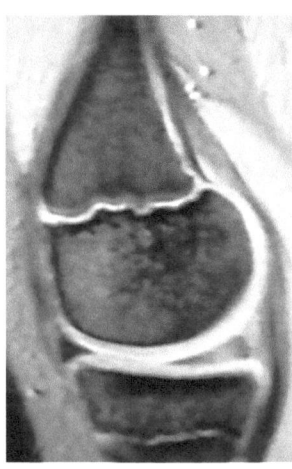

Fig. 8.21 MRI showing a normal bright signal within the posterior horn of the paediatric medial meniscus, potentially mistaken for degeneration or a tear

where they are usually an incidental finding but can cause a deep ache, often confused with anterior knee pain. The most common site is in association with a lateral meniscal radial tear which allows synovial fluid to leak out into the subcutaneous layer. These do occur in adolescence and even younger children and pathologically they are indistinguishable from a ganglion. They are easily palpable, typically when the knee is in extension, and they disappear when the knee is flexed. Treatment is by excising the tear and decompressing the cyst arthroscopically from inside the knee [59].

The real concern is that the diagnosis is correct. Occasionally, the cause of a lump in or around the knee will be pigmented villonodular synovitis, synovial chondromatosis, or even a hemangioma. MRI is then essential before exploring these lesions.

Meniscal Lesions

Meniscal Tears

Meniscal tears in childhood are rare, accounting for 2% of all meniscal tears [60]. The paediatric incidence does appear to be increasing with more participation in contact sports, often combined with anterior cruciate ligament (ACL) rupture [61]. Careful clinical examination will establish the diagnosis but can be difficult if the knee is swollen. MRI has greatly improved the diagnosis but a high signal associated with increased vascularity seen within the substance of the meniscus can resemble mucoid degeneration (Fig. 8.21). It should not be mistaken for a tear, especially at the menisco-synovial junction, or for a hypermobile lateral meniscus.

Arthroscopy still has a place in the diagnosis if the symptoms cannot be accounted for or if the knee is swollen and locked. Meniscal tears in childhood should be treated very conservatively. Minor tears, less than 1 cm long, and partial thickness tears, heal. More extensive tears should be repaired. The increased vascularity and cell population of the meniscus will facilitate healing but the idea that the meniscus can regenerate in childhood is a myth.

McNicholas et al. [62] reviewed clinically 63 adolescents 30 years after open meniscectomy. While 71% said they were satisfied with their knees, 36% had significant joint narrowing. These findings reinforce the earlier views of King [63] and Fairbank [64] who were the first to recognize the importance of the menisci and the relationship between meniscectomy and later osteoarthritis.

Meniscal repair is now an accepted procedure for the appropriate tear. The indications can be extended in children where the increased vascularity, biochemical factors, and histological structure of the meniscus give greater scope for healing. The blood supply of the outer one-third of the meniscus and the concept of red and white zones is attributed to Arnoczky and Warren [65]. They showed that the vascularity of the adult meniscus does not extend more than 5 mm from the menisco-capsular junction. This is the white–white zone and repair will not succeed. Less than 3 mm from the junction is the red–red zone and repair is very likely to succeed. Between 3 and 5 mm is the red–white zone where repairs have a reasonable chance of healing, especially in younger patients [66].

The prime indications for meniscal repair are as follows:

- an unstable longitudinal tear in the red/white zone within 3–5 mm of the rim (tears less than 1 cm long can be expected to heal without suturing)
- an injury less than 8 weeks old
- a patient aged less than 20 years old

- a stable knee (an associated ruptured ACL is an absolute indication for ligament reconstruction)

A variety of techniques for repair are recognized. Open repair was popularized by De Haven and Hales [67]. An arthroscopic inside-out technique was the next to be developed and is still the best tried and most successful (Fig. 8.22). Recently, all-inside techniques using toggle devices and self-tying sutures have been advocated. The results of meniscal repair are still not established although healing rates as high as 75% for the standard inside-out suture repair can be expected [68].

In general terms, preservation of meniscal tissue is the main priority. The place of meniscal allograft in the skeletally immature is not established. It is as yet an unproven procedure [69].

The hypoplastic, hypermobile medial meniscus is an occasional cause of pain with activity, caused by the femoral condyle contacting the tibial plateau in extension. Modification of activity is all that is required.

Discoid Meniscus

The discoid meniscus is a true congenital malformation that occurs in 0.4–5% of the population although the incidence may be as high as 16.6% in the Japanese [70, 71]. It is often bilateral and almost always involves the lateral meniscus although it has been reported, very rarely, in the medial meniscus. Three types have been described by Watanabe [72] and this classification largely determines the treatment:

- Type I Complete: the meniscus is a round disc completely covering the tibial plateau. It has normal attachments and so is stable.
- Type II Incomplete: this is simply a thicker and wider than normal meniscus but leaves some of the tibial plateau uncovered. It also has normal attachments and is stable.
- Type III Wrisberg type: this often causes confusion. It may be complete or incomplete and is distinguishable at arthroscopy by its thickened posterior edge. Its main feature is that it is only attached posteriorly by the Wrisberg ligament and has no attachment to the posterior capsule. So during flexion, the meniscus can move forward and laterally [73] (Fig. 8.23).

The cause is not known. It is a myth that all menisci start as discs and develop into the normal crescent shape [74]. Histologically, there is always some mucoid degeneration which will develop into a horizontal tear making preservation of meniscal tissue, when treated, difficult.

The first indication that a child has a discoid meniscus may come as young as 3 years old. Classically, the knee starts to "clunk" on flexing and extending. It can be dramatic and cause distress although it is not particularly painful. This tends to stop happening as the physiological valgus of the knee decreases, and the child is symptom-free until a tear

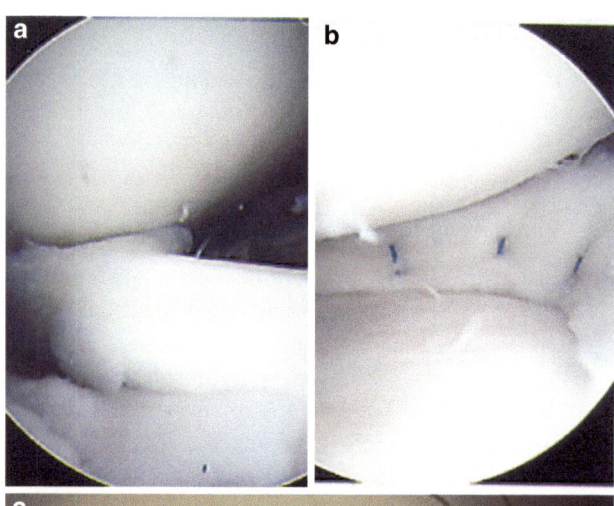
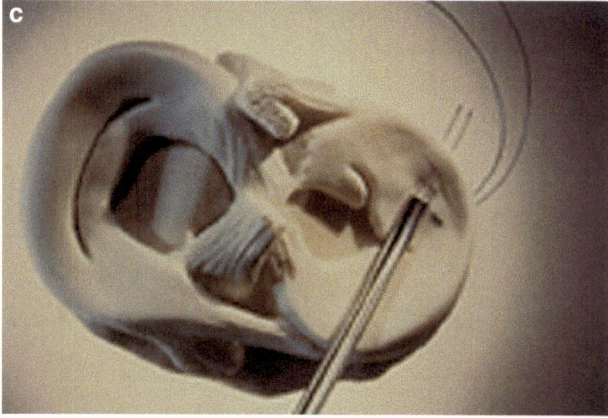

Fig. 8.22 (**a**) A displaced bucket handle tear of the medial meniscus. (**b**) Tear reduced and held with three inside-out sutures. (**c**) The technique of inside-out meniscal repair (courtesy Smith and Nephew)

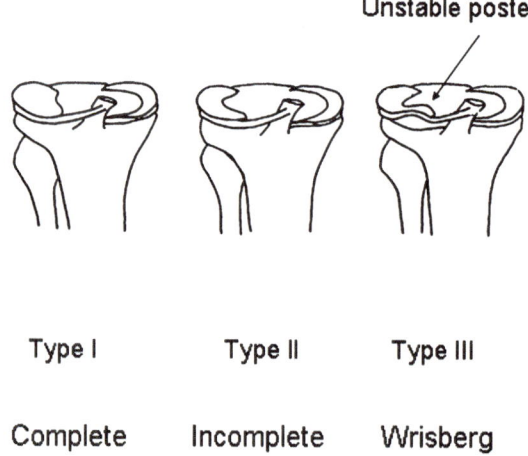

Fig. 8.23 The Watanabe classification of discoid lateral menisci

Fig. 8.24 (**a**) MRI appearances and (**b**) specimen of a discoid torn meniscus

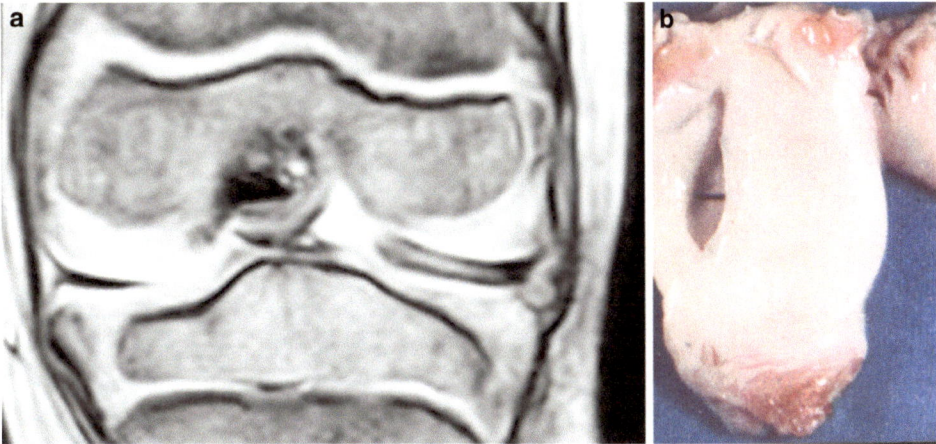

develops or the knee locks due to an unstable meniscus later in childhood or more usually in adolescence.

MRI scan is often diagnostic although a discoid meniscus can be missed (Fig. 8.24). The radiographic appearance is unreliable; widening of the lateral joint space, flattening of the lateral femoral condyle, and cupping of the lateral tibial plateau are not specific.

Management depends upon the type and the degree of symptoms. Treatment of discoid menisci found incidentally on MRI is not justified unless the symptoms are appropriate. At arthroscopy, visualization of the meniscus can be difficult as the lateral compartment is filled with tissue. Probing will reveal a tear but it is the posterior rim which needs to be carefully inspected and probed to test for stability. This will be easier after a tear has been excised. The rim is usually thickened and very mobile, easily pulled into the intercondylar notch or under the femoral condyle. It is then clear there are no posterior capsular attachments. If this is the case a subtotal meniscectomy is still recommended. Attempting to stabilize an unstable posterior horn is hazardous and success is most unlikely. If the meniscus is stable, the tear is excised arthroscopically and the rim saucerized.

While preservation of meniscal tissue is the ideal, the tears are often horizontal and the remaining meniscus is of poor quality. Relatively short-term outcomes at about 5 years are good following total meniscectomy whereas at 20 years most have symptoms and radiographic signs of osteoarthritis [75]. It remains to be seen if partial meniscectomy and repair of the unstable and abnormal meniscal tissue will achieve healing, thus providing some protection and possibly improving this outcome.

Ligament Problems

Congenital absence of the ACL is rare and usually seen only in association with congenital dislocation of the patella or lower limb dysplasias such as congenital short femur or tibia with a hypoplastic fibula and absent lateral rays of the foot [76]. Patients tolerate the instability surprisingly well, but if a leg-lengthening procedure is undertaken deformity and laxity are likely to become worse. Modern bracing techniques can provide an acceptable alternative to reconstruction.

Ligament injury is rare in childhood because the ligaments are stronger than the bones and their attachments blend directly with epiphyseal cartilage or periosteum. The proximal tibial epiphysis is relatively protected by the collateral ligaments which cross the growth plate, whereas at the femur the attachment is to the epiphysis (Fig. 8.25). A severe injury will cause a fracture separation through the lower femoral or, rarely, the upper tibial growth plate in childhood.

A typical injury likely to rupture a ligament in an adult will then result in just a sprain or avulsion of a fragment of cartilage and bone in childhood, for example, avulsion of the tibial spine or a fracture of the tibial tuberosity (Fig. 8.26). Meyers and McKeever [77] classified tibial spine avulsions according to the degree of displacement, stressing the importance of accurate reduction to preserve stability (Table 8.3) (see Chapter 38).

Ligament injuries, including mid-substance rupture of the ACL rather than the more common avulsion of the tibial spine, are increasing in frequency in juveniles [78]. This reflects increased involvement in intense sporting activities. The results of conservative treatment of ACL injuries have the same poor outlook as in adults [79]. Fear of damaging the physis, producing deformity or even growth arrest, is the reason for reluctance to reconstruct ligaments in the immature although increasingly reconstruction is undertaken, particularly if there is a meniscal tear which has been repaired. Extra-articular and non-anatomical reconstructive operations are generally unsatisfactory. A standard hamstring reconstruction drilling across both the tibial and femoral physes, using fixation placed well away

Fig. 8.25 (**a**) The collateral ligaments showing the attachments in relation to the epiphyses. (**b**) The incidence of fracture types and ligament injuries in relation to age

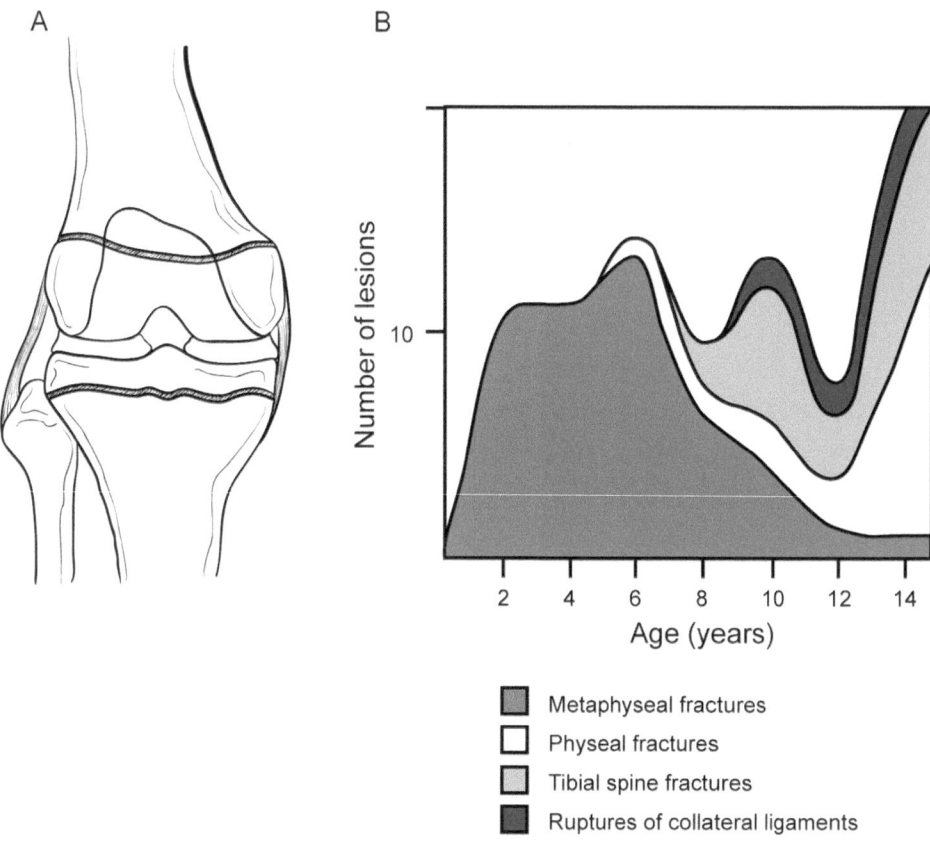

Fig. 8.26 (**a**) Tibial spine avulsion fracture. (**b**) Fragment fixed back with a small cannulated screw

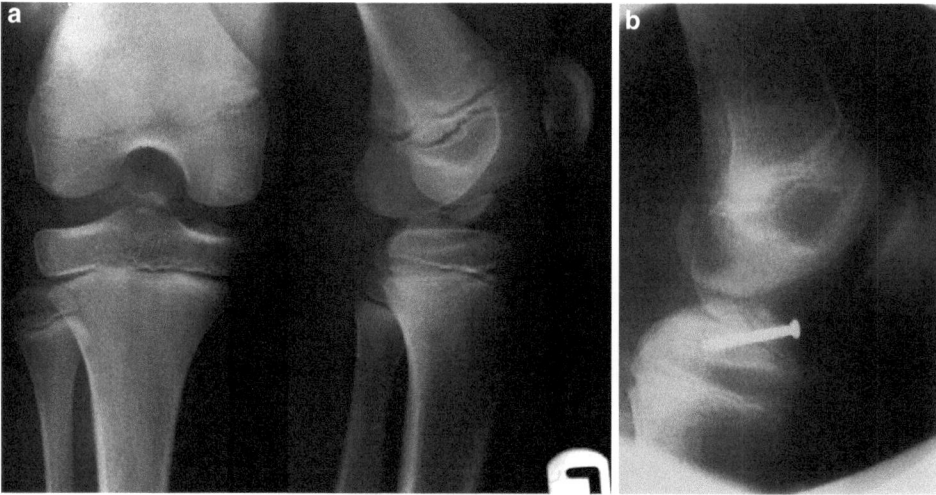

from the growth plate, does seem to be effective and carries a minimal risk of growth disturbance. Reconstruction should only be recommended when there is an appreciable risk of the child sustaining further damage such as a meniscal tear.

A standard four-strand hamstring graft is taken and should fill the tunnel as fully as possible. At arthroscopy, the remnant of the ACL is removed and if the notch is considered narrow, a notchplasty performed. Reconstruction is performed by a standard arthroscopic technique using the same guides as in the adult. The drill holes are made slowly to minimize heating and destruction of tissue at the physis. The holes are cleared of loose bone. A closed loop endobutton is used proximally. The graft is inserted and the button flipped. Distally, a screw placed alongside the graft should not be used as there is a small risk of it crossing the growth plate. A washer and screw placed transversely across the tibia

Table 8.3 Classification of tibial spine avulsion injuries. Meyers and Mckeever [77]

Grade 1. Undisplaced
Grade 2. Partially displaced (up to 50%)
Grade 3. Completely displaced + rotation
Grade 4. Comminuted

is recommended (Fig. 8.27). Postoperatively, a brace may be used but is not essential although it does emphasize the need for gradual rehabilitation. Children will tend to progress too rapidly if the knee feels comfortable.

The complications of this procedure are no different from those of the same procedure in adults. The real concerns are growth disturbance with leg length discrepancy or a valgus deformity caused by tethering. The grafts grow with the child (Fig. 8.28) and reports of growth disturbance are largely anecdotal, usually associated with injudicious placement of a fixation device [80]. If possible, sporting activity should be modified until maturity because of the risk and the consequences of re-rupture. The results are comparable to those in adults but with a slightly higher rate of re-rupture and meniscal tears [81].

Posterior cruciate ligament injuries in childhood are very rare and more likely to be the pull-off or avulsion type accompanied by a bony fragment. This should be reattached back if displaced more than 5 mm or if the tibia drops back markedly. With the increased use of domestic trampolines and participation in extreme sports, mid-substance ruptures are being seen more often. The principle is to delay reconstruction until skeletal maturity and it is unusual for an immature patient to require reconstruction. The drill hole through the tibia is necessarily very close to the back of the tibia at the level of the physis and damage will be more extensive than the more direct tunnel for anterior cruciate reconstruction. The risk of growth disturbance is therefore much greater and not justified in most cases [82].

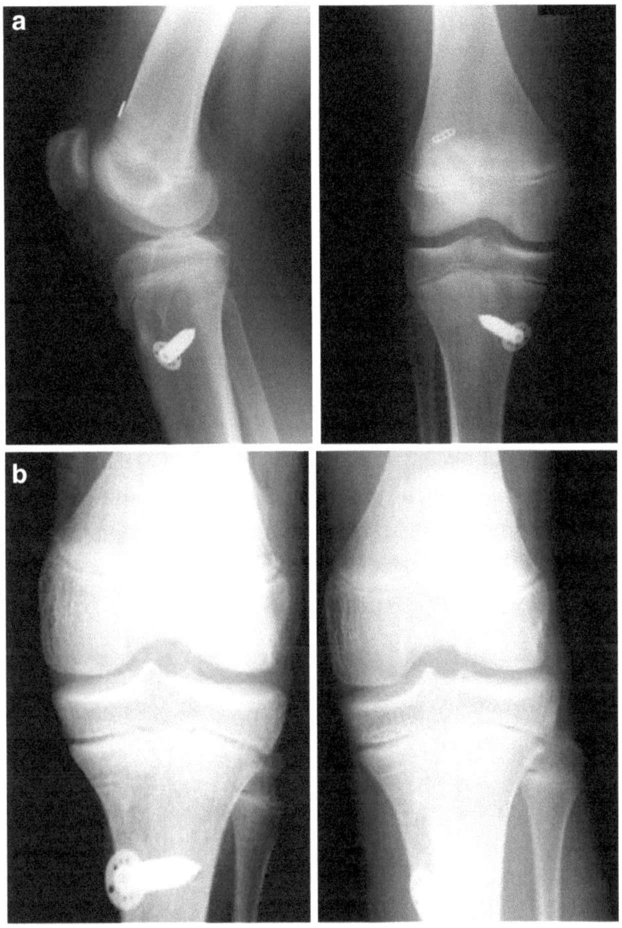

Fig. 8.28 (**a**) Immediate postoperative radiograph. (**b**) The same view, 2 years later, showing considerable growth of the whole graft length

Multiple ligament injury associated with a dislocated knee is fortunately very rare in children. A conservative approach should be adopted with good results being obtained using simple plaster cast immobilization following reduction.

Other Distinct Causes

There are a number of other diagnoses which cause knee pain which are rare in children and so not appropriate for inclusion in this chapter. These are patellar tendinitis (jumper's knee), quadriceps tendinitis, and Hoffa's fat pad syndrome. A foreign body such as glass or a needle, or a neuroma, causes knee pain, which is usually, but not always, obvious from the history. Other causes of pain which are covered elsewhere in this book include bone tumors which have a predilection for the region of the knee (Chapter 14) and skeletal dysplasias (Chapter 7 and Chapter 8). Bone and joint infection and inflammatory arthritis are also common in the knee and are covered in Chapter 10 and 13, respectively.

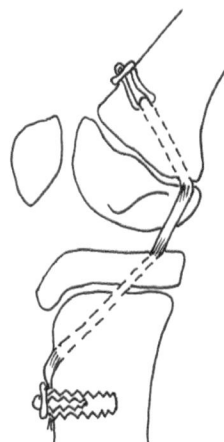

Fig. 8.27 Line drawing of transphyseal anterior cruciate ligament reconstruction in a child

Obscure Causes of Anterior Knee Pain

Idiopathic Knee Pain

This is knee pain for which no distinct cause can be found. It is most commonly associated with malalignment with or without chondral damage and is known as chondromalacia. The two conditions are often related. Anterior knee pain is specific. It is an aching pain, felt over the medial side of the patella, which is made worse by loading the joint such as going up stairs or after prolonged sitting. It causes catching, crepitus, or even locking in extension.

In a deep squat, up to 17 times the body weight is loaded through the patella. Additionally, the patella bears the brunt of overuse or repetitive stressing so it is not surprising that pain is common, occurring in 15% of army recruits [83].

Malalignment

The terms malalignment, maltracking, and patella instability are often used loosely and interchangeably to describe patellofemoral problems with or without pain. This leads to confusion. Each needs to be defined and used specifically. Malalignment is a description of lower limb morphology which results in excessive compression of the patella in the trochlea groove. It occurs with varus or valgus knees, recurvatum, persistent femoral anteversion, compensatory external tibial torsion, and patella alta. A feature is an increased Q angle, a consequence of internal torsion of the femur compensated for by external torsion of the tibia as the child grows. It is measured by dropping a line from the anterior superior iliac spine to the center of the patella and then from the center of the patella to the tibial tuberosity (Fig. 8.29). Although normally less than 10°, it is not an indicator of maltracking which can occur with or without malalignment. It is also a poor indicator of patellar instability. An unstable patella can occur in the presence of malalignment, maltracking, or both. It can also occur in the absence of both. It is perfectly possible for a normally aligned, normally tracking patella to dislocate although this is usually a significantly traumatic event. It is of no surprise that there is confusion about the terminology used in this condition.

Recurvatum, genu valgum, femoral anteversion, and increased Q angle are as common in patients without symptoms as they are in those with pain. Malalignment is, however, a cause of anterior knee pain when there is tightness of the quadriceps and hamstrings and when femoral anteversion and an increased Q angle are combined [84]. There has been no proven connection between forefoot pronation or valgus flat foot and anterior knee pain.

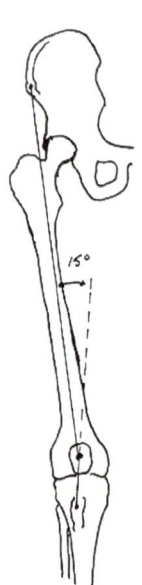
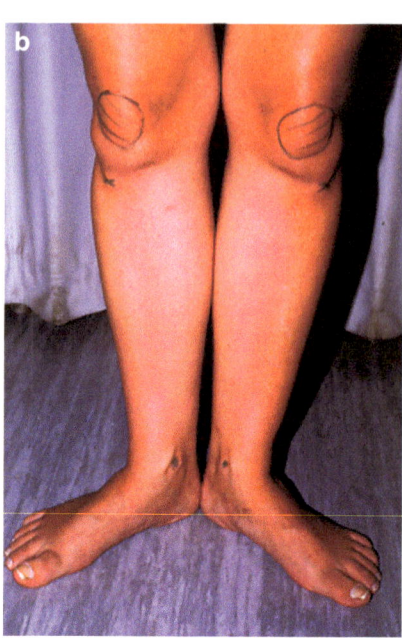

Fig. 8.29 (**a**) The Q angle. The angle between line from the superior iliac spine to the center of the patella and from the center of the patella to the tibial tuberosity. (**b**) An increased Q angle as a result of compensatory lateral tibial torsion for persistent femoral anteversion causing intoeing in childhood

Maltracking

This refers, again specifically, to a patella that fails to track symmetrically in the femoral trochlear groove during flexion and extension. This phenomenon has been extensively studied by Fulkerson [85]. He introduced the concept of "subluxation" and "tilt" of the patella (Figs. 8.30 and 8.31). This is measured on a simple sky-line patellar radiograph in 30° of flexion or in extension on a computed tomography (CT) cut. Shift alone, tilt alone, and a combination of both occur and treatment should be directed specifically to treating which of these is present.

Maltracking in extension is almost always lateral and can be demonstrated on clinical examination. The patient, sitting on the edge of a couch, extends the knee against gravity and, as the patella disengages from a position of stability in the trochlear groove, it shifts laterally. This physical sign is usually seen as the knee extends from 20° of flexion to full extension, and may be associated with and inhibited by pain. It may also be seen by simply asking the patient to contract the quadriceps with the knee extended when the patella will jump laterally, sometimes known as the "inverted J" sign. The confusion with this pattern of maltracking is that when mild it may be a cause of anterior knee pain and the skyline view will be normal; when more severe it can cause recurrent dislocation of the patella, especially in childhood and

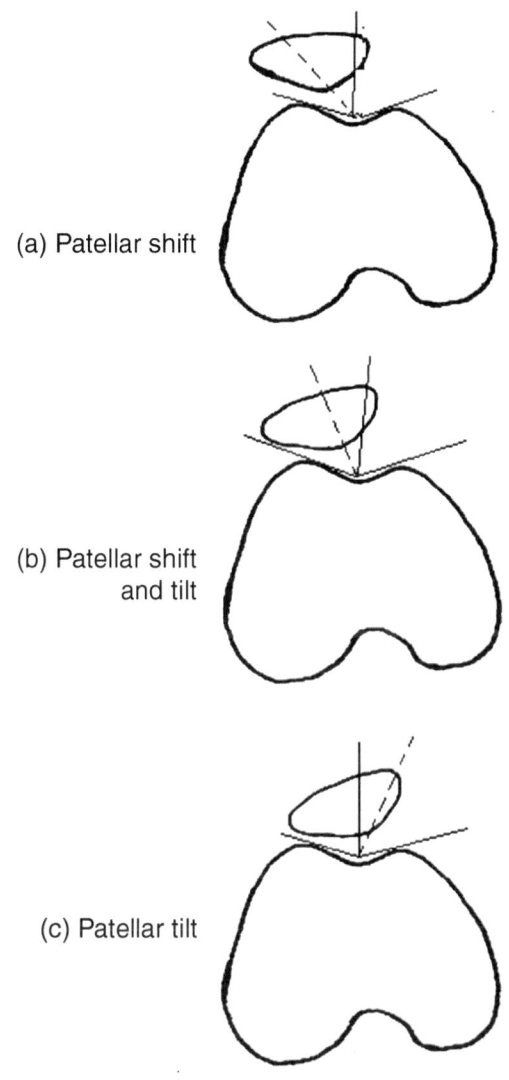

(a) Patellar shift

(b) Patellar shift
and tilt

(c) Patellar tilt

Fig. 8.30 Patellar shift and tilt

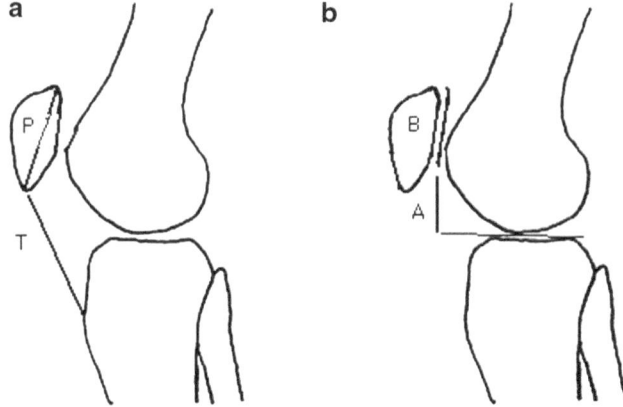

Fig. 8.31 (**a, b**) Measurements of patellar height

adolescence. At its most extreme, the patella dislocates laterally in extension, relocating on flexing the knee. It is caused by quadriceps tightness. The lateral retinaculum may or may not be tight. Again, the skyline view may be normal but there is likely to be some evidence of either tilt or subluxation or even both. There will often be patella alta on a lateral view. Associated femoral anteversion and an increased Q angle are incidental and not diagnostic.

Maltracking in flexion is difficult to see clinically but, by definition, present on the skyline view. The usual finding is lateral tilt, due to a tight lateral retinaculum. It is often a cause of lateral patellar pain but if severe and in the hypermobile, it can cause dislocation in flexion.

Patellar Dislocation and Instability

The anatomical relationship of the patella to the femoral sulcus or trochlea is complex, extension producing contact between the lower pole of the patella and the trochlea, and flexion a deeper engagement with the upper pole. Static soft tissue restraints include the medial patellofemoral ligament which contributes 60% of medial stability [86], the lateral fascial superficial oblique and deep transverse (lateral patellar ligament) components of the retinaculum, and the patellar inferior pull which may be compromised by patella alta and lateral condylar "conflict" or abnormal impingement. Medial patellomeniscal and lateral patellotibial ligaments are also recognized.

Dynamic control is achieved by the vastus medialis oblique muscle which works in tandem with the medial patellofemoral ligament and further contributions from the remaining components of the quadriceps mechanism. With a history of patellar subluxation or dislocation there is a 50% likelihood of further episodes of instability; after acute dislocation the risk of further maltracking is approximately one in five. The presence of ligament laxity, lower limb torsional abnormalities (Chapter 2), increased Q angle, and patella alta worsen the prognosis, as do overt maltracking, patellar tilt, and apprehension (Figs. 8.29, 8.30, and 8.31).

Imaging of the knee in the older adolescent includes:

1. Radiographic views:

   a. anteroposterior (osteochondral lesions/ loose bodies and lateral femoral condylar lesions)
   b. lateral (patella alta, trochlea dysplasia) (Fig. 8.31).
   c. skyline (taken in 30–40° of flexion, with or without weight-bearing stress, to show subluxation or tilting of the patella and the congruence angle, trochlear dysplasia, and other patellofemoral relationships in largely static positions) (Fig. 8.30).

2. MR scans (bone bruising, chondral defects, avulsed osteochondral fragments, the medial patellofemoral ligament, and further morphological details of the patellofemoral joint).
3. CT scans (axial views are preferred to potentially misleading sagittal images and depict the tibial tubercle–trochlear groove offset [87] (Fig. 8.32) and the rotational profile of the lower limb).

Soft tissues procedures include percutaneous or open, extra-articular lateral release, medial retinacular imbrication or medial patellofemoral ligament reconstruction, and V–Y quadricepsplasty for severe patella alta with habitual dislocation or congenital knee dislocation. Habitual or obligatory lateral dislocation occurs every time the knee flexes. The condition is a manifestation of a shortened quadriceps mechanism, often in association with genu valgum. Tension along the anterior structures causes the patella to sublux or dislocate laterally repeatedly. With time the intrinsic stability of the patella is lost as it becomes increasingly dysplastic and the sulcus flattens laterally. The pathological anatomical changes are comparable to the progressive deformity of untreated developmental dysplasia of the hip.

Arthroscopic lateral release may prove sufficient although other augmentation procedures are usually indicated. Distally, a patellar tendon medialization by the Roux–Goldthwaite procedure or alternative soft tissue realignment is effective for lateral dislocation in extension (Fig. 8.33). Very occasionally, proximal or distal femoral rotational osteotomy is necessary but skeletal procedures such as

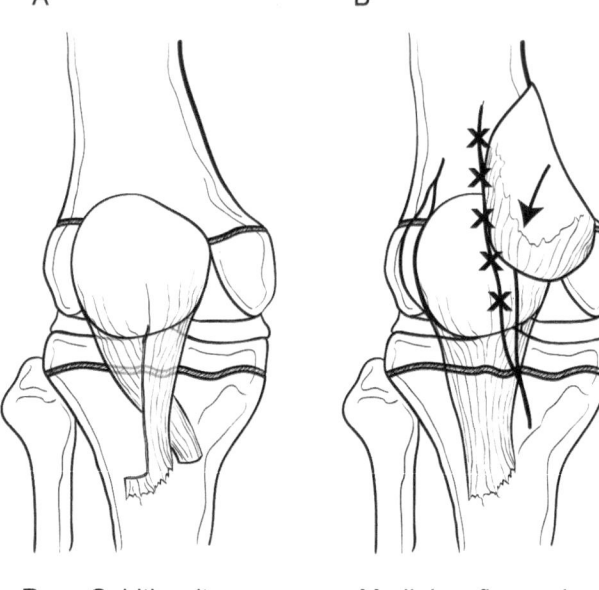

A B

Roux-Goldthwaite
split patellar tendon
medial transfer

Medial reefing and
lateral release

Fig. 8.33 (**a**) The Roux–Goldthwaite procedure is safe and generally effective in the older child or adolescent. (**b**) Lateral release and medial reefing for post-traumatic recurrent dislocation. Note cutting off of top of Roux-Goldthwaite

trochleoplasty or tibial tubercle transfer should not be undertaken until the end of growth.

Unfortunately, most interventions do not retard the degenerative changes which follow chronic patellofemoral instability. Osteoarthritis may take more than 5 years to develop but the condition tends to progress, perhaps offering some patellar stability with time. Microfracturing or drilling of cartilage defects and chondral grafting do not have a role in patellofemoral instability syndromes during childhood. In osteochondritis dissecans, however (see above), there is a place for these techniques.

Excessive Lateral Pressure Syndrome

This is a consequence of maltracking and a tight lateral retinaculum, causing excessive wear on the lateral facet of the patella. It is a very specific and identifiable cause of anterior knee pain.

Chondromalacia Patellae

Chondromalacia patellae remain a difficult subject. It is helpful to remember that it is a physical sign and not a symptom or a diagnosis in itself although it is commonly used as

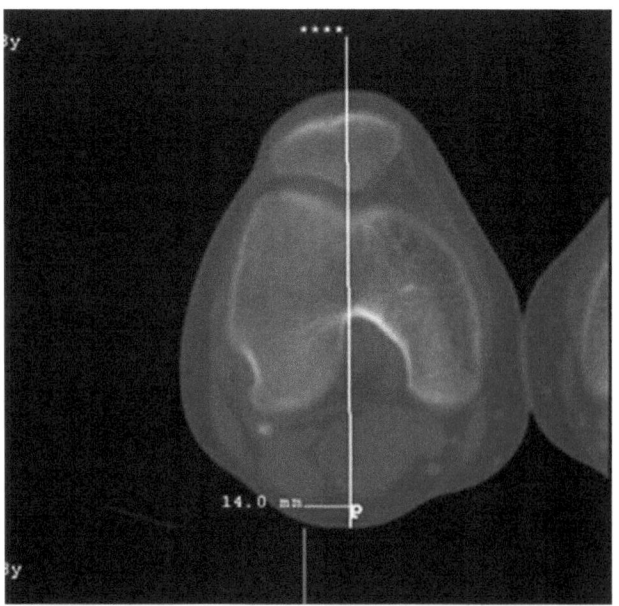

Fig. 8.32 A CT scan showing the tibial tubercle-trochlear groove "offset," a predisposing factor for patellar instability if greater than 15 mm

such. It describes softening of the articular cartilage, recognized by crepitus on compression of the patella against the femur or pain when the quadriceps are contracted while the examiner's index finger is held across the insertion into the upper pole of the patella as in Clarke's test. The confusion is because it has multiple causes which may be idiopathic, post-traumatic, or secondary to maltracking or malalignment. The term describes a pathological lesion of articular cartilage, which when mild may be reversible, but when severe merges with osteoarthritis. As chondromalacia is most often seen in the medial facet of the patella and osteoarthritis on the lateral it is concluded that the one does not necessarily lead to the other. As with osteoarthritis the symptoms are not always proportional to the macroscopic appearance. Standard radiographs may appear normal but MRI scanning is the most useful test and can show the changes well.

Management

Treatment of all the conditions giving rise to obscure anterior knee pain should be conservative. This means physiotherapy and, where there is overuse, activity modification. Physiotherapy consists initially of a comprehensive stretching program for the quadriceps, hamstrings, iliotibial band, and lateral retinaculum. This will include patellar mobilizations. Then isometric and inner range strengthening exercises are added, concentrating on the inner quadriceps and vastus medialis obliquus. Taping, the use of a patellar brace and foot orthoses can all be tried for symptomatic relief but the results are variable. This regimen will be successful in 80% [88]. In the remaining 20%, arthroscopic irrigation may prove beneficial. The patella is inspected and tracking can be further assessed by flexing and extending the knee while examining the patella. Tracking is best seen from a lateral suprapatellar portal.

The modified Outerbridge classification is used to record the damage to the articular surface of the patella [89]:

* Grade I: "closed disease": the articular surface is intact. There may be a slightly blistered appearance or a soft bulky feel when the area is probed with a hook.
* Grade II: "open disease": the probe will now reveal fibrillation and fissures that may or may not be obvious at first sight.
* Grade III: wide spread fibrillation or "cauliflower" appearance.
* Grade IV: the fibrillation is full thickness and erosive changes extend down to the bone which may be exposed.

The size of the lesion should also be recorded using the hook of the probe as a measure.

When there is a definite diagnosis such as excessive lateral pressure syndrome, surgery directed toward correction of this is indicated if physiotherapy has failed. In this instance, there will always be tilt, with or without subluxation. The lateral retinaculum is tight and lateral release may be effective. It should be stressed that the indications for lateral release are very few and it must only be undertaken when there is tilt. It can be done open or arthroscopically but an adequate release must be performed to allow the lateral border of the patella to be elevated perpendicular to the trochlea by the end of the procedure.

Neuropathic Pain

Children with chronic or recurrent pain often locate their symptoms to the knee [90]. The commonest conditions causing pain are post-traumatic or post-surgical peripheral neuropathic pain such as a scar neuroma, complex regional pain syndromes types 1 and 2, and neuropathic pain due to a nerve tumor.

The diagnosis of a scar neuroma is usually straightforward. It is then strictly a "distinct diagnosis" but it is not a cause of knee pain, hence its inclusion as an "obscure diagnosis." Scars around the knee are often complicated by areas of numbness as cutaneous nerves are difficult to avoid and so neuromas in the scars also occur. The management is the same as for any neuroma with the use of local anesthetic patches to confirm the diagnosis and excision if troublesome (see Chapter 23: Part II).

Similarly, nerve tumors are a distinct diagnosis but are included as they may present as knee pain. There may be a palpable tumor which can be confused with a popliteal cyst or ganglion. Very occasionally a glomus tumor is responsible so this emphasizes the importance of a neurological examination in the assessment of knee pain. These unusual causes of knee pain need to be considered before a generic diagnosis of anterior knee pain is made and no treatment offered.

Complex Regional Pain Syndrome

Complex regional pain syndrome (CRPS) incorporates the previous name of reflex sympathetic dystrophy (RSD) and causalgia or neurogenic pain. CRPS type I is RSD and type II is causalgia [91]. Type I comprises a characteristic, spontaneous pain with the sensations of burning, hypersensitivity, and paresthesia. The limb is cold, mottled, and swollen with waxy skin. There is muscle wasting and stiffness. In type

II, all the above are present but there is also evidence of peripheral nerve damage.

CRPS does occur in children. Recent awareness of this has led to earlier diagnosis and more successful treatment [92]. It is very rare under the age of 6 years, commonly affects the lower limb, and is six times more frequent in girls. This is different from adults where the ratio is more equal.

The usual treatment of antidepressants, sympathetic blockade or local anesthetic, and corticosteroid injections are unpredictable in children. The potential for recovery is much better than in adults and a rehabilitation program of physiotherapy combined with cognitive behavioral therapy can be very successful.

The Swollen Knee

The acutely swollen knee may be a manifestation of a range of conditions, foremost of which will be infection. This raises the question of aspiration and even exploration as an emergency. Children are prone to fall on their knees and whereas metallic foreign bodies such as needles or glass are obvious on radiograph, penetrating pieces of wood and other radiographically less obvious material may be present. In the acute stage, air may be seen within the joint, and this can give a clue to the depth of the injury. An acute and transient synovitis is quite common in the juvenile knee as a response to trauma, especially if there is joint laxity. The possibility of a missed patellar dislocation with spontaneous relocation should always be remembered.

Synovial chondromatosis in childhood is extremely rare and when it does occur there may be hundreds of tiny cartilaginous "rice particles" within the knee [93]. As these loose bodies are not ossified, the diagnosis will not be made radiologically but by MRI. The multiple, tiny loose bodies must all be washed out; repeat arthroscopy is sometimes required.

Pigmented villo-nodular synovitis is an inflammatory process of unknown cause, although an auto-immune reaction seems likely. The knee is painful, swollen, and stiff. Locking and crepitus may be present if the synovial proliferation is exuberant. The synovium is brown, thickened, and nodular. Subchondral erosions develop secondary to the release of proteolytic enzymes, and these erosions are seen on both sides of the joint. Histological examination reveals multinucleate giant cells and deposits of hemosiderin, which gives the tissue its color. The treatment is arthroscopic synovectomy.

Septic arthritis, an important cause of a swollen knee, must be recognized and drained early if permanent damage and stiffness are to be minimized. The diagnosis depends upon the history, the appearance of the child who is pyrexial and unwell, and a swollen and tender knee that is too painful to move. Immuno-deficiency and sickle cell disease should not be forgotten, and the vaccination history should be checked. The initial radiograph is usually unhelpful, but may show a pre-existing osteomyelitic focus. Late in the disease, articular changes may become apparent.

Arthroscopy offers a most effective method of obtaining synovial fluid and tissue for bacteriological culture and histological review. The joint can be thoroughly inspected and irrigated, and the procedure avoids the greater morbidity of arthrotomy. Arthroscopy should be repeated every 2 days until the knee is no longer swollen and the serum markers of infection are normal. Although at first the knee should be splinted and the child rested in bed, gentle movement of the knee and protected weight bearing should then be encouraged. Systemic antibiotics remain the mainstay of early treatment, depending upon the culture and the sensitivity of the organisms identified. *Staphylococcus aureus* remains the most common organism. Effective initial cover for both staphylococci and streptococci would be flucloxacillin 200 mg/kg per day (given as four equal doses) and ceftriaxone 80 mg/kg per day (see Chapter 10).

Chronic swelling of the knee suggests low-grade inflammation, such as tuberculosis or juvenile arthritis. When faced with a knee that is warm, boggy, and intermittently swollen in a child, it is important to obtain a family history and to examine the child completely. All other joints should be assessed for reduced range of movement and synovitis. A paediatric rheumatology opinion is essential. Surgical intervention, even in the form of arthroscopy, should be resisted as it is likely to make the joint stiffer. This can cause difficulty if there is a question of infection but the chronic nature of the swelling, the thickening of the synovium, and a very high C-reactive protein (CRP) in the absence of fever are against the diagnosis of infection.

The acute, traumatic, swollen knee in children is as likely to be associated with pathology as it is in the adult (Fig. 8.34). A hemarthrosis may be due to an avulsion or shear fracture of articular cartilage with or without a bony fragment attached. Mid-substance rupture of the anterior cruciate and, rarely, the posterior cruciate ligament are being increasingly diagnosed [63].

Psychogenic Pain

A sensitive knee, in the absence of the signs of chronic regional pain syndrome, swelling, or appropriate trauma, can be the site of pain of psychological origin. It tends to occur in early adolescence and the symptoms are out of proportion to the history which may not even include trauma. The child limps badly or may even be in a wheelchair. School avoidance, depression, anxiety, and family dysfunction are

Fig. 8.34 The causes of hemarthrosis in a child

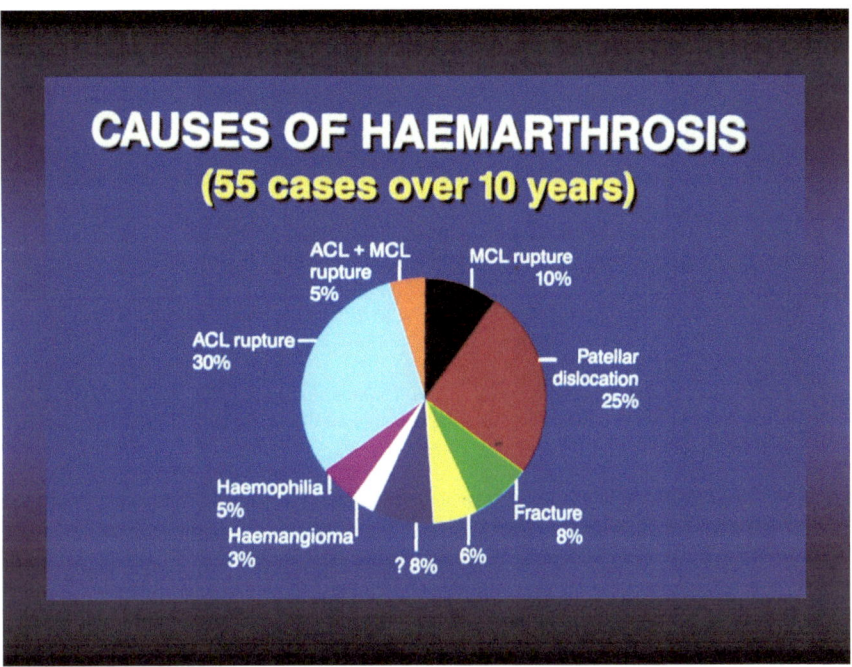

all causes. There may be excessive pressure on a child to perform. A thorough history and examination are vital to be absolutely sure there is no physical cause. Examination may yield important clues. There may be a different range of movement of joints when examined lying down rather than standing up. The limp may disappear when the child walks backward or the child may not be able to do so. The child may stand on the leg when still but avoid taking weight when walking and will resist all attempts to examine the joint although it may appear normal to inspection. There may, rarely, be artifactual marks of self abuse. Once a physical cause is excluded physiotherapists, paediatricians, and psychologists with an interest in this range of conditions can be very successful in treating these children with a combination of physiotherapy, cognitive behavioral therapy, and video feedback.

Tumors

Tumors in childhood (see Chapter 14) show a predilection for the knee, perhaps because the knee is frequently injured. One should therefore have a low threshold for requesting radiographs, especially when the history is short and there is no clear precipitant of the symptoms. As cancer is the second most common cause of death in childhood, bone and soft tissue tumors are of considerable concern particularly as their presentation may be mistaken for other conditions.

Gebhardt et al. reviewed 1999 cases of tumors affecting the knee in childhood and found that knee neoplasia was more common the older the child [94]. Benign bone tumors

comprise 50% of referrals and the most common lesion is the osteochondroma, which can cause a variety of problems. A large posterior swelling will limit knee flexion, whereas medial and lateral excrescences can be the cause of snapping knee and attrition of the hamstring tendons. Multiple lesions may be associated with a growth disturbance and consequent knee deformity of a degree that requires correction. Large lesions may be painful because they are always being knocked during games.

The risk of limb angulation secondary to the osteochondroma is probably not more than 1% and not in itself is considered a reason for excision. Other lesions in decreasing order of frequency are non-ossifying fibroma, chondroblastoma, osteoid osteoma, aneurysmal bone cyst, giant cell tumor, chondromyxoid fibroma, simple bone cyst, and fibrous dysplasia. Osteosarcoma and Ewing's tumor are the principal malignant tumors, and infiltrative conditions such as leukemia and histiocytosis X can occasionally affect the knee. Soft tissue tumors should always be considered as potentially malignant but, fortunately, they are rare and easy to distinguish from popliteal and meniscal cysts.

References

1. Macnicol MF. The Problem Knee, 2nd edition. Oxford: Butterworth Heineman; 1995:8–13.
2. Jacobsen K, Vopalecky F. Congenital dislocation of the knee. Acta Orthop 1985; 7:194–9.
3. Curtis BH, Fisher RL. Congenital hyperextension with anterior subluxation of the knee: surgical treatment and long-term observations. J Bone Joint Surg [Am] 1969; 51A:255–8.

4. Parsch K, Ultrasound diagnosis of congenital knee dislocation. Orthopade. 2002 Mar, 31(3):306–7

5. Katz MP, Grogono BJS, Soper KC. The etiology and treatment of congenital dislocation of the knee. J Bone Joint Surg [Br] 1967; 49B:112–20.

6. Curtis BH, Fisher RL. Heritable congenital tibiofemoral subluxation: clinical features and surgical treatment. J Bone Joint Surg [Am] 1970; 52A:1104–14.

7. Ferris BD, Jackson AM. Congenital snapping knee (habitual anterior subluxation of the tibia in extension) J Bone Joint Surg [Br] 1990; 72B:453–6.

8. Pappas AM, Anas P, Toczylowski HM. Asymmetrical arrest of the proximal tibial physis and genu recurvatum deformity. J Bone Joint Surg [Am] 1984; 66A:575–81.

9. Moroni A, Pezzuto V, Pompili M, Zinghi G. Proximal osteotomy of the tibia for the treatment of genu recurvatum in adults. J Bone Joint Surg [Am] 1992; 74A: 577–86.

10. Bowen JR, Morley DC, McInverny V, MacEwen GD. Treatment of genu recurvatum by proximal tibial closing-wedge anterior displacement osteotomy. Clin Orthop 1983; 179:194–9.

11. Choi JH, Chung CY, Cho TJ, Park SS. Correction of genu recurvatum by the Ilizarov method. J Bone Joint Surg [Br] 1999; 81B:769–74.

12. Stein H, Dickson RA. Reversed dynamic slings for knee flexion contractures in the haemophiliac. J Bone Joint Surg [Br] 1975; 57B:282–3.

13. Del Bello DA, Watts HG. Distal femoral extension osteotomy for knee flexion contracture in patients with arthrogryposis. J Pediatr Orthop 1996; 16:122–6.

14. Murray C, Fixsen JA. Management of knee deformity in clinical arthrogryposis multiplex congenita (amyoplasia congenita). J Pediatr Orthop B 1997; 6:186–91.

15. Brunner R, Hefti F, Tgetgel JD. Arthrogrypotic joint contracture at the knee and foot: correction with a circular frame. J Pediatr Orthop B 1997; 6:192–7.

16. Salenius P, Vankka E. The development of the tibiofemoral angle in children. J Bone Joint Surg [Am] 1975; 57A:259–61.

17. Fraser RK, Dickens DR, Cole WG. Medial physeal stapling for primary and secondary genu valgum in late childhood and adolescence. J Bone Joint Surg [Br] 1995; 77B:733–5.

18. Stevens PM, Maguire M, Dales MD, Robins AJ. Physeal stapling for idiopathic genu valgum. J Pediatr Orthop 1999; 19:645–9.

19. Bowen JR, Leahy JL, Zheng Z, MacEwen GD. Partial epiphysiodesis at the knee to correct angular deformity. Clin Orthop 1985; 198:184–9.

20. Volpon JB. Idiopathic genu valgum treated by epiphysiodesis in adolescence. Int Orthop 1997; 21:228–31.

21. Macnicol MF. The correction of lesser leg length inequalities. Curr Orthop 1999; 13:212–7.

22. Edgerton BC, Mariani EM, Morrey BF. Distal femoral varus osteotomy for painful genu valgum. A 5–11 year follow-up study. Clin Orthop 1993; 288:263–9.

23. Healy WL, Anglen JO, Wasilewski SA, Krackow KA. Distal femoral varus osteotomy. J Bone Joint Surg [Am] 1983; 70A:102–9.

24. Ogden JA, Ogden RN, Pugh L, et al. Tibia valga after proximal metaphyseal fractures in childhood: a normal biologic response. J Pediatr Orthop 1995; 15:489–93.

25. Blount WP. Tibia vara. Osteochondrosis deformans tibiae. J Bone Joint Surg [Am] 1937; 19A:1–10.

26. Erlacher P. Deformierende Prozesse de Epiphysengenend bei Kindern. Arch Orthop Unfallchir 1922; 20:81–4.

27. Langenskiold A. Tibia vara. Acta Chir 1952; 103:9–14.

28. Levine AM, Drennan JC. Physiological bowing and tibia vara: the metaphyseal-diaphyseal angle in the measurement of bow-leg deformities. J Bone Joint Surg [Am] 1982; 64A:1158–63.

29. Bateson EM. The relationship between Blount's disease and bow legs. Brit J Radiol 1968; 41:107–14.

30. Ferriter P, Shapiro F. Infantile tibia vara: factors affecting outcome following proximal tibial osteotomy. J Pediatr Orthop 1987; 7: 1–7.

31. Langenskiold A. Tibia vara: osteochondrosis deformans tibiae. Blount's disease. Clin Orthop 1981; 158:77–81.

32. Siffert RS. Intra-epiphyseal osteotomy for progressive tibia vara: a case report and rationale of management. J Pediatr Orthop 1982; 2:81–3.

33. van Huyssteen AL, Hastings CJ, Olesak M, Hoffman EB. Double-elevating osteotomy for late-presenting infantile Blount's disease: the importance of concomitant lateral epiphysiodesis. J Bone Joint Surg [Br] 2005; 87B:710–5.

34. Monticelli G, Spinelli R. A new method of treating the advanced stages of tibia vara (Blount's disease). Ital J Orthop Traumatol 1984; 10:245–303.

35. Coogan PG, Fox JA, Fitch RD. Treatment of adolescent Blount's disease with the circular external fixation device and distraction osteogenesis. J Pediatr Orthop 1996; 16:450–4.

36. Morrissy RT. Atlas of Pediatric Orthopaedic Surgery. Philadelphia: JB Lippincott; 1992:455–64.

37. Miller S, Radomisli T, Ulin R. Inverted arcuate osteotomy and external fixation for adolescent tibia vara. J Pediatr Orthop 2000; 20:450–4.

38. Van Olm JMJ, Gillespie R. Proximal tibial osteotomy for angular knee deformity in children. J Bone Joint Surg [Br] 1984; 66B:301–6.

39. Rab GT. Oblique tibial osteotomy for Blount's disease (tibia vara). J Pediatr Orthop 1988; 8:715–20.

40. Hayek S, Segev E, Ezra E, et al. Serrated W/M osteotomy. Results using a new technique for the correction of infantile tibia vara. J Bone Joint Surg [Br] 2000; 82B:1026–9.

41. Laurencin CT, Ferriter PJ, Millis MB. Oblique proximal tibial osteotomy for the correction of tibia vara in the young. Clin Orthop 1996; 327:218–24.

42. Dietz FR, Weinstein SL. Spike osteotomy for angular deformities of the long bones in children. J Bone Joint Surg [Am] 1988; 70-A:848–52.

43. Macnicol MF. Realignment osteotomy for knee deformity in childhood. Knee 2002; 4:113–20.

44. Steel HH, Sandrow RE, Sullivan PD. Complications of tibial osteotomy in children for genu varum or valgum. J Bone Joint Surg [Am] 1971; 53A:1629–35.

45. Macnicol MF. Focal fibrocartilaginous dysplasia of the femur. J Pediatr Orthop B 1997; 8:661–3.

46. Aglietti P, Buzzi R, Insall JN. Disorders of the patellofemoral joint. In: Insall JN, Scott WN, eds. Surgery of the Knee, 3rd ed. Philadelphia: Churchill Livingstone; 2001:929.

47. Jackson AM. Anterior knee pain. J. Bone Jt. Surg [Br] 2001; 83-B:937–948.

48. Ogden JA. Radiology of postnatal skeletal development. Patella and tibial tuberosity. Skeletal Radiol 1984; 1:246–57.

49. Hunt DM, Somashaker N. A review of sleeve fractures of the patella in children. Knee 2005; 12:3–7.

50. Lloyd Roberts GC, Jackson AM, Albert JS. Avulsion of the distal pole of the patella in cerebral palsy. J Bone Joint Surg [Br] 1985; 67-B:252–4.

51. Enneking WF. Clinical Musculoskeletal Pathology, 3rd ed. Gainesville FL: University of Florida Press; 1990:166.

52. Cahill BR, Berg BC. 99 m-Technetium phosphate compound joint scintigraphy in the management of juvenile osteochondritis dissecans of the femoral condyles. Am J Sports Med 1983; 11:329–35.

53. De Smet AA, Ilahi OA, Graf BK. Untreated osteochondritis of the femoral condyles: prediction of patient outcome using

radiographic and MR findings. Skeletal Radiol 1997; 26(8): 463–7.

54. Ramappa AJ, Gill TJ, Bradford CH, et al. MRI to assess knee cartilage repair tissue after microfracture of chondral defects. J Knee Surg 2007; 20:228–34.

55. Petersen L, Minas T, Brittberg M, Lindahl A. Treatment of osteochondritis dissecans of the knee with autologous chondrocyte transplantation: results at two to ten years. J Bone Joint Surg [Am] 2007; 85-A (Suppl 2):17–24.

56. Twyman RS, Desai K, Aichroth PM. Osteochondritis dissecans of the knee. A long term study. J Bone Joint Surg [Br] 1991; 73-B:461–4.

57. Linden B. Osteochondritis dissecans of the femoral condyles: a long term follow -up study. J Bone Joint Surg [Am] 1997; 53:769–76.

58. Dinham JM. Popliteal cysts in children. J Bone Joint Surg [Br] 1975; 57:69–71.

59. Glasgow MMS, Allen PW, Blakeway C. Arthroscopic treatment of cysts of the lateral meniscus. J Bone Joint Surg [Br] 1993; 75-B:299–302.

60. Henry JH, Craven PR Jr. Traumatic meniscal lesions in children. South Med J 1981; 74:1336–7.

61. Stanitski CL, Harvell JC, Fu F. Observations on acute knee hemarthrosis in children and adolescents. J Paed Orthop 1993; 13:506–10.

62. McNicholas MJ, Rowley DI, McGurty D, et al. Total meniscectomy in adolescence. A 30-year follow-up. J. Bone Joint Surg [Br] 2000; 82-B:217–21.

63. King D. The healing of semilunar cartilages. J Bone Joint Surg [Br] 1936; 18-B:333–42.

64. Fairbank HA. Knee joint changes after meniscectomy. J Bone Joint Surg [Br] 1948; 30-B:664–70.

65. Arnoczky SP, Warren RF. Microvasculature of the human meniscus. Am J Sports Med 1982; 10:90–5.

66. Noyes FR, Barber-Westin SD. Arthroscopic repair of meniscal tears extending into the avascular zone in patients younger than twenty years of age. Am J Sports Med 2002; 30: 589–600.

67. De Haven KE, Hales W. Peripheral meniscal repair; an alternative to meniscectomy. Orthop Transact 1981; 5:399–400.

68. Steenbrugge F, Verdonk R, Verstraete K. Long-term assessment of arthroscopic meniscal repair: a 13 year follow-up study. Knee 2002; 9:181–7.

69. Peters G, Wirth CJ. The current status of meniscal allograft transplantation and replacement. Knee 2003; 10:19–31.

70. Noble J, Hamblen DL. The pathology of the degenerate meniscus. J Bone Joint Surg [Br] 1975; 57-B:180–6.

71. Ikeuchi H. Arthroscopic treatment of discoid lateral meniscus; technique and long term results. Clin Orth Rel Res 1982; 167:19–28.

72. Watanabe M, Takeda S, Ikeuchi H. Atlas of Arthroscopy. Tokyo: Igakushan; 1979.

73. Kaplan EB. Discoid lateral meniscus of the knee joint: nature, mechanism and operative treatment. J Bone Joint Surg [Am] 1957; 39A:77–87.

74. Clark CR, Ogden JA. Development of the menisci of the human knee joint. J Bone Joint Surg [Am] 1983; 65-A:538–47.

75. Räber DA, Friederich NF, Hefti F. Discoid lateral meniscus in children. J Bone Joint Surg [Am] 1998; 80-A:1579–86.

76. Thomas NP, Jackson AM, Aichroth PM. Congenital absence of the anterior cruciate ligament. J Bone Joint Surg [Br] 1985; 67-B:572–5.

77. Meyers MH, McKeever FM. Fractures of the intercondylar eminence of the tibia. J Bone Joint Surg [Am] 1970; 52-A:1677–84.

78. Dorizas JA, Stanitski CL. Anterior cruciate ligament injury in the skeletally immature. Orthop Clin North Am 2003; 34:355–63.

79. Aichroth PM, Patel DV, Zorilla P. The natural history and treatment of rupture of the anterior cruciate ligament in children and adolescents. J Bone Joint Surg (Br) 2002; 84-B:38–41.

80. Kocher MS, Saxon HS, Hovis WD, Hawkins RJ. Management and complications of anterior cruciate ligament injuries in skeletally immature patients: Survey of the Herodicus Society and the ACL Study Group. J Paediatr Orthop 2002; 22:452–57.

81. Kocher MS, Smith JT, Zoric BJ, et al. Transphyseal anterior cruciate ligament reconstruction in the skeletally immature pubescent adolescents. J Bone Joint Surg [Am] 2007; 89-A:2632–9.

82. Harner CD. Posterior Cruciate ligament repair and reconstruction. In Micheli LJ, Kocher MS, eds. The Pediatric Knee. Philadelphia: Saunders Elsevier; 2006:389.

83. Milstrom C, Finestone A, Shlamkovitch N, et al. Anterior knee pain caused by overactivity: a long term prospective follow up. Clin Orth Rel Res. 1996; 331:256–60.

84. Hvid I, Anderson LI. The quadriceps and its relation to femoral torsion. Acta Orthop Scand 1982; 53:577–9

85. Fulkerson JP, Shea KP. Disorders of patello-femoral alignment. J Bone Joint Surg [Am] 1990; 72-A:1424–29.

86. Amis AA, Firer P, Mountney J, et al. Anatomy and biomechanics of the medial patellofemoral ligament. Knee 2003; 10:215–20.

87. Mulford JS. Assessment and management of chronic patellofemoral instability. J Bone Joint Surg [Br] 2007; 89B:709–16.

88. Kannus P, Natri A, Paakklala T, Järvinnen M. An outcome study of chronic patellofemoral pain syndrome. 7-year follow-up of patients in a randomised, controlled trial. J Bone Joint Surg [Am] 1999; 81-A:355–63.

89. Outerbridge RE. The etiology of chondromalacia patellae. J Bone Joint Surg [Br] 1961; 43-B:752–7

90. McGrath P. Chronic pain in children. In Crombie IK, Croft PR, Linton SJ, eds. Epidemiology of Pain. Seattle WA: IASP Press; 1999:81–82.

91. Stanton-Hicks M, Janig W, Hassenbuch S, et al. Reflex sympathetic dystrophy: changing concepts and taxonomy. Pain 1995; 63:127–33.

92. Wilder RT, Berde CB, Wolohan M, et al. Reflex sympathetic dystrophy in children. Characteristics and follow up of 70 patients. J Bone Joint Surg [A] 1992; 74:910–19.

93. Carey RPL. Synovial chondromatosis of the knee in childhood. J Bone Joint Surg [B] 1983; 65:444–7.

94. Gebhardt MC, Ready JE, Mankin HJ. Tumors about the knee in children. Clin Orth Rel Res 1990; 255:86–110.

Chapter 9

The Foot

John A. Fixsen

Introduction

Foot deformities such as in-toeing, curly toes, and flat feet are common causes of parental anxiety. As a result, they make up a large part of the routine referrals to a children's orthopaedic clinic. The orthopaedic surgeon must not only understand the condition and its natural history but also be able to explain it to the parents and allay their anxiety. A careful history including details of pregnancy, birth, and development, together with examination of the child, both statically on the couch and actively—walking and running—is essential. Time spent explaining the position carefully at the first interview is well spent, particularly if it saves unnecessary follow-up appointments, which tend to reinforce the parents' anxiety that something is wrong as the doctor continues to want to see their child. Clearly, if the parents remain unconvinced or the surgeon unsure as to the outcome or nature of the condition, then continued follow-up is necessary.

The surgeon should remember that there are very few foot deformities that actually prevent walking. If a child's motor development is delayed, parents will nearly always blame the obvious in-toeing gait or flat foot that they can see. The surgeon must look beyond the obvious for the real cause of the problem, such as cerebral palsy, spina bifida occulta, or Down syndrome. It is often a difficult and delicate task to persuade parents that the obvious foot deformity is not the root cause of the problem. Treatment of the foot may not only be unnecessary but will not solve the child's developmental or coordination problems.

In-Toe Gait

In-toeing is probably the single most common cause of referral of a child to a children's orthopaedic clinic. It may arise in the foot itself, in the lower leg, at the hip, or be secondary to a central problem or a combination of some or all of these.

Metatarsus Varus, Adductus, or Adductovarus

In the foot itself, metatarsus varus, adductus, or adductovarus comprise the most common entity producing an in-toe gait. It is essential to differentiate this benign, largely self-resolving condition from congenital talipes equinovarus [1]. In club foot, both the forefoot and the hindfoot are in equinus and varus, whereas in metatarsus varus the forefoot is in varus but the hindfoot is in neutral or valgus, with normal posterior skin creases (Fig. 9.1).

The condition is rarely noted at birth but usually becomes obvious in the first few months of life or when the child starts to walk. The forefoot is in varus or adduction, very often with some supination but no equinus. The hindfoot is in neutral or valgus. The deformity is often best seen from the sole of the foot, and in mild and moderate cases is easily correctable by simple finger pressure on the first ray. It is essential to examine the whole child carefully because metatarsus varus can be associated with neurological conditions such as spina bifida occulta or spinal muscular atrophy, in which case there is usually evidence of muscle wasting and lack of normal movements in the lower limb. There is a very rare rigid form of the condition called serpentine, skew, or "Z-foot" (see below), in which the forefoot is in fixed valgus (Fig. 9.2).

The etiology of metatarsus varus is unknown, although Harris [2] suggested that it could be associated with a persistent prone-lying sleeping position. Recently, prone lying for infants has been associated with the "cot death" syndrome; as a result supine lying has been encouraged, and the incidence of metatarsus varus appears to have reduced considerably.

J.A. Fixsen (✉)
Orthopaedic Department, Great Ormond Street Hospital for Sick Children, London, UK

Fig. 9.1 Clinical photographs showing (**a**) anterior and (**b**) posterior views of a patient with metatarsus varus aged 18 months. Note the forefoot and hallux varus but both heels are in slight valgus. There is no equinus and the posterior creases are normal

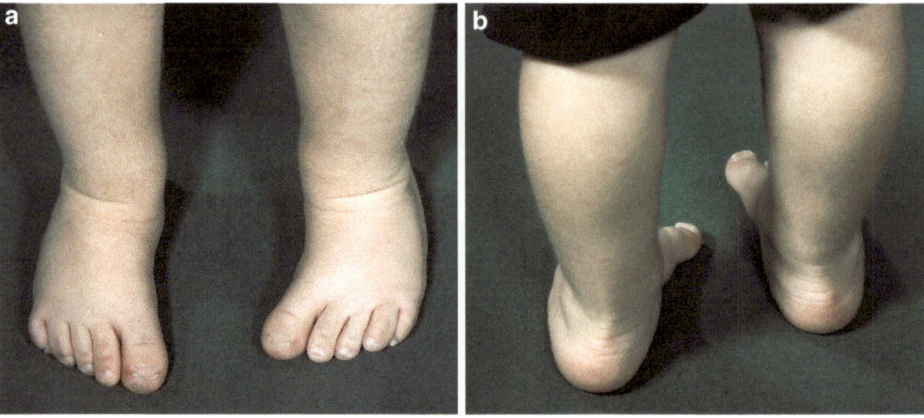

Fig. 9.2 Clinical photographs showing (**a**) anterior and (**b**) posterior views of serpentine, skew, or "Z-feet" in a child aged 4 years

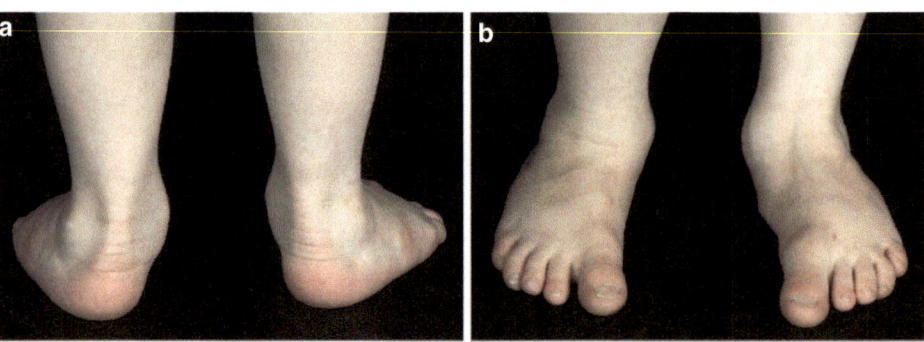

Radiographs show that the metatarsals are adducted relative to the mid- and hindfoot and the talocalcaneal angles are normal or increased in the anteroposterior view (Fig. 9.3). In the rare serpentine, Z, or "skew" foot, the navicular and cuboid are laterally displaced on the talus and the calcaneum (Fig. 9.4).

Treatment

There is considerable argument about the treatment of this common condition. The natural history has been reported by Ponseti and Becker [3] and Rushforth [4], both of whom found that in the majority of patients the condition corrected spontaneously with or without treatment. The former reported that approximately one in nine patients needed treatment. They used plasters, which they pointed out were difficult to apply, and because they worked in a special center for children's orthopaedics they probably had a greater number of difficult cases than average. In Rushforth's series of 130 feet which received no treatment and were followed up for 7 years, 86% corrected completely, 10% showed mild persistence of the deformity, which did not worry the patient or their parents in any way, and only 4% showed persistence of the deformity. Rushforth was unable to predict, until the child reached the age of 3–4 years, which feet were not going to correct. This puts the orthopaedic surgeon in

a considerable dilemma: at least four in five feet will correct spontaneously without any treatment, and it is very difficult to identify those patients requiring treatment. In general, any patient in whom the foot corrects easily to neutral or beyond will probably correct spontaneously. The child with a very rigid deformity and a deep medial crease should be treated initially with stretching by the mother (Fig. 9.5). Ponseti and Becker [3] advised that plastering above the knee was necessary to control the whole leg. They emphasized the difficulty of applying these plasters. They advised that the plasters were changed every 2–3 weeks and that correction was usually obtained within 8–10 weeks, but in some patients relapse occurred after the plasters were removed. Farsetti et al. [5] published a long-term follow-up of untreated and non-surgically treated metatarsus adductus and reported good results in all 16 untreated feet and in 90% of those treated with long leg plasters. Recently, Katz el al. [6] reported treating 85 inflexible feet with below-knee plasters, achieving satisfactory results.

In order to avoid excessive overtreatment of this generally benign condition, the vast majority of these feet should be left alone or, if inflexible, treated with plasters. If, at the age of 3–4 years, there is a persistent deformity, operative correction can be considered. Browne and Paton [7] described an anomalous insertion of the tibialis posterior and noted that the main bulk of the tendon did not attach to the navicular bone, but extended into the forefoot. This was released

Fig. 9.3 Anteroposterior radiographs of both feet in a patient with metatarsus varus (**a**) at 9 months and (**b**) at 3 years 3 months. No treatment was given

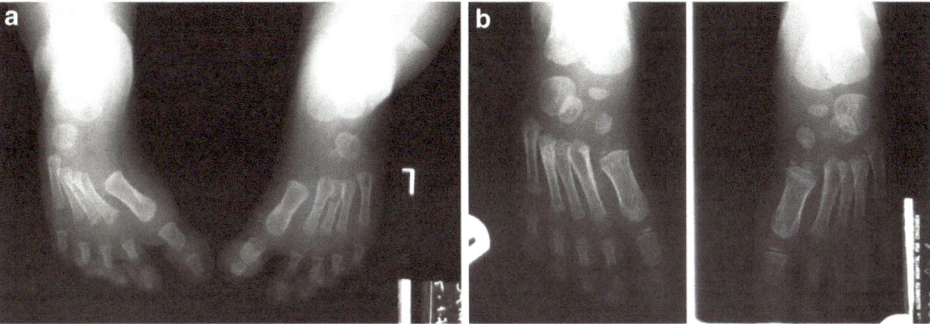

Fig. 9.4 (**a**) Anteroposterior and (**b**) lateral radiographs of true serpentine feet in a boy aged 5 years 4 months. Note the lateral shift of the mid-tarsus on the hindfoot and supination of the forefoot

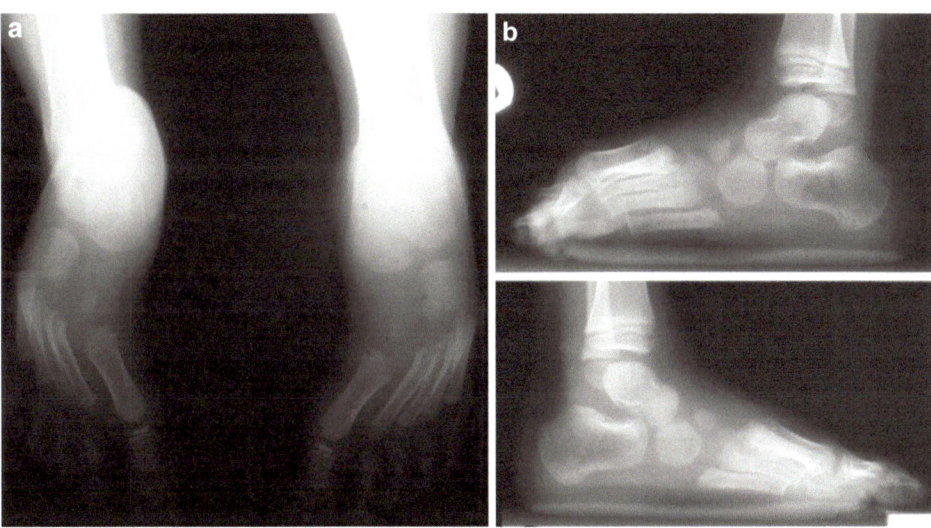

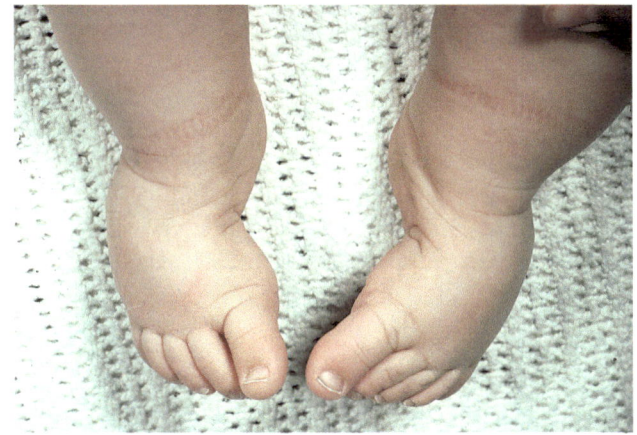

Fig. 9.5 Clinical photograph of a child aged 9 months with severe metatarsus varus showing a marked medial crease. The deformity was rigid and not passively correctable

together with the abductor hallucis and the deformity corrected by plaster. Heyman et al. [8] recommended the more extensive procedure of tarsometatarsal capsulotomies. Stark et al. [9] reported a 41% overall failure rate and a 50% incidence of a painful dorsal prominence at the site of the surgical scar, in a review of this procedure performed over an 18-year period. The author's own limited experience of this operation is similar to that described by Stark et al. [9]. After the child has reached the age of 6 years, multiple metatarsal osteotomies as described by Berman and Gartland [10] can be used. Again, there are significant complications associated with this operation, with failure of correction and damage to the growth plate (physis) of the first metatarsal causing shortening and progressive deformity indicating that this operation should be used with great care. It is extremely rare to see an adult with persistent symptomatic metatarsus varus. On this basis, and the evidence that the majority of these feet correct with time, it is important not to overtreat this condition. In particular, surgery should be avoided unless it is absolutely necessary because it is quite clear that operation can produce symptoms and deformity of greater severity than the condition itself.

Bleck [11] advocated a more radical early approach to conservative treatment with serial plasters. However, he accepted that the results of his study did not make it possible to predict with certainty which feet must be treated and acknowledged the influence of "the public attitude toward deformity" among his treatment population.

Fig. 9.6 (**a**) Clinical photograph of the feet and lower legs of a patient with Larsen's syndrome. Note the serpentine feet and dislocated knees. (**b**) AP radiograph of the left foot showing the severe Z-shaped deformity

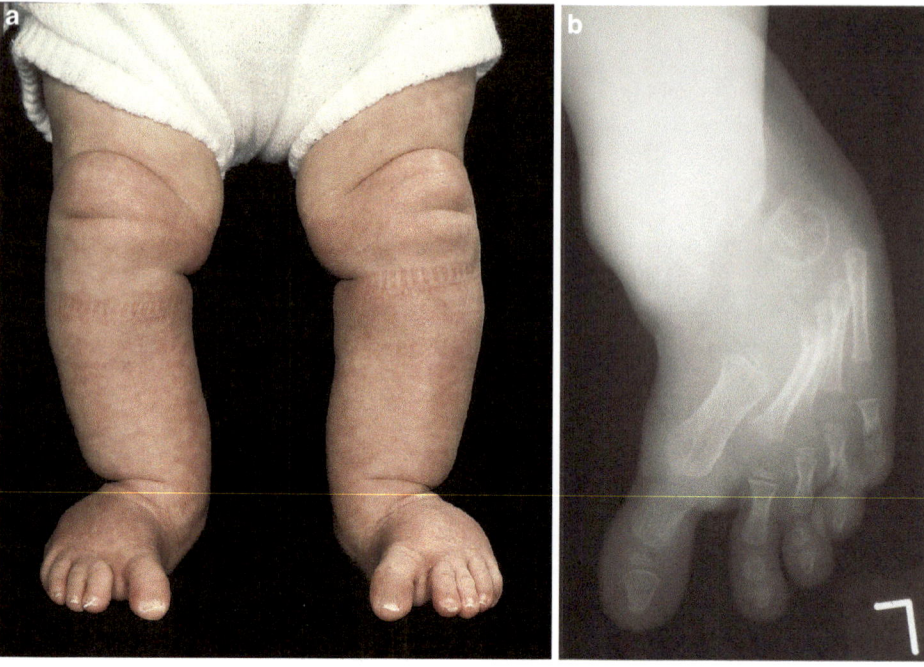

Serpentine, Skew, or "Z-Foot"

A true serpentine, skew, or "Z-foot" is a very rare entity. Kite [12] described 12 examples among a total of 2818 cases of metatarsus varus, an incidence of 0.43%. In this condition the forefoot varus and adduction is fixed and the hindfoot is in fixed valgus. The radiographs show that the navicular and cuboid bones are laterally displaced on the talus and calcaneum with the metatarsals in varus, giving rise to the classical "Z- or S-shaped" foot (Fig. 9.4). This is extremely difficult to treat because all three components of the deformity require correction. Lloyd-Roberts and Clark [13] pointed out that this rare condition may be associated with a ball-and-socket ankle joint, so that fusing the subtalar joint may not correct the valgus. It is important to look at the whole patient, as this condition may be associated with other anomalies such as Larsen's syndrome (Fig. 9.6). Mosca [14], in an important review of skew foot, suggested that, in infants and young children, management should follow that of metatarsus adductus: in older children and adults, only those with symptoms should be treated. In 1995, he described satisfactory short-term results in 10 symptomatic skew feet operated on to correct all three components of the deformity. The operation was performed at an average age of 10 years. The operation combined a reversed Evans [15] type of calcaneal lengthening procedure to correct the hindfoot and midfoot and a medial cuneiform opening wedge osteotomy, as described by Fowler et al. [16], to correct the forefoot. The tendo-Achilles, which was always short, was also lengthened.

Congenital Talipes Calcaneo-Valgus

Postural calcaneo-valgus is the most common position of the foot in the newborn (Fig. 9.7). It is normal to be able to dorsiflex the foot of the neonate so that the dorsum touches the anterior aspect of the tibia; however, there should be a full range of plantar flexion. In congenital talipes calcaneo-valgus the foot is markedly dorsiflexed and everted, but plantar flexion is limited, often to only the neutral position. The condition is more common in firstborn children. It is associated with oligohydramnios and the "molded baby syndrome" described by Lloyd-Roberts and Pilcher [17]. It is said to be associated with congenital dislocation of the hip in 5% of cases, and instability of the hip must be looked for in patients with this deformity. It is very important to look for any suggestion of neuromuscular abnormality, both

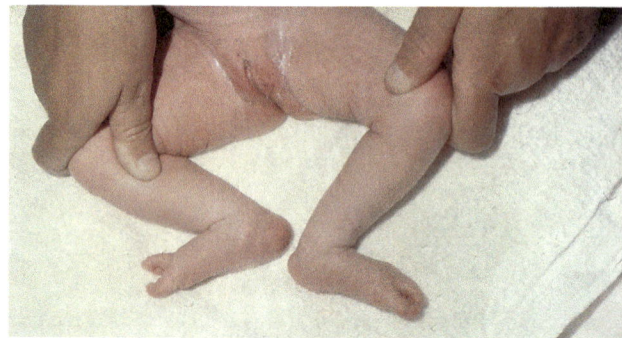

Fig. 9.7 Clinical photograph of typical calcaneo-valgus feet in a newborn infant

in the spine and in the leg, typically wasting or a difference in size between the two legs. The condition must be distinguished from congenital vertical talus (congenital convex pes valgus), in which the forefoot is dorsiflexed and valgus, but the hindfoot is in fixed equinus (see Chapter 33).

If there is no evidence of an underlying abnormality, this condition nearly always responds to simple stretching into plantar flexion and inversion by the mother under instruction from the physiotherapist. This should be done regularly several times a day, probably when the baby is being fed and the nappy changed. In the vast majority of patients, the condition will correct by the age of 3 months. If there is failure to correct by this age, the patient should be looked at very carefully for evidence of any underlying neuromuscular abnormality or generalized condition. It is probably wise to follow-up the child until walking is established.

Parents are often very worried by this condition and believe that their child will have an abnormal foot or difficulty with walking. Some orthopaedic surgeons such as Giannestras [18] advocate a more aggressive policy, with serial plasters followed by modifications to shoe wear. In the author's experience, this type of treatment has not been necessary unless the deformity has been associated with an underlying neuromuscular or skeletal deformity.

Tip-Toe Walking

Persistent Tip-Toe Walking or Persistent Equinus

The mature heel–toe pattern of gait should normally be adopted by the age of 2 years [19]. One of the most important things for an orthopaedic surgeon to recognize is the child who had developed a mature heel–toe pattern of gait but then reverted to a toe–heel or toe–toe gait. This is nearly always pathological, and conditions such as muscular dystrophy, spinal dysraphism, peroneal muscular atrophy (hereditary motor and sensory neuropathy), and spinal tumor must be looked for.

Idiopathic Tip-Toe Walking

In this situation the child persistently walks up on the toes, although when standing may bring the heels to the ground. There may be a degree of hyperextension of the knee and also external rotation of the feet in order to bring the heels to the ground more easily. Typically, the tip-toe gait is more noticeable in bare feet than when wearing shoes. On the couch, dorsiflexion of the foot with the knee extended is sometimes limited, but can be normal with no evidence of

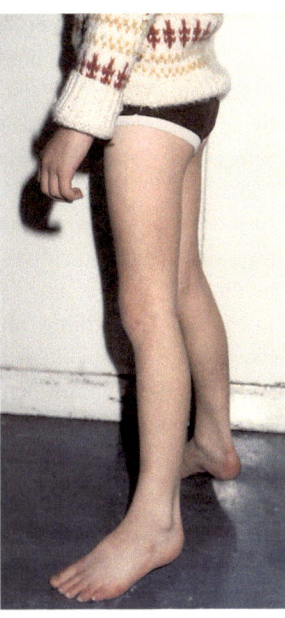

Fig. 9.8 Clinical photograph of a persistent tip-toe walker aged 7 years. Note the heels are well off the ground, the knees extended, and the legs externally rotated

tendo-Achilles shortening. Occasionally true shortening of the tendo-Achilles with fixed equinus is present. Hall et al. [20] described this as idiopathic shortening of the tendo-Achilles. They pointed out that this condition was often not recognized until the child was at school, as it had been accepted that the child habitually walked like this, and that it would correct with time (Fig. 9.8). They advised surgical lengthening of the tendo-Achilles.

Idiopathic tip-toe walking is a diagnosis of exclusion. Neuromuscular disorders such as spastic diplegia and other forms of cerebral palsy should be considered. For a period all patients referred to the orthopaedic department at The Hospital for Sick Children, London, were referred to a paediatric neurologist to determine if it was possible to make a neurological diagnosis in every case of tip-toe walking. A skilled paediatric neurologist was able to find some underlying neurological cause in approximately 50% of tip-toe walkers. This gait is also associated with hyperactive children, learning disorders, autism, and schizophrenia.

In the past, physiotherapy in the form of stretching by the mother or under the supervision of the physiotherapist, plaster casting, and braces have been advised for the treatment of persistent idiopathic tip-toe walking. However, Eastwood et al. [21] showed that tendo-Achilles lengthening (TAL) was significantly better than conservative forms of treatment. In their series of patients, 16% had a positive family history of tip-toe walking and 50% had suffered significant neonatal jaundice. In 20%, muscle biopsies were performed and these showed features suggestive of a neuropathic process, including a predominance of type I muscle fibers. In 1998 Stricker and Angulo [22] also showed that casts and bracing were really no better than no treatment and that surgery gave better results. It was interesting that

32% of their 80 patients had a family history of toe walking, 28% were born prematurely, 16% reported delay in psychomotor development or speech, and 31% had perinatal hyperbilirubinemia. Muscle biopsy was not performed in this series. The investigators concluded that the origin of idiopathic tip-toe walking was unclear in the majority of cases. In those children who showed persistent heel cord contracture, surgical treatment was more effective than conservative methods.

In a maturity follow-up using gait analysis of idiopathic toe walkers treated either by plasters or by TAL, there were still changes in ankle kinematics and kinetics but this was not detectable visually in most subjects [23].

The Painful Heel

Kohler's Disease (Osteochondritis of the Navicular)

Kohler [24] described a painful self-limiting disease of the tarsal navicular that showed flattening, sclerosis, and fragmentation of the navicular on radiograph (Fig. 9.9). The tarsal navicular ossifies between the ages of 2.5 and 3.5 years. There are considerable variations in the development and pattern of its ossification, so the radiographic appearances may be irrelevant unless the child also has symptoms and local signs. The condition commonly occurs between the age of 4 and 7 years and, in up to 33% of patients, both feet may be involved. The patient presents with pain, limp, and tenderness over the tarsal navicular. Sometimes there is sufficient local swelling redness and warmth for the diagnosis of infection to be considered. Waugh [25], in a careful study of 52 feet, showed the ossification of the tarsal navicular occurred later in boys than in girls. Abnormalities of ossification were more frequent in boys. He was of the opinion that abnormal ossification resulted from compression of the bony nucleus at the critical phase of growth of the navicular bone. Biopsy performed when the question of infection or tumor had been raised showed areas of necrosis and resorption of dead bone, with the formation of new bone similar to that seen in Perthes' disease. Waugh also showed that, within 2–3 years, the appearances of the navicular had returned to normal. Cox [26], in a long-term review of 55 patients, found no evidence of permanent deformity or disability after this disease.

Treatment depends upon the severity of the symptoms. Often, no treatment is necessary and the child will recover spontaneously. Occasionally pain is sufficiently severe to require immobilization of the foot in a below-knee walking plaster or the use of an orthosis for 6 weeks.

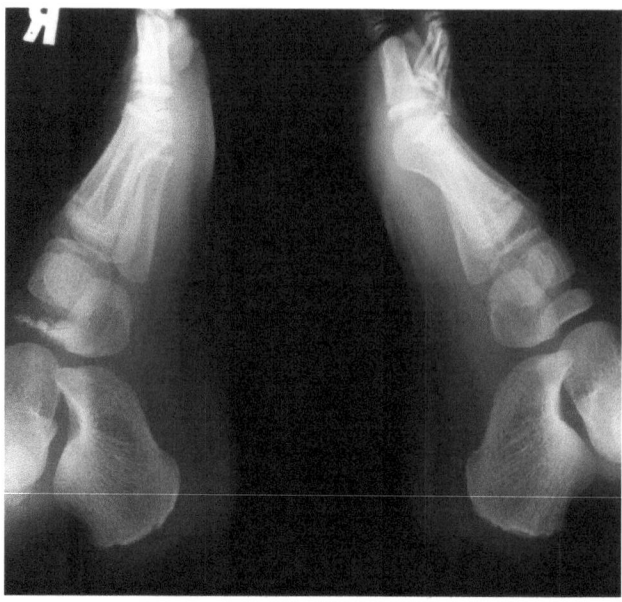

Fig. 9.9 Lateral radiographs of the feet in a 5-year-old child. (Left) Kohler's disease (osteochondritis of the tarsal navicular) in the right foot with flattening, fragmentation, and sclerosis. (Right) The normal left foot for comparison

Calcaneal Apophysitis (Sever's Disease)

Sever described this condition in 1912 [27]. He believed it to be a form of osteochondritis of the calcaneal apophysis. However, the appearance of increased density and fragmentation of the calcaneal apophysis is now known to be a normal radiographic finding in the age group concerned (Fig. 9.10).

The child, usually between the ages of 7 and 12 years and more commonly a boy than a girl, presents with pain and tenderness over the insertion of the tendo-Achilles into the calcaneus. The patient commonly finds it more comfortable to wear a shoe with a heel than to walk barefoot. The child is often a keen footballer or gymnast, and the tenderness is accurately localized to the insertion of the tendo-Achilles. This condition is now believed to be a strain of the insertion of the tendo-Achilles. It must be distinguished from Achilles tendonitis, which can also occur in children, particularly keen sportsmen, but is associated with pain and swelling over the tendo-Achilles above the calcaneus. It is also possible to develop a bursitis in which the small bursa between the posterosuperior corner of the calcaneus and the tendo-Achilles becomes inflamed. The rare subacute osteomyelitis of the calcaneus should also be considered (see below: under *Other Cause of Pain in the Heel*).

Treatment usually consists of temporarily fitting a lift under the heel of the shoe, gentle calf stretching, and reduced activity. If this is not sufficient, a short period in plaster may be necessary, although this is rarely necessary. However, it

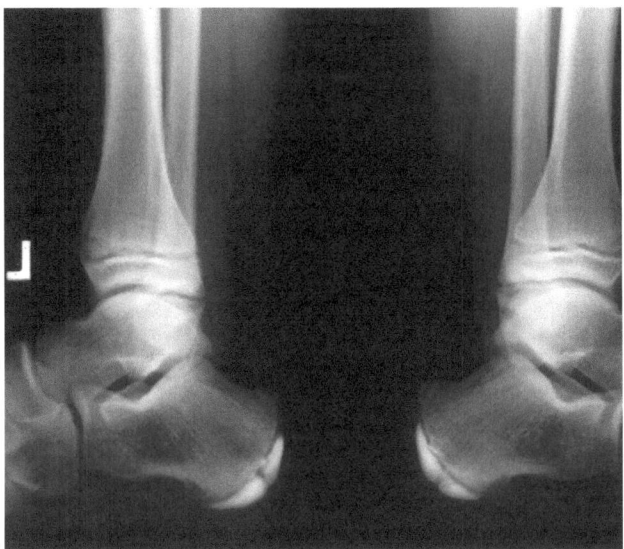

Fig. 9.10 Lateral radiograph of both hindfeet of a child aged 11 years with so-called Sever's disease. The sclerosis and fragmentation of the calcaneal apophysis are normal radiographic appearances at this age. The patient was complaining of pain over the insertion of the tendo-Achilles on the right side only

is important to regulate activity carefully when the plaster is removed, otherwise the symptoms will recur. This condition can be a considerable nuisance in children who are keen on sport, particularly football and gymnastics.

Calcaneal Boss

This condition is almost entirely confined to adolescent girls, who develop a painful bony swelling over the superolateral corner of the calcaneus. This is almost always associated with wearing a high-heeled court shoe, which causes pressure over this area, resulting in a bursa over the normal prominence of the calcaneus at this site. With time, the feet become accustomed to the pressure of the shoes and the condition settles. Sometimes there is sufficient anxiety and pressure to do something about it that the surgeon may be persuaded to operate. However, it is much better to change the design of shoe and take the pressure off the heel or pad the heel and wait for the condition to subside. If the surgeon is persuaded to remove the bony lump that underlies the swelling, this involves removing a substantial portion of the posterosuperior corner of the calcaneus. Great care must be taken not to damage the terminal branches of the sural nerve and to avoid a painful neuroma which can cause more troublesome symptoms than the original lump. Almost all these patients will respond to modification of footwear and time.

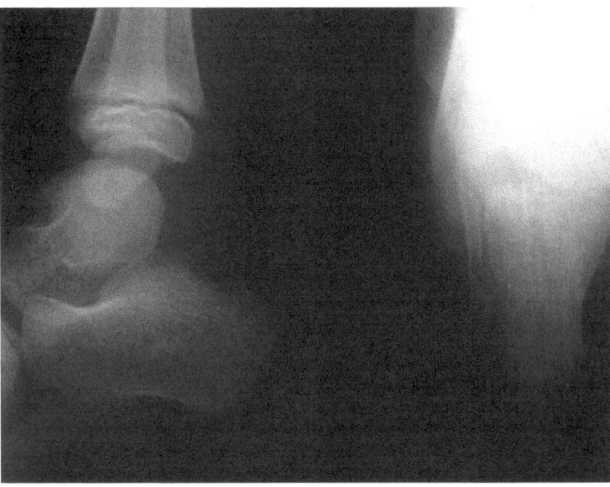

Fig. 9.11 Lateral (*left*) and axial (*right*) radiographs of a child with a fracture of the calcaneus causing a limp. The fracture is only visible on the axial view

Other Cause of Pain in the Heel

There are a number of other interesting causes of pain in the heel. A child may traumatize the heel by jumping from a height. Fractures of the calcaneus are notoriously difficult to see on radiographs unless an axial view of the os calcis is taken in addition to the conventional anteroposterior (AP) and lateral views (Fig. 9.11).

Infection in the calcaneus often runs an unusual subacute course (see Chapter 10) and has been misdiagnosed as a sprain, ligamentous injury, or Sever's disease [28] (Fig. 9.12).

Generalized bony conditions such as fibrous dysplasia and neurofibromatosis can also present with pain in the heel, as can bone tumors such as bone cysts and osteoid osteoma (Fig. 9.13). The latter may be very difficult to see, and a bone scan can be very useful in the investigation of obscure pain in the heel region.

Flat Feet

Flat Foot (Pes Planus)

In the past there has been great concern among parents and doctors about flat feet. However, a knowledge of the natural history of foot development in the child and the awareness that the ordinary flexible flat foot associated with joint laxity should be considered a normal variant and not a disability have led to a much more rational attitude to this very common condition.

Fig. 9.12 Lateral radiographs showing subacute osteomyelitis of the calcaneus. (*Left*) The initial radiograph was taken 2 months before the second (*right*). Note the development of the lytic lesion (abscess) with time. The patient was initially treated for a strain of the tendo-Achilles at the time of the first radiograph

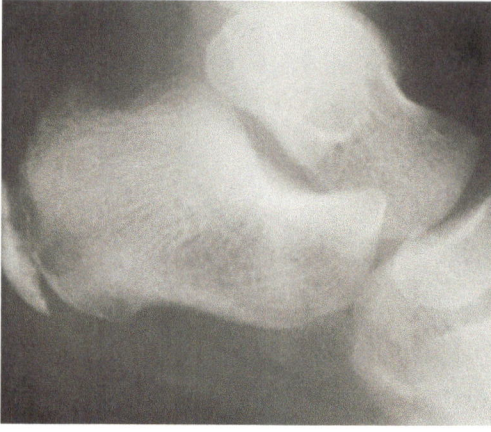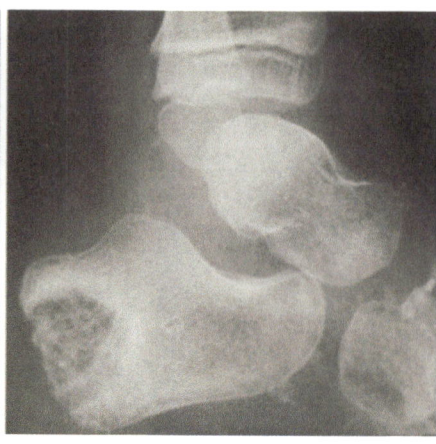

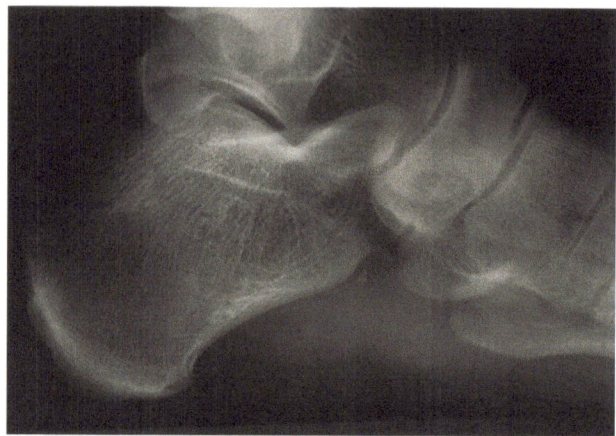

Fig. 9.13 Lateral radiograph of a child with pain in the hindfoot showing a lytic lesion with a central nidus in the tarsal navicular which proved to be an osteoid osteoma

Natural History

Staheli et al. [29] made an important contribution to our understanding of the natural history of foot development in the child.

At birth, the most common position for the foot is in slight dorsiflexion and eversion, a mild calcaneo-valgus. At the end of the first year, when the child begins to stand, the foot nearly always looks flat, particularly because there is a large pad of fat on the medial side of the foot beneath the navicular. This is a normal fat pad, although it can look quite large and sometimes has a considerable vascular element. Between the ages of 1 and 2 years, walking becomes established and the child characteristically stands with the feet everted and externally rotated. As a result the feet look very flat, but this should not be considered an abnormality (Fig. 9.14). Between the ages of 2 and 3 years, the medial arch starts to appear. If, at this stage, a child's feet remain significantly flat, with the medial arch resting near or on the ground, it is most important to test for the presence of joint laxity. The majority of these feet will be so-called flexible flat feet, which are asymptomatic and require no treatment. The assessment of join laxity can be difficult, particularly as it varies considerably between races. Carter and Wilkinson [30] described five tests for joint laxity in the upper and lower limbs that have become accepted as evidence of familial joint laxity (Fig. 9.15), but these do not take into account considerable racial variations. Cheng et al. [31] have shown that among Chinese children, the tests of Carter and Wilkinson are not sufficiently sensitive for children in Hong Kong because they are generally far more flexible than the European children tested by Carter and Wilkinson.

Diagnosis

In the diagnosis of flat foot, the problem is to distinguish the normal variant, usually associated with joint laxity, for which no treatment is necessary, from patients who have a

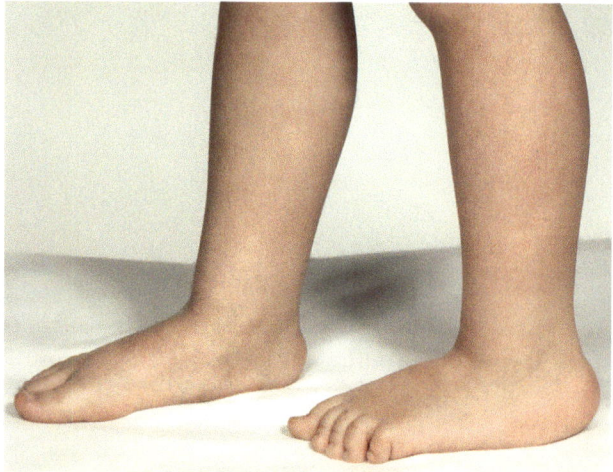

Fig. 9.14 Clinical photograph of a child aged 18 months showing the normal weight-bearing appearance of the feet at this age with flattening of the medial arch

Fig. 9.15 Line drawings from Carter and Wilkinson of the five tests for joint laxity. (**a**) Hyperextension of the elbows. (**b**) Thumb can be placed on the flexor surface of the forearm. (**c**) Fingers extend parallel to the dorsum of the forearm. (**d**) Feet dorsiflex above 30°. (**e**) Knees hyperextend. Adapted with permission and copyright of the British Editorial Society of Bone and Joint Surgery [30]

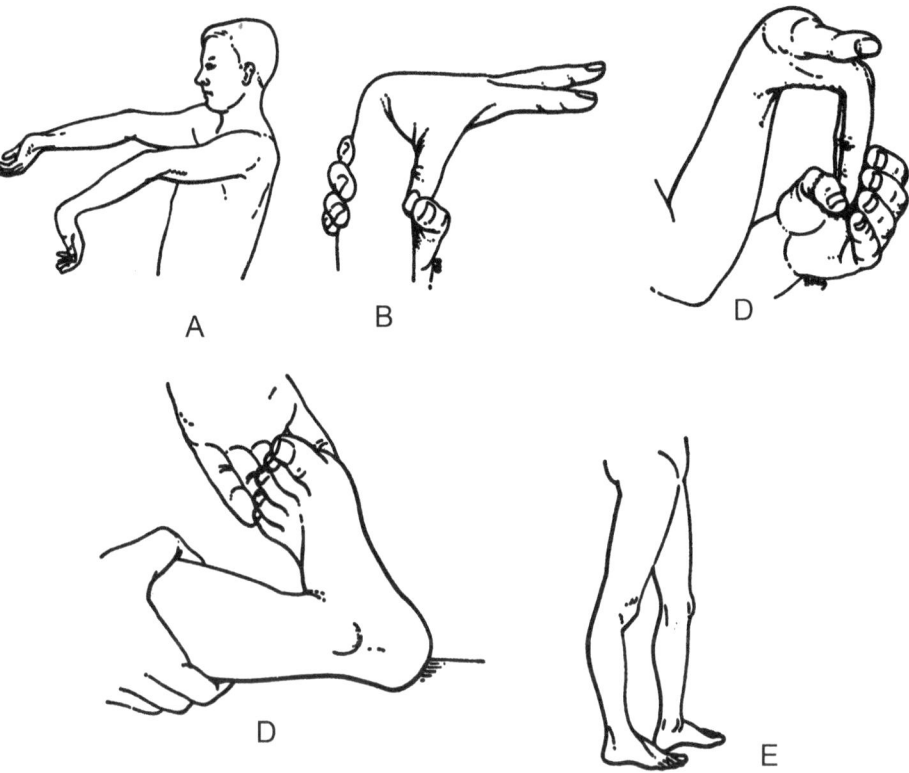

significant abnormality causing symptoms for which treatment is necessary and which are often due to some underlying cause not arising in the foot. Morley [32], in an unselected series of patients attending routine health clinics, showed that 97% of children younger than 18 months had apparent flat feet. By the age of 10 years, only 4% of children had any evidence of flat feet. In this series, there was no evidence that any treatment such as shoe modifications, insoles, or exercises made any difference to the natural evolution of the feet. Rose et al. in 1986 [33] published the results of an important 25-year study designed to distinguish normal anatomical variants from pathological conditions. They stated that tests for flat foot should relate to function and should be dynamic rather than static. They accepted that all except markedly valgus, everted feet in young children were normal and showed that children progressively developed an arch with time, so that initially broad feet in pre-school children became normal with time, irrespective of whether they had any treatment or not.

Rose et al. [33] pointed out that the great toe extension test is the most useful test for dynamic function of the medial arch. In this test, when the big toe is actively dorsiflexed the medial arch should rise and the tibia externally rotate (Fig. 9.16). The simplest way of testing whether a child has normal flexible flat feet that require no treatment is to get the child to stand on tip-toe. If the arches are restored by this action, the tibia rotates laterally and the heel goes into varus, the feet are normal. Wenger et al. [34], in a most important

prospective study, asked the question: "Can flexible flat feet in children be influenced by treatment?" The conclusion of this study was that flexible flat feet in young children improve with growth. Treatment with corrective shoes, inserts, or specially designed insoles did not alter the natural history of the condition. Rao and Joseph [35] in an interesting study of shod and un-shod children in India suggested that shoe wear in early childhood was detrimental to the development of a normal longitudinal arch, particularly in children with marked joint laxity. However, Echam and Forriol [36] in a similar study of shod and un-shod children in the Congo concluded that footwear made little difference.

Management

In light of the above, as far as management is concerned, there are two types of flat feet:

a. *The common flexible flat foot* is pain-free, associated with normal muscle power and mobility, and has a normal great toe extension test. This type of foot should be considered a normal variant. Frequently it is familial and associated with joint laxity. These feet require no treatment, and there is no evidence that conservative treatment of any sort alters the natural history of the condition.

b. *The pathological type of flat foot*. This is often painful. It may have abnormal muscle power being either weak

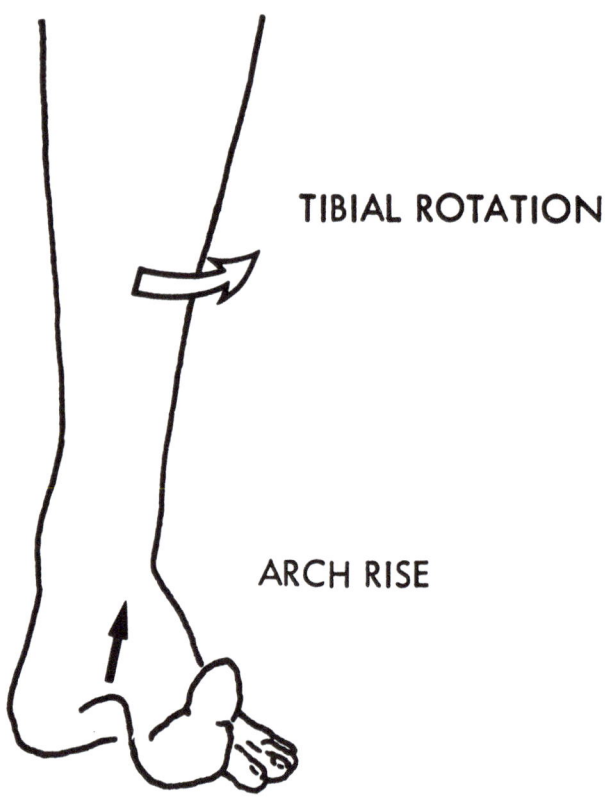

TIBIAL ROTATION

ARCH RISE

The great toe extension test.

Fig. 9.16 Line drawing from showing the great toe extension test. Reproduced with permission and copyright © of the British Editorial Society of Bone and Joint Surgery [33]

operation, described by Evans in 1975 [15] and recently popularized by Mosca [14], in which the lateral border of the foot is lengthened by inserting a wedge of bone in the anterior end of the calcaneus, has produced good results. Finally, medial displacement osteotomy of the calcaneus, described by Koutsogiannis [38], was successful in the short term in some cases.

Tarsal Coalition (Peroneal Spastic Flat Foot)

Sir Robert Jones in 1897 [39] drew attention to a form of rigid valgus everted foot in which the peroneal muscles were in spasm. This condition became known as "peroneal spastic flat foot." The association of this clinical syndrome with tarsal coalition was first described by Slomann in 1921 [40] and Badgely in 1927 [41], who reported the presence of a partial or complete calcaneo-navicular bar in association with peroneal spastic flat foot. In 1948 Harris and Beath [42] described talocalcaneal coalition, and a wide variety of forms of tarsal coalition have been described since then. The patient, who is usually in the second decade, presents with characteristic clinical signs, often after minor trauma to the foot or ankle, which are initially diagnosed as a simple twist or sprain. However, the symptoms persist. The patient continues to complain of disability, difficulty with walking and running, and, if the peroneal spasm is not recognized, may be accused of exaggerating the symptoms and a functional overlay. There are usually clear-cut clinical signs: the foot is held flat and in valgus (Fig. 9.17); the medial arch is not restored when the patient attempts to stand on tip-toe; any attempt to invert the foot at the subtalar joint causes pain, usually over the lateral side of the foot, with spasm of the peronei. Rarely, spasm of the tibialis posterior may occur with an inversion deformity [43]. Plain AP and lateral radiographs

or hypertonic and may be associated with abnormal mobility, i.e., excessive movement or rigidity. These feet require careful investigation before treatment. Frequently the problem is due to a generalized condition, often neuromuscular in origin, or to some local condition arising in the foot. Treatment with insoles, shoe modifications, or exercises may be helpful in this type of foot problem, but it is essential to diagnose the underlying cause if possible.

In the rare severe idiopathic flat foot without any underlying cause, but which is developing symptoms, orthopaedic treatment may be necessary. Supporting the foot with insoles, surgical footwear, or an orthosis may relieve both symptoms and excessive shoe wear. In the older child with severe talocalcaneal hypermobility, the Grice type of subtalar arthrodesis will stabilize the subtalar joint very satisfactorily, but at the expense of permanent stiffening of the joint and possible later problems in the ankle. Localized naviculocuneiform fusion to restore the medial arch has not been successful in the long term [37]. The so-called reverse Evans

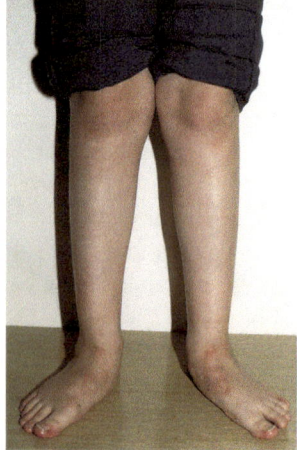

Fig. 9.17 Clinical photograph of a patient with bilateral peroneal spastic flat feet due to bilateral calcaneo-navicular bars

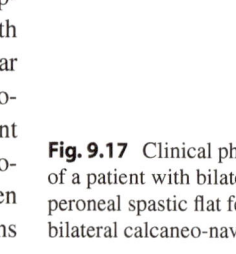

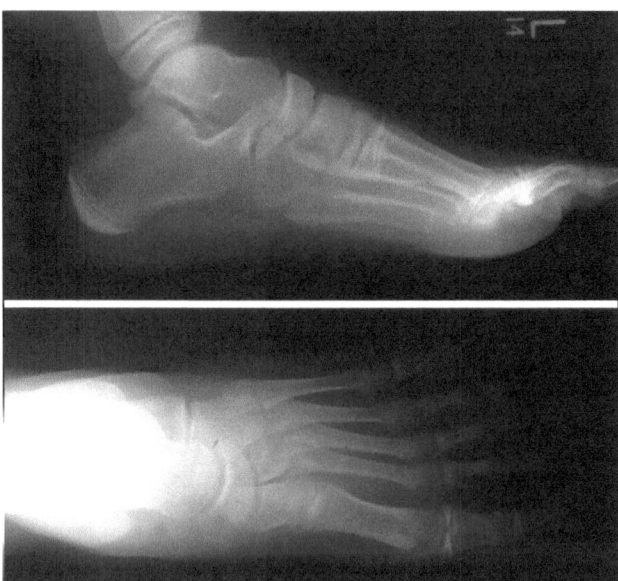

Fig. 9.18 (*Upper*) Lateral radiograph of the foot showing a partial calcaneo-navicular bar and the "anteater's nose" sign. (*Lower*) AP radiograph. Note that the calcaneo-navicular bar is very difficult to see on this view

demonstrate the valgus deformity of the foot. A useful sign of calcaneo-navicular coalition, "The anteater's nose," was reported in 1987 by Oestreich et al. [44]. A 45° oblique radiograph is also very useful when looking for a talonavicular bar. Harris and Beath [42] recommended a 45° axial view for talocalcaneal coalition. A computed tomography (CT) scan is very helpful in the assessment of all forms of tarsal coalition, and particularly talocalcaneal bars (Fig. 9.18).

The inheritance of this condition is interesting. Leonard [45] reported that, among 98 first-degree relatives of 31 patients, 39% had totally asymptomatic tarsal coalition on radiographic examination. The incidence of tarsal coalition in the population is therefore unknown as it is frequently entirely asymptomatic. Leonard postulated an autosomal dominant inheritance of almost full penetrance.

Treatment

The management of this condition can be very difficult. If a patient presents with minor symptoms, a medial arch support or medial wedge on the heel may be sufficient to support the medial arch of the foot and relieve the spasm. Frequently, however, the spasm persists. A manipulation under anesthesia, with or without local injection of hydrocortisone and local anesthetic into the subtalar region, followed by a below-knee plaster with the foot held in neutral for a period of 6–8

weeks, may be necessary. This often relieves the pain while the patient is in plaster, but it commonly relapses when the plaster is removed. Some surgeons, therefore, recommend prolonged splintage for up to 6 months using a carefully molded plastic ankle–foot orthosis. Braddock [46] published the results of conservative treatment in 56 feet followed up for 21 years. This important review showed that about 50% of the patients had suffered minor symptoms, which did not bother them significantly. Only 10% had had persistent symptoms requiring triple arthrodesis. The prognosis for the foot and the response to treatment bore no relation to the radiographic appearances, and symptomatic tarsal arthritis was rare in the long term.

From the surgical point of view, Mitchell and Gibson [47] recommended excision of the calcaneo-navicular bar in patients aged between 10 and 14 years who did not show any secondary changes in other tarsal joints. Macnicol et al. [48] reviewed 16 feet in 11 patients at an average of 23 years after excision of their calcaneo-navicular bars; 67% had had a good or excellent result. Five feet had poor results that responded well to triple arthrodesis. The so-called beaking of the talus on the preoperative radiograph correlated with a poor result from excision of the calcaneo-navicular bar. Dwyer [49] suggested calcaneal osteotomy to treat the valgus hindfoot. Cain and Hyman [50] reported the results of a closing medial wedge osteotomy of the calcaneus with satisfactory relief of pain and improved movement in the majority of the 40 feet operated upon in their series.

CT scanning has made talocalcaneal bars much easier to diagnose and assess. Olney and Asher [51] published an early report recommending resection of the persistently symptomatic talocalcaneal middle facet coalition, even in the present of talar beaking. In 1997 McCormack et al. [52] reported a 10-year follow-up of eight of these patients who had operations in nine feet. Eight of the nine feet had done well, particularly those with smaller coalitions, and none had required further surgery. The authors pointed out that this technique allows the option of a later arthrodesis if the resection does not relieve symptoms.

It is important to remember that a tarsal coalition is not always the cause of a painful peroneal spastic flat foot. It can occur after previous surgery, in particular, overcorrection of the foot in club foot, and in association with juvenile idiopathic arthritis, which frequently affects the subtalar joint in children. It may also be seen in association with infection in the hindfoot and tumors such as an osteoid osteoma. Blockey [53] drew attention to the fact that peroneal spasm can occur without a tarsal anomaly and that the presence of a tarsal anomaly does not mean that the foot is inevitably stiff. He postulated that a tarsal coalition makes the foot more liable to break down under stress and that a minor injury may precipitate peroneal spasm. It is important for the orthopaedic surgeon to recognize this condition and treat it energetically, before the spasm becomes established.

The Toes

Curly Toes

The majority of babies at birth show significant flexion of the toes, particularly the lateral three toes which may also adopt a varus alignment (Fig. 9.19). This often causes anxiety among parents, even before the child starts to walk, particularly if one of the adults in the family or a close relative has recently had problems from toe deformities. In general, if the toe can be passively straightened and there is no fixed deformity, it is most unlikely to cause any symptoms. However, if there is a fixed deformity this may require treatment once the child is established in walking. Many years ago, Trethowan [54] recommended over- and understrapping. Sweetnam [55] was unable to find any evidence that this type of conservative treatment influenced the natural history of the disorder. Most parents found it extremely difficult to persist with this treatment for more than a few months. In the majority of patients curly toes do not cause any symptoms and should be left alone. In the few cases in which there is persistent deformity causing symptoms, surgical correction by simple tenotomy of the flexor tendon, as reported by Menelaus and Ross [56], has given good results from a simple procedure that can be performed on a day-case basis and allows the patient to walk within 24 hours of the operation. Some surgeons recommend the insertion of an axial K wire to hold the digit straight while the tenotomized tendon heals in a lengthened position. This is much simpler than formal transfer of the long-toe flexor into the extensor as described by Taylor [57], which is probably best reserved for patients with severe clawing of the toes associated with neuromuscular imbalance.

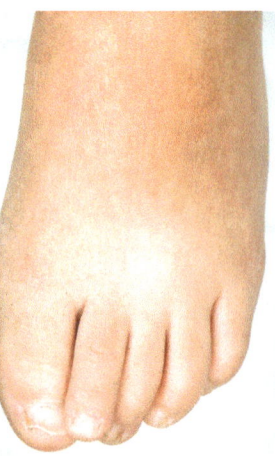

Fig. 9.19 Clinical photograph of an infant showing typical, curly lateral three toes

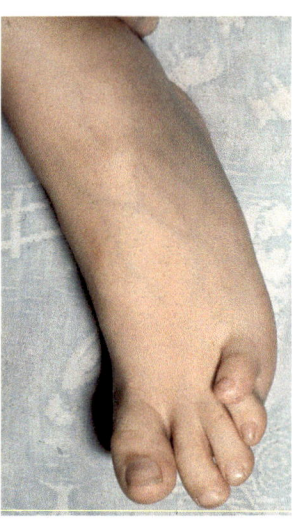

Fig. 9.20 Clinical photograph showing an overlapping fifth toe (congenital elevation of the fifth toe)

Overriding Fifth Toe (Congenital Elevation of the Fifth Toe)

This is a true congenital deformity of the fifth toe which is hypoplastic, elevated, and rotated medially. It overlies the fourth toe (Fig. 9.20). The deformity is fixed and does not correct spontaneously with time. Treatment is required if problems with shoe wear and pressure from the shoes on the toe become troublesome. Conservative measures are rarely successful, and a number of surgical procedures have been described. A simple V-Y plasty, described by Wilson [58], releases the dorsal contracture, but often the toe will not remain corrected after this procedure and the deformity recurs. The double V-Y plasty, described by Butler and reported by Cockin [59], combines a V-Y plasty on the dorsum of the foot and a Y-V plasty on the sole of the foot, connecting the two so that the toe is not only released dorsally but also pulled down into the plantigrade position by the Y-V plasty on the sole. This can provide good correction but must be performed with care to avoid damage to the neuromuscular bundles. Unfortunately, the new, lateralized position of the fifth toe may increase shoe pressure from the side, with resurgence of the deformity. More radical bony procedures such as proximal phalangectomy or even amputation of the fifth toe should be reserved for patients who have failed previous soft tissue surgery.

Hallux Valgus

Hallux valgus in the young child is rare unless it is associated with other major congenital anomalies affecting the foot, such as Apert's syndrome (acrocephalosyndactyly). However, it becomes increasingly common in teenagers. In

Fig. 9.21 Clinical photograph of bilateral hallux valgus in an adolescent. Note the broad forefoot, prominent medial bunion, and fifth metatarsal bunionette

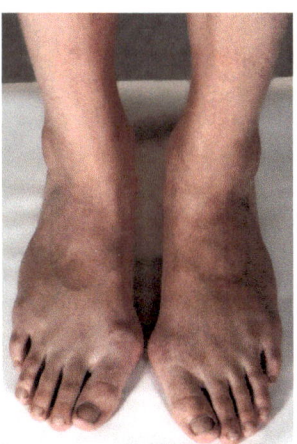

Corrective Procedures

More than 100 procedures have been described for the correction of hallux valgus. Bony procedures performed before the end of growth in the foot, at 13–14 years of age, are likely to fail because of recurrent deformity. Therefore, in the very rare case in which it is necessary to consider surgery before skeletal maturity, McBride's [61] so-called conservative operation is indicated. If at all possible, the surgeon should try to delay operation until skeletal maturity. Unfortunately, splints, insoles, and physiotherapy have little effect upon hallux valgus, and the only reasonable conservative treatment is to ensure that adequately fitting shoes are worn that do not press on the toes or the bunion.

Once skeletal maturity is reached, there is a bewildering array of osteotomies. Helal et al. [62] reviewed the results of a number of procedures and came to the conclusion that the oblique or Wilson osteotomy gave the most consistent results. The problem with this oblique osteotomy is that it can shorten the first metatarsal and so it is unsuitable if the second toe is particularly long. As in all metatarsal osteotomies, it is absolutely essential that the metatarsal head is not allowed to displace dorsally, thus reducing weight bearing on the first metatarsal head and increasing the pressure on the second metatarsal head, leading to metatarsalgia and, occasionally, stress fracture. The Chevron osteotomy, described by Johnson et al. in 1979 [63], is aimed at reducing the amount of shortening and holding the metatarsal head more firmly. This operation undoubtedly controls the metatarsal head well, but it is important not to damage the blood supply to the metatarsal head and to avoid avascular necrosis, which leads to pain and joint degeneration. Other popular forms of metatarsal osteotomy are the Homann-Thomason, described by Mygind [64] in which a peg is used to hold the head in position, the Mitchell [65], and more recently the scarf osteotomy [66]. Most surgeons will try a variety of these distal osteotomies and then settle on the one which they find works best for them.

In many ways proximal osteotomy at the base of the first metatarsal seems more logical. Clearly, this should be used with great care before skeletal maturity, because the growth plate is proximal and not distal, and must not be damaged. However, although good results have been reported by Simmonds and Menelaus [67], it is a more difficult procedure. It is harder to correct the metatarsal alignment and obtain long-term satisfactory results. It may be necessary, in severe cases, to combine the McBride procedure with a basal osteotomy to obtain full control of the deformity. Mann et al. [68] reported satisfactory results in 93% of patients in whom the combination of a basal crescentic first metatarsal osteotomy was combined with a modified McBride procedure. However, only 7 of 75 patients were younger than 20

the past, it was frequently assumed that this condition was caused by poorly fitting shoes, and parents were blamed for their child's hallux valgus. However, the condition is much more likely to be familial rather than acquired. Patients with this type of foot have a characteristically supple, broad forefoot with hallux valgus and a bunion on the medial side and often a bunionette or fifth metatarsal bunion on the lateral side (Fig. 9.21). Ill-fitting shoes do not cause the deformity, but they can cause symptoms by pressure over the medial side of the metatarsal head, leading to development of a bunion and crowding of the toes.

Medial deviation of the first metatarsal (metatarsus primus varus) is common and may be associated with a lateral deviation of the fifth metatarsal and a bunionette. Metatarsus varus is very common in young children and it is tempting to suggest that hallux valgus is the long-term result; however, there is no good evidence for this. Farsetti et al. [5], in their long-term review of metatarsus varus, found only one case of mild hallux valgus in one foot. In 1960, Piggot [60] in a very useful review showed that up to 20° of valgus at the first metatarsophalangeal joint is within normal limits. Between 20 and 25° of valgus, the big toe is deviated but does not necessarily progress to hallux valgus. Adolescents and young adults with this degree of valgus should be watched. However, once the valgus angle is greater than 25° progressive deformity is almost inevitable. Similarly, lateral subluxation of the proximal phalanx of the big toe on the first metatarsal head leads to inevitable progression of the deformity and, ultimately, degenerative change. The paper by Piggott [60] provides a rational basis for advising surgical correction: up to 20° there is no indication for surgery on account of the deformity itself; between 20 and 25° the situation should be watched; when there is more than 25° of deformity or lateral subluxation of the proximal phalanx on the metatarsal head, it is reasonable to offer surgical correction to prevent further progression and ultimately osteoarthritis in the joint.

Fig. 9.22 Clinical photograph of an overriding second toe. Note inward curling of the third, fourth, and fifth toes

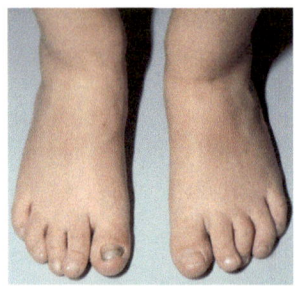

Fig. 9.23 Clinical photograph of severe hallux varus in association with a localized fibrous band

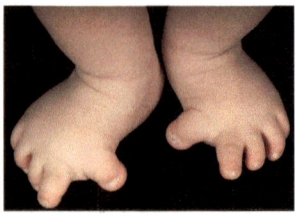

years, and the authors have made no special mention, in the description of the operative technique, of the care necessary to avoid damage to the epiphyseal plate at the base of the first metatarsal in patients in whom it is still open. Recently Davids et al. [69] have reported lateral hemiepiphysiodesis of the great toe for juvenile hallux valgus, with encouraging early results.

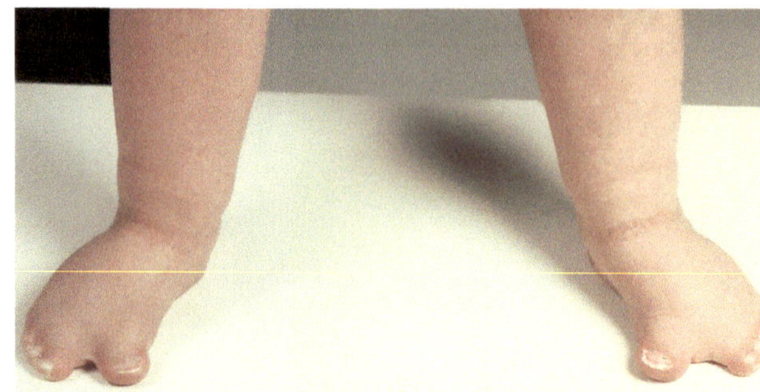

Overriding Second Toe

This condition is commonly seen in children's feet, particularly in association with curly third, fourth, and fifth toes (Fig. 9.22). The hallux is in mild valgus and the lateral three toes curl medially, so that the second toe is displaced dorsally and lies at a higher level than the first metatarsal and other toes. The condition is nearly always fully correctable passively and corrects spontaneously when the child starts to walk. Provided there is no fixed deformity, no treatment is indicated and parents can be reassured that, if shoes of adequate width are fitted, once the child starts to walk the condition should not cause any further problems. Very occasionally there is a persistent fixed contracture and tenotomy of the extensor tendon is indicated. Fixed flexion deformity of the third toe can also occur. If this does not correct with passive stretching by the mother, then a fixed hammer toe deformity can develop, causing problems with shoe wear and the development of the toenail. Simple flexor tenotomy or, occasionally, flexor-to-extensor transfer may be necessary if the deformity is symptomatic.

Hallux Varus

Minor forms of this condition are very common in association with metatarsus varus. Provided the deformity is fully correctable passively, the hallux varus should correct as the forefoot varus corrects, without any specific treatment. It can also occur as an isolated phenomenon in association with a localized fibrous band on the medial side of the foot (Fig. 9.23). If this fails to respond to passive stretching, the contracted fibrous band on the medial side of the

Fig. 9.24 Clinical photograph of the feet of a child with Apert's syndrome and hallux varus. Note syndactyly of the other toes

great toe, the tight abductor hallucis, and shortened medial capsule of the metatarsophalangeal joint of the big toe can be released. Finally, hallux varus may be associated with localized bony anomalies such as abnormal phalanges, duplication and accessory toes, congenital short first metatarsal, and with generalized conditions such as Apert's syndrome (acrocephalosyndactyly) (Fig. 9.24), diastrophic dwarfism, and myositis ossificans progressiva. Quite extensive and complex soft tissue and bony surgery may be necessary to correct hallux varus in these patients. [70, 71].

Hallux Rigidus

Hallux rigidus occurs in children and adolescents. Unlike the condition in adults, it is more common in girls than in boys. McMaster [72] has suggested an acute pathogenesis, or that chronic trauma associated with stubbing or stress on the big toe may cause a chondral or osteochondral injury to the head of the first metatarsal. Radiographically this is often not seen because it is largely or entirely a chondral lesion. As a result of the injury, the patient develops so-called metatarsus primus elevatus from spasm of the flexor of the big toe, with loss of dorsiflexion of the big toe and tenderness over the dorsum of the metatarsophalangeal joint. The patient walks awkwardly on the outer side of the foot as a result of loss of the normal "rock-over" at the first metatarsophalangeal joint. Protection of the joint by a rocker bar may relieve the symptoms, as may a short period of rest in a plaster. If, however, this fails, a dorsal closing wedge osteotomy of the proximal phalanx of the big toe as described by Bonney and MacNab

[73] can produce good results, provided the patient has 30° of plantar flexion before surgery. Citron and Neil [74] reported good long-term results at an average follow-up of 22 years in nine of ten toes treated with dorsal wedge osteotomy of the proximal phalanx. Radiographically the usual changes of degenerative arthritis are not seen in children, but sometimes a defect similar to that of osteochondritis of the knee may be seen on the metatarsal head, as has been reported by Kessel and Bonney [75].

Metatarsus Primus Elevatus

This condition was believed by Lambrinudi [76] to be a primary developmental abnormality. Nowadays, most surgeons would consider this to be secondary to plantar flexor spasm of the big toe. This may be seen in association with hallux rigidus and after surgical procedures on the mid- or hindfoot that cause supination of the foot so that the first metatarsal is elevated and the big toe has to be held in flexion in order to reach the ground. This is seen after surgery for congenital talipes equinovarus and also in neuromuscular conditions such as poliomyelitis and spina bifida. The patient develops pain over the dorsal bunion and also from the flexion of the big toe. It can be a difficult condition to treat unless muscle balance can be restored. This imbalance is commonly associated with a strong tibialis anterior, elevating the first metatarsal, and weakness of the peroneus longus. Lapidus [77] described transfer of flexor hallucis longus through a tunnel in the first metatarsal into the dorsum of the proximal phalanx, with a basal osteotomy of the first metatarsal, for this deformity.

Interphalangeal Valgus of the Big Toe

Sometimes valgus of the big toe occurs, not at the metatarsophalangeal joint but at the interphalangeal joint, usually associated with a congenital anomaly of the distal phalanx. This can cause problems with the distal phalanx pressing on the second toe, or even lying underneath it. Radiographs may show a malformation of the interphalangeal joint, the epiphysis of the distal phalanx often appearing wedge shaped, the base of the wedge being on the medial side. If symptoms are sufficient, the deformity can be corrected either by osteotomy of the proximal phalanx, removing a medially based wedge, or after growth has finished by fusion of the interphalangeal joint, provided there is a full range of pain-free movement at the first metatarsophalangeal joint.

Duplication, Syndactyly, and Accessory Toes

Minor anomalies such as duplication, syndactyly, and accessory toes are quite common. They may occur on their own or in association with generalized conditions such as chondroectodermal dysplasia (Ellis–Van Creveld syndrome) and Apert's syndrome (Fig. 9.24) and also with local abnormalities such as tibial dysplasia. Congenital shortening of the first metatarsal is seen in fibrodysplasia (myositis) ossificans progressiva (Chapter 7) and dysplastic nails in the nail-patella syndrome (onycho-osteodystrophy). It is very important to look at the entire patient in addition to the feet.

Syndactyly frequently needs no treatment. Duplications and accessory toes can sometimes be simply reduced or removed, but occasionally the skeletal architecture is very complex and careful planning and meticulous surgery are necessary. Both Phelps and Grogan [78] and Turra et al. [79] in important reviews of surgery for polydactyly reported good long-term results in the majority of post-axial polydactyly patients but more problems in pre-axial polydactyly due to recurrent hallux varus. Parents may frequently ask for the surgery to be performed early, before the child starts to walk, but often it is better to wait until the child has reached at least the age of 1 year, so that the bony architecture of the foot can be more accurately assessed before surgery is decided upon.

The Accessory Navicular

The accessory navicular (prehallux; os tibiale externum) is one of many benign ossicles which may be detected radiographically in relation to the midfoot and hindfoot. It is the most likely to become symptomatic, particularly in later childhood, and may be familial [80]. The type 1 ossicle is very small, residing within the tibialis posterior tendon; it rarely requires excision. The type 2 is larger (approximately 1 cm in diameter) and is joined to the main navicular through cartilage. The lump is analogous with a bipartite patellar ossicle. Stress, trauma, skeletal growth, and pressure from the inner border of the shoes have all been implicated in the onset of symptoms.

Kidner [81] considered that the accessory navicular was associated with, or even causative of, flat foot. This is now disproved and his relatively complex and potentially hazardous rerouting of the tibialis posterior tendon was shown by Macnicol and Voutsinas [80] to be no better than simple excision of the accessory bone and careful contouring of the residual navicular medially.

The majority of symptomatic feet can be managed conservatively, with reassurance of the child and parents and minor adjustment of the shoes. A magnetic resonance (MR) scan reveals marrow edema [82] and helps to define the extent of the skeletal reaction. If symptoms and scan changes persist, excision of the lesion is achieved through a curved, skin crease incision and longitudinal splitting of the tendon, leaving intact the various attachments of the tibialis tendon to the tarsal bones. Unlike the postoperative splintage advised following the Kidner procedure, the lesser procedure of excision allows partial weight bearing with crutches for a few weeks and a relatively rapid resumption of normal activity.

Symptoms may recur to some extent as the child completes the adolescent growth spurt. It is therefore important to ensure that supportive and comfortable shoes do not give way to fashionable but symptom-provoking footwear.

Congenital Split or Cleft Foot (Lobster Claw Foot)

This is a rare congenital anomaly characterized by failure of development of the central two or three rays of the foot (Fig. 9.25). The first metatarsal may be normal or enlarged and the hallux is usually in valgus. There is then a large cleft and the remainder of the foot is made up of the lateral fourth or fifth rays, with the phalanges deviating medially. The hindfoot is usually normal. The common form is bilateral and inherited as an autosomal dominant with incomplete penetrance. There is a more rare unilateral form, in which there is usually no family history. The condition can occur on its own or in association with clefts of the hands. It can also be associated with cleft lip and cleft palate and deafness.

Surgery may be considered to improve footwear and cosmesis. Abraham et al. [83], in a useful review, classified the deformity into three groups according to severity: type I in which a central partial forefoot cleft is present and can be treated by a soft tissue syndactylism with correction of the hallux valgus if necessary; type II, a complete forefoot cleft involving the tarsus, can be treated by a soft tissue syndactylism with osteotomy of the first ray to aid the soft tissue

closure; and type III in which there is complete absence of the first to the fourth rays, so the patients did not require surgery and managed well in normal shoes with a shoe filler or "false foot."

References

1. Bankart ASB. Metatarsus varus. Brit Med J 1921; 2: 685.
2. Harris NH. Rotational deformities and their secondary effects in the lower extremities in children. J Bone Joint Surg 1972; 54B: 172
3. Ponseti IV, Becker JR. Congenital metatarsus varus. The results of treatment. J Bone Joint Surg 1966; 48A: 702–711.
4. Rushforth GF. The natural history of hooked forefoot. J Bone Joint Surg 1978; 60B: 530–542.
5. Farsetti P, Weinstein L, Ponseti IV. The long term functional and radiographic outcomes of untreated and non-operatively treated metatarsus adductus. J Bone Joint Surg 1994; 76A: 257–265.
6. Katz K, David R, Soudry M. Below knee plaster cast for the treatment of metatarsus adductus. J Paediatr Orthop 1999; 19: 49–50.
7. Browne RS, Paton DF. Anomalous insertion of the tibialis posterior in congenital metatarsus varus. J Bone Joint Surg 1979; 61B: 74–76.
8. Heyman CH, Herndon CH, Strong JM. Mobilisation of the tarso-metatarsal and intermetatarsal joints for the correction of resistant adduction of the forepart of the foot in congenital club foot or congenital metatarsus varus. J Bone Joint Surg 1986; 40A: 299–310.
9. Stark KG, Johanson JE, Winter RB. The Heyman-Hendon tarsometatarsal capsulotomy for metatarsus adductus; results in 48 feet. J Paediatr Orthop 1987; 7: 305–310.
10. Berman A, Gartland J. Metatarsal osteotomy for the correction of adduction of the forepart of the foot in children. J Bone Joint Surg 1971; 53A: 498–506.
11. Bleck EE. Metatarsus adductus: classification and relationship to outcomes of treatment. J Paediatr Orthop 1983; 3: 2–9.
12. Kite JH. Congenital metatarsus varus. J Bone Joint Surg 1967; 46A: 388–397.
13. Lloyd-Roberts GC, Clark RC. Ball and socket ankle joint in metatarsus adductus varus. J Bone Joint Surg 1973; 55B: 193–196.
14. Mosca VA. Flexible flat foot and skew foot. J Bone Joint Surg 1995; 77A: 1937–1945.
15. Evans D. Calcaneovalgus deformity. J Bone Joint Surg 1975; 57B: 170–278.
16. Fowler SB, Banks AL, Parrish TF. The cavovarus foot. J Bone Joint Surg 1959; 41A: 757.
17. Lloyd-Roberts GC, Pilcher MF. Structural idiopathic scoliosis in infancy. J Bone Joint Surg 1965; 47B: 520–523.
18. Giannestras J. Foot Disorders, Medical and Surgical Management, 2nd ed. London: Henry Kimpton; 1973.
19. Sutherland DM, Olsehn R, Cooper L, Woo SLY. The development of mature gait. J Bone Joint Surg 1980; 62A: 336–353.
20. Hall JE, Salter RB, Bhalla SK. Congenital short tendo calcaneus. J Bone Joint Surg 1967; 49B: 695–697.
21. Eastwood DM, Cole G, Dickens DRD. Idiopathic toe walking: is this a neurological problem "solved" by surgery? Proceedings of the British Society of Children's Orthopaedic Surgery. J Bone Join Surg 1996; 78B:(Suppl 1) 11.
22. Stricker SJ, Angulo JC. Idiopathic toe-walking: a comparison of treatment methods. J Paediatr Orthop 1998; 18: 289–293.
23. Stott NS, Walt SE, Lobb GA, et al. Treatment for idiopathic toe-walking: results at skeletal maturity. J Pediatr Orthop 2004; 24: 63–69.

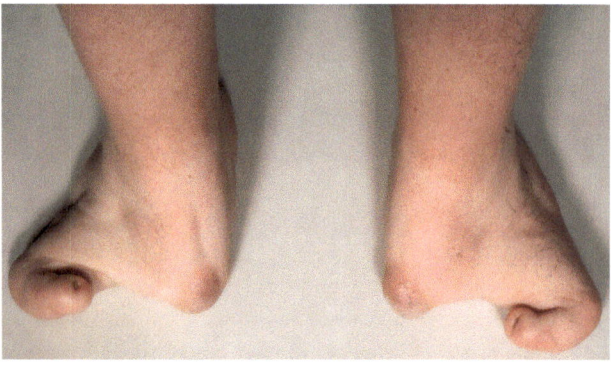

Fig. 9.25 Clinical photograph of the severe form of cleft (lobster claw) foot (Abrahams et al. [78] type III)

24. Kohler A. Uber einer haufige bisher ansheinend uberkannte Erkrankung einzeiner kindlicher Knocken Munchen. Medizinische Wochtenschrift 1908; 55: 1923.

25. Waugh W. The ossification and vascularisation of the tarsal navicular and their relation to Kohler's disease. J Bone Joint Surg 1958; 40B: 765–777.

26. Cox MJ. Kohler's disease. Postgrad Med J 1958; 34: 58–59.

27. Sever JW. Apophysitis of the os calcis. NY Med J 1912; 95: 1025–1029.

28. Antoniou D, Connor AM. Osteomyelitis of the calcaneus and talus. J Bone Joint Surg 1974; 56A: 338–345.

29. Staheli LT, Chew BE, Corbett M. The longitudinal arch. A survey of 882 feet in normal children. J Bone Joint Surg 1987; 69A: 426–428.

30. Carter C, Wilkinson J. Persistent joint laxity and congenital dislocation of the hip. J Bone Joint Surg 1964; 46B: 40–45.

31. Cheng JCY, Chan PS, Hui PW. Joint laxity in children. J Paediatr Orthop 1991; 11: 752–756.

32. Morley AJM. Knock knee in children. Brit Med J 1957; 2: 976–979.

33. Rose GK, Welton CA, Marshal T. The diagnosis of flat foot in the child. J Bone Joint Surg 1986; 67B: 71–78.

34. Wenger DR, Maudlin D, Speck G, et al. Corrective shoes and inserts as treatment for flexible flat foot in infants and children J Bone Joint Surg 1989; 71A: 800–810.

35. Rao UB, Joseph B. The influence of footwear on the prevalence of flat foot. J Bone Joint Surg 1992; 74B: 525–527.

36. Echam JJ, Forriol F. The development in foot print morphology in 1851 Congolese children from urban and rural areas and the relationship between this and wearing shoes. J Pediatr Orthop B 2003; 12: 141–146.

37. Seymour N. The late results of naviculo-cuneiform fusion. J Bone Joint Surg 1967; 49B: 558–559.

38. Koutsogiannis E. Treatment of mobile flat feet by displacement osteotomy of the calcaneus. J Bone Joint Surg 1971; 53B: 96–100.

39. Jones Sir R. Peroneal spasm and its treatment. Report on a meeting of the Liverpool Medical Institution Journal 1897; 17: 442.

40. Slomann MC. Coalition calcaneo navicularis. J Orthop Surg 1921; 3: 586–602.

41. Badgely CE. Coalition of the calcaneus and the navicular. Arch Surg 1927; 15: 75–88.

42. Harris RI, Beath T. Etiology of peroneal spastic flat foot. J Bone Joint Surg 1948; 30B: 624–634.

43. Simmons EH. Tibialis posterior varus foot with tarsal coalition. J Bone Joint Surg 1965; 47B: 533–536.

44. Oestreich E, Mize WA, Crawford AH, Morgan RB. The "anteater's nose." A direct sign of calcaneo navicular coalition on the lateral radiograph. J Paediatr Orthop 1987; 7: 709–711.

45. Leonard MA. The inheritance of tarsal coalition and its relationship to spastic flat foot. J Bone Joint Surg 1974; 56B: 520–525.

46. Braddock GTF. A prolonged follow up of peroneal spastic flat foot. J Bone Joint Surg 1961; 43B: 734–737.

47. Mitchell GP, Gibson JMC. Excision of calcaneonavicular bar for painful spasmodic flat foot. J Bone Joint Surg 1967; 49B: 281–287.

48. Macnicol MF, Inglis G, Buxton RA. Symptomatic calcaneonavicular bars. J Bone Joint Surg 1986; 68B: 128–131.

49. Dwyer FC. Causes, significance and treatment of stiffness of the subtaloid joint. Proc Royal Soc Med 1976; 69: 97–102.

50. Cain TJ, Hyman S. Peroneal spastic flat foot. J Bone Joint Surg 1978; 60B: 527–529.

51. Olney BW, Asher MA. Excision of symptomatic coalition of the middle facet of the talo-calcaneal joint. J Bone Joint Surg 1987; 69A: 539–544.

52. McCormack J, Olney B, Asher M. Talo-calcaneal coalition resection: a 10-year follow up. J Paediatr Orthop 1997; 17: 13–15.

53. Blockey NJ. Peroneal spastic flat foot. J Bone Joint Surg 1959; 37B: 191–202.

54. Trethowan WH. Treatment of hammer toes. Lancet 1925; 1: 1257–1258.

55. Sweetnam DR. Congenital curly toes. An investigation into the value of treatment. Lancet 1958; 2: 398–400.

56. Meneiaus MB, Ross ERS. Open flexor tenotomy for hammer toes and curly toes in childhood. J Bone Joint Surg 1984; 66B: 770–771.

57. Taylor RG. The treatment of claw toes by multiple transfers and flexor to extensor tendons. J Bone Joint Surg 1951; 35B: 539–542.

58. Wilson JN. V-Y correction for varus deformity of the 5th toe. Br J Surg 1953; 41: 133–135.

59. Cockin J. Butler's operation for overriding 5th toe. J Bone Joint Surg 1968; 60B: 78–81.

60. Piggot H. The natural history of hallux valgus in adolescents and early adult life. J Bone Joint Surg 1960; 42B: 749–760.

61. McBride ED. A conservative operation for bunions. J Bone Joint Surg 1928; 10B: 735–739.

62. Helal B, Gupta SK, Gojaseni P. Surgery for adolescent hallux valgus. Acta Orthop Scand 1974; 45: 271–295.

63. Johnson KA, Cofield RH, Morrey BF. Chevron osteotomy for hallux valgus. Clin Orthop Rel Res 1979; 142: 44–47.

64. Mygind H. Operations for hallux valgus. Report of Danish Orthopaedic Association. J Bone Joint Surg 1952; 34B: 529.

65. Mitchell CL, Fleming JL, Allen R, et al. Osteotomy bunionectomy for hallux valgus. J Bone Joint Surg 1958; 40A: 41–49.

66. Crevoisier X, Mouhsine E, Ortolano V, et al. The scarf osteotomy for the treatment of hallux valgus deformity: a review of 84 cases. Foot Ankle Int 2001; 22: 970–976.

67. Simmonds FA, Menelaus MB. Hallux valgus in adolescence. J Bone Joint Surg 1960; 42B: 761–768.

68. Mann RA, Rudicel S, Grabes SC. Repair of hallux valgus with a distal soft tissue procedure and proximal metatarsal osteotomy. J Bone Joint Surg 1992; 74A: 124–129.

69. Davids JR, McBrayer D, Blackhurst DW. Juvenile Hallux Valgus Deformity, Surgical Manager by lateral hemiepiphyseodesis of the great toe metatarsal. J Pediatr Orthop 2007; 27: 826–70.

70. Mubarak SJ, O'Brien J, Davids JR. Metatarsal epiphyseal bracket: treatment by central physiolysis. J Paediatr Orthop 1993; 13: 5–8.

71. Anderson PJ, Hall CM, Evans RD, et al. The feet in Apert's syndrome. J Paediatr Orthop 1999; 19: 504–507.

72. McMaster MJ. The pathogenesis of hallux rigidus. J Bone Joint Surg 1978; 60B: 82–87.

73. Bonney G, MacNab I. Hallux valgus and hallux rigidus. A critical survey of operative results. J Bone Joint Surg 1952; 34B: 366–385.

74. Citron N, Neil M. Dorsal wedge osteotomy of the proximal phalanx for hallux rigidus. J Bone Joint Surg 1987; 69B: 835–837.

75. Kessel I, Bonney G. Hallux rigidus in the adolescent. J Bone Joint Surg 1958; 40B: 668–673.

76. Lambrinudi C. Metatarsus primus elevatus. Proc Royal Soc Med 1938; 31: 1273.

77. Lapidus PW. "Dorsal Bunion": its mechanics and operative correction. J Bone Joint Surg 1940; 22: 627–637.

78. Phelps DA, Grogan DP. Polydactyly of the foot. J Pediatr Orthop 1985; 5: 448–451.

79. Turra S, Gigante C, Businella G. Polydactyly of the foot. J Pediatr Orthop 2007; B 16: 216–220.

80. Macnicol MF, Voutsinas S. Surgical treatment of the symptomatic accessory navicular. J Bone Joint Surg 1984; 66B: 218–222.

81. Kidner FC. The prehallux (accessory scaphoid) in its relation to flat foot. J Bone Joint Surg 1929; 11: 831–834.

82. Miller TT, Staron RB, Feldman F, et al. The symptomatic accessory tarsal navicular bone: assessment with MR imaging. Radiology 1995; 195: 849–53.

83. Abraham E, Waxman B, Shirali S, Durkin M. Congenital cleft foot deformity treatment. J Paediatr Orthop 1999; 19: 404–430.

Chapter 10

The Clubfoot: Congenital Talipes Equinovarus

Deborah M. Eastwood

The clubfoot is a common, classic, paediatric orthopaedic problem. Every orthopaedic surgeon knows what the deformity looks like but most find it more difficult to describe or to define. The etiology is still largely unknown but ideas about treatment have changed considerably over the last few years.

The overall picture of a talipes equinovarus deformity is one of ankle equinus, hindfoot varus, and forefoot adduction with pronation of the first ray giving the appearance of cavus (Fig. 10.1a). The typical, isolated clubfoot is congenital and idiopathic in origin. Some cases are positional or postural in which case the deformity, by definition, resolves completely by 3 months with minimal treatment. At the other end of the spectrum some examples of rigid clubfoot are associated with syndromic conditions and more generalized musculoskeletal problems (Fig. 10.1b). A further subgroup of foot problems are seen in neuromuscular disorders such as spina bifida where the deformity may worsen with time as the neuromuscular imbalance develops (Table 10.1).

Incidence

The incidence of isolated clubfoot varies between racial groups: in Caucasians the rate of idiopathic cases is approximately 1:1000 live births; in Asians, slightly lower at 0.7:1000; and in Aboriginals, Polynesians, Maoris, and native Hawaiians, the rate of 4–6:1000 is significantly higher. All studies agree that boys are more commonly affected than girls: the ratio is usually quoted as 2:1 but rising to 4:1 in the Aboriginal groups. Among live births, approximately 50% of cases are bilateral.

D.M. Eastwood (✉)
Department of Paediatric Orthopaedics, Great Ormond Street Hospital, London, UK

A familial tendency is apparent among first-degree relatives but inheritance is considered by most to be multifactorial (Table 10.2) [1–3].

The complex clubfoot, one that is associated with other congenital anomalies, has an incidence of 0.7–0.9:1000 births and is significantly more likely to be bilateral.

Other factors associated with an increased incidence are first-trimester amniocentesis [4], maternal smoking [5, 6], hyperemesis, and maternal anemia [3].

Antenatal Diagnosis

In developed countries, antenatal ultrasound scans are now used almost universally in the management of the mother and child during pregnancy. Increasingly, ultrasonography is also being used to detect fetal anomalies such as a clubfoot but the false-positive rates can be high, depending upon the timing of the scan, the skill of the operator, and whether or not the scan is primarily assessing the pregnancy or the fetus. The detection of these anomalies has obvious implications for the parents and the medical staff as both groups require accurate information regarding the condition and its prognosis in order to plan management. In certain cases, termination of the pregnancy may be an option.

The overall detection rate of talipes equinovarus foot deformities in utero has improved with time and, currently, in a large non-selected Norwegian population, 77% of cases were identified antenatally [7]. The earliest such cases that can be identified is at 12 weeks but "new" cases can be seen as late as the third trimester [8]. Bar-Hava et al. [9] have noted that the clubfoot deformity can appear as a transient phenomenon and others have noted that the diagnosis, or the complexity of the case, can change during pregnancy in up to 25% of cases [10]. Many authors have stressed the need for sequential and detailed fetal anomaly scans (DFAS) in order to reduce the false-positive rate. Bar-On et al. report a positive predictive value of 83% (a false-positive rate of 17%) [10]. Generally, it is easier to detect bilateral cases

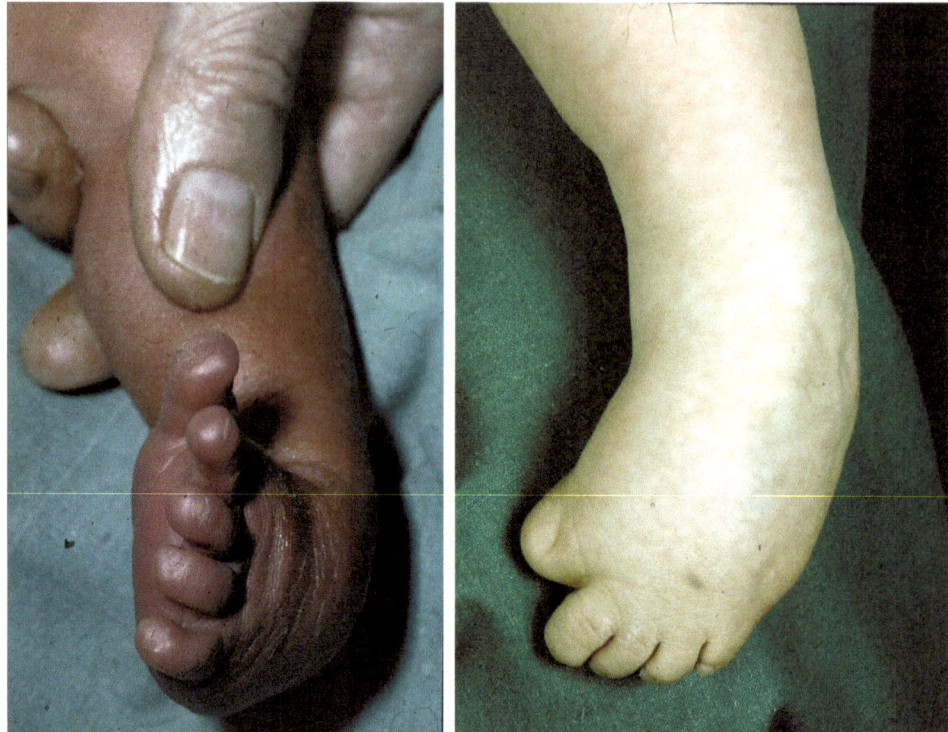

Fig. 10.1 (**a**) Clinical photograph of a unilateral idiopathic clubfoot deformity. (**b**) Clinical photograph of a unilateral syndromic clubfoot deformity

Table 10.1 Types of clubfoot

Type	Characteristic	Other features	Example
Idiopathic	Rigid foot	Isolated finding	
Postural	More supple	Associated with other "moulding" affects, e.g., plagiocephaly	
Neuromuscular	Often rigid but not necessarily so	Altered muscle tone and reflexes. Sensory changes and muscle imbalance	Spina bifida or myelomeningocele
Syndromic	Very rigid	Associated with widespread musculoskeletal abnormalities and often anomalies affecting other systems	Constriction bands; Arthrogryposis; Tibial dysplasia; Larsen syndrome; Pierre Robin; syndrome; diastrophic dwarfism

and these are more likely to be the complex cases [7]. Thus, correspondingly, the false-positive rate is higher in the isolated cases [11]. It is therefore important not only to detect cases but also to classify them accurately. Bar-On et al. [10] reported an accuracy of 73% in obtaining a specific diagnosis of an isolated versus a complex deformity and they noted that all errors were ones of overdiagnosis.

It is important to recognize that the in utero diagnosis of a clubfoot deformity does not correlate with the severity of the condition at birth. Indeed, in some studies a postural clubfoot at birth is considered as a positive finding, while in others such a case is labeled as a false positive: perhaps, the term *functional false positive* should be used for

these cases [12]. Certainly, when counseling parents antenatally, it is important to recognize that some apparently severe foot deformities may require minimal or indeed no postnatal treatment [12, 13]. The rates of surgical intervention quoted almost all predate the widespread use of the Ponseti technique and in terms of contemporary management are probably meaningless. While it is likely that more detailed scans and advancing technology will improve our understanding of the prenatal foot deformity, there is no suggestion as yet that fetal surgery in utero would be helpful.

At present, there is no indication for amniocentesis and karyotyping when an isolated clubfoot is diagnosed by DFAS [14].

Table 10.2 Familial influences on the presentation of clubfoot

Parent(s)	Affected child	% Chance of sibling CTEV
Normal	Male	2.5
	Female	6.5 if male 2.5 if female
Affected	Male or Female	10–25
	Monozygotic twins	Concordance rate 32.5
	Dizygotic twins	Concordance rate 3

Pathoanatomy

The primary pathology in the clubfoot is subluxation of the talonavicular joint. There are associated, similar abnormalities of the calcaneocuboid and talocalcaneal joints. The talar head is readily palpable on the dorsolateral aspect of the foot. Anatomical dissections and radiographic studies [15–17] have shown that the talus is plantarflexed and, with respect to the ankle mortise, the anterior end of the long axis of the talus has rotated laterally even though the actual talar head and neck are tilted medially and plantarward. The calcaneus is also plantarflexed and its long axis is rotated through the subtalar joint but in the opposite direction to that of the talus. This medial spin means that the anterior end of the calcaneus lies medially, while the posterior part lies adjacent to the lateral malleolus. (Fig. 10.2). Both the navicular and cuboid lie medially. All these joint subluxations are held by capsular, ligamentous, or musculotendinous contractures. The structures most commonly identified as being tight are the sheaths of the tibialis posterior tendon and the peroneal tendons, the plantar-based talocalcaneonavicular (or spring) ligament, and the calcaneofibular ligament. These ligaments contain more collagen fibers and increased cellularity on histological examination [18, 19]. Several authors [20, 21] have identified cells with myofibroblastic characteristics on electron microscopy of the medial structures of the clubfoot and consider that these may contribute to the deformities. However, a more recent paper [22] suggested that collagen crosslinking was normal and failed to identify myofibroblasts. Recently, Hattori et al. [23] have shown reduced elasticity in the lateral ligaments and capsule compared to the medial structures, adding weight to the concept of the posterolateral tether.

Abnormalities of muscle infrastructure and insertion have also been identified. There is evidence of intramuscular fibrosis and limited muscle excursion with a predominance of type 1 muscle fibers in the posteromedial muscle groups, noted along with other histological features that suggest a local or regional neurological abnormality [24–26].

The dorsalis pedis artery may be absent or its supply to the foot altered in patients with clubfoot [27, 28]. Recently, Katz et al. [29] have shown a deficient blood flow in this vessel in almost half of clubfoot cases compared with only 8% of

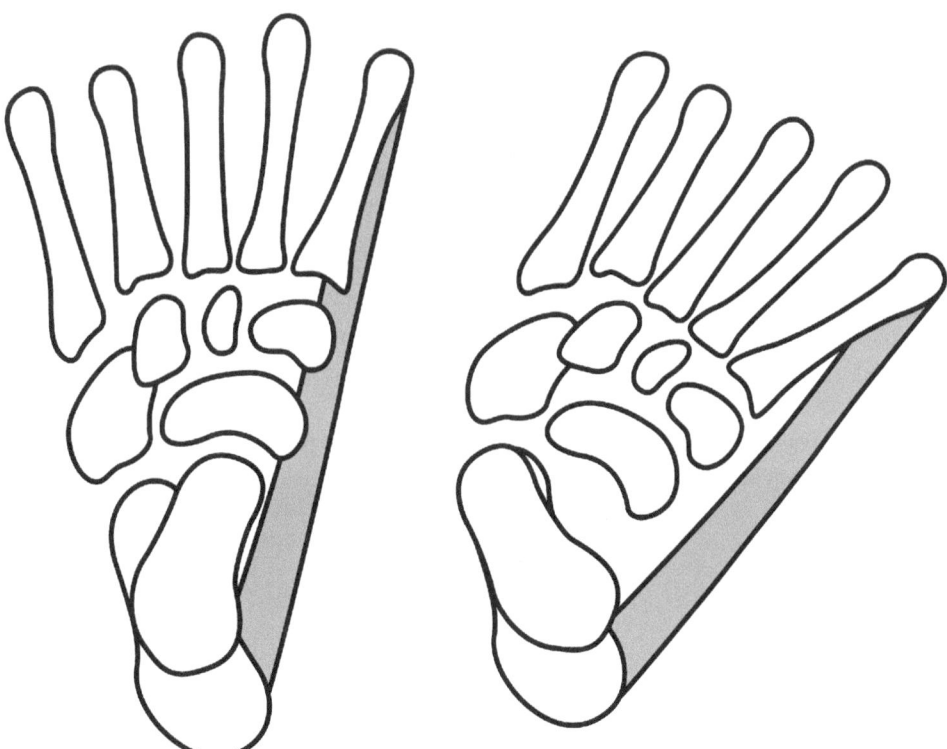

Fig. 10.2 Line diagram of the relationships between the talus and the calcaneus (and the associated tarsal bones) in the normal and the club foot

normal feet. They suggest that the severity of the deformity relates to this.

While, overall, there is agreement regarding these descriptions of the pathological changes associated with a clubfoot deformity, there is still considerable disagreement about their etiology and whether any individual anomaly is a cause or an effect. Many of the histological studies are small and have not been repeated and in the case of fetal dissections, the data may not be representative of the more general example of a clubfoot.

Etiological Theories

Genetic Influences

Many papers [30, 31] have studied the familial incidence of idiopathic talipes equinovarus and noted the different incidence in first-degree versus second- and third-degree relatives and the lack of complete concordance in monozygotic twins. They have concluded that inheritance must be multifactorial. Twin studies have characterized the increased incidence and suggested that the risk for the second monozygotic twin is 1:3 [32, 33]. Recent genetic studies are beginning to identify possible candidate genes. Ester et al. [34] noted that certain chromosomal deletions (on the long arm of chromosome 2) were associated with the clubfoot phenotype. Previous linkage studies have also implicated this region and it may harbor genes that contribute to the development of clubfoot. Single nucleotide polymorphisms (SNPs) in three apoptotic genes were investigated. Programmed cell death that is regulated by these genes is important during growth and development, and the study suggests that apoptotic genetic variation may play a role in clubfoot etiology. The same group of researchers [35] also noted the association of clubfoot with maternal smoking and investigated the biotransformation of environmental exogenous substances such as tobacco smoke which can be modulated by genes such as the N-acetylation genes (NAT1 & 2). Slow NAT2 acetylation may be a risk factor for idiopathic clubfoot with NAT2 being a possible biotransformation candidate gene.

Other Theories

Some long-standing theories on the etiology are now becoming discredited. The increased use of antenatal ultrasound scans has shown that intrauterine fetal *molding* is not a common cause of idiopathic clubfoot deformity although it may account for some of the "late" cases that develop in previously normal fetuses when the relative lack of amniotic fluid in late pregnancy may contribute to a postural clubfoot deformity. Early amniocentesis is associated with an increased incidence of clubfoot, particularly when accompanied by an amniotic fluid leak. Molding at this early stage may have a role in some cases [4].

There is an obvious association between clubfoot deformities and certain *neuromuscular* conditions such as spina bifida, and in these feet, neuromuscular imbalance must be an important factor. Much more subtle or more short-lived episodes of imbalance may be a factor in other idiopathic cases and some of the pathological muscle changes identified would support a resolving neuropathic process [25]. It is difficult to know whether the changes seen are primary or adaptive and more recent studies have failed to substantiate these theories [36].

The primary abnormality may be with the initial formation of the cartilage anlage or a *failure of the normal maturation process* during fetal development. The fetal foot position changes from one of equinovarus to one of calcaneovalgus at about the same time as changes in blood supply to the fetal limb occur. Problems with this maturation process may account for those cases in which the dorsalis pedis pulse is absent and the deformity severe [29].

It is well recognized that the clubfoot is often small and the calf thin and possibly short. Shimode et al. [37] confirmed these findings and quantified the field change that affects growth of the whole lower limb including the femur and thigh. Changes in limb length and girth were more obvious distally than proximally and were significantly more obvious in the operatively treated cases compared to those treated conservatively.

It is unlikely that one single etiological agent or theory can account for all cases of clubfoot deformity. The etiology is probably multifactorial, different influences affecting foot development at different stages with potentially a summative effect on the severity of the deformity. Thus a genetic tendency allied to a mild, temporary neuromuscular imbalance may lead to a foot deformity that could be significantly exacerbated in the later stages of pregnancy by a period of intrauterine molding.

If the relevant influences producing any individual deformity could be identified, this might help to establish a better individual prognosis and affect the choice of treatment.

Clinical Assessment

The diagnosis of a clubfoot deformity is clinical. A full assessment of the child will help to distinguish the idiopathic foot from the "syndromic" foot (Table 10.1) and identify any obvious underlying neuromuscular imbalance. Careful note should be made of skin or soft tissue dimples or signs of an amniotic band as these features are indicative of a "syndromic" foot and are associated with a poorer response to treatment.

The flexibility of the foot is an important feature and the fixed deformities at each level should be identified and quantified as this helps the clinician to understand which tight structures are limiting joint movement and may influence treatment. Deep posterior and medial skin creases are universal in the idiopathic clubfoot and may distinguish this foot from a simple postural deformity.

Classification Systems

Although several systems exist it is becoming apparent that only two are useful in terms of ease of application and communication, reliability, and as a guide to prognosis.

Both of the commonly used systems of Dimeglio [38] (Fig. 10.3) and Pirani [39] (Table 10.3) apply a point score to various physical findings which when summated differentiate between mildly affected feet that require little or no treatment and the more severely affected foot that is likely to require treatment. Flynn et al. [40] showed good inter- and intra-observer correlation with both systems and noted that there was a significant improvement in correlation once the learning curve had been "completed." The Pirani score has been modified, but not revalidated, since this study. Wainwright et al. [41] looked at four commonly used classification systems in the United Kingdom and found the Dimeglio system to be the most reliable.

It is hoped that such systems will be used increasingly to quantify the severity of the clubfoot being treated in order to allow a more valid comparison of treatment methods.

Imaging

Traditionally, plain radiographs have formed part of the baseline evaluation of the clubfoot deformity but often the information obtained was of limited value. Standard radiographic views are difficult to obtain so this tends to invalidate attempts at radiographic measurement, as does the observation that the ossific nuclei may be more eccentrically placed within the cartilage anlage in the clubfoot than in the normal infantile foot. Stress radiographs that theoretically might quantify the flexibility of the infant foot are also difficult to obtain. Radiographs may be useful in simple terms to exclude any obvious bony abnormality such as a tibial dysplasia masquerading as a clubfoot deformity (Fig. 10.4). The lateral and anteroposterior (AP) talocalcaneal angles should diverge: parallelism in one or both views, particularly on simulated weight bearing, suggests persistent deformity. Radiographs can also identify "false correction" when dorsiflexion is occurring as a result of a midfoot breech.

Computed tomography (CT) and magnetic resonance (MR) scans define the pathoanatomy of the deformity and have been used to document the effects of treatment on the foot, but neither technique is used for primary assessment of the infant clubfoot.

Ultrasound does show promise in evaluating the clubfoot. Several studies have identified ultrasonographic features that are reliably different in the clubfoot and the normal foot and these can be used to assess the foot and monitor the effect of treatment. The most commonly used measurement is the medial malleolar to navicular (MMN) distance which is significantly lower in clubfeet than in normal feet and although the distance increases in both feet with age, the rate of change is significantly less in the clubfoot [42].

Management of the Idiopathic Foot

Over recent years, there has been a reversal in philosophy concerning the most effective treatment of the infant clubfoot deformity with a complete swing away from the extensive surgical approach that all too often seemed to follow "traditional" conservative regimes [43]. Manipulative techniques have been in use for several centuries, the Thomas wrench being an early, extreme example of this, and Kite's method, a more acceptable and popular method in the mid-20th century. Dissatisfaction with the results of these relatively lengthy treatment protocols led to a swing toward surgical releases but the long-term results of such surgery have been disappointing [44]. Not surprisingly, this encouraged a trend back to conservative methods just at the time when one particular technique was reporting improved long-term results. This happened simultaneously with the development of the simple, effective scoring systems mentioned above that allowed practitioners to document the type of foot they were seeing and, to a certain extent, the influence of treatment upon it.

Ponseti Method

The Ponseti [45] method of treatment corrects the clubfoot by a process of serial manipulations and cast applications that sequentially correct the three essential deformities of the foot namely the cavus, the adduction, and the equinovarus. Several minutes of manipulation are required at every cast

Classification			Assessment of Clubfoot by Severity Scale			
Classification grade	Type	Score	Characteristics: Deformity	Points (pts)	Characteristics: Other parameters	Points (pts)
I	Benign	(<5)	90-45°	4	Posterior crease	1
II	Moderate	(=5<10)	45-20°	3	Medial crease	1
III	Severe	(=10<15)	20-0°	2	Cavus	1
IV	Very severe	(=15<20)	<20 to −20°	1	Poor muscle condition	1

Sagittal plane evaluation of equinus

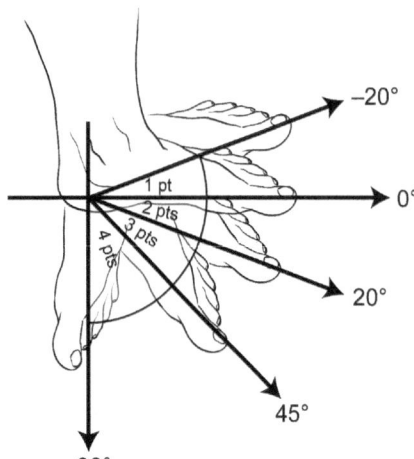

Frontal plane evaluation of varus

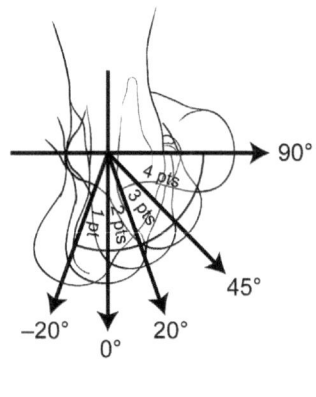

Horizontal plane evaluation of derotation of the calcaneopedal block

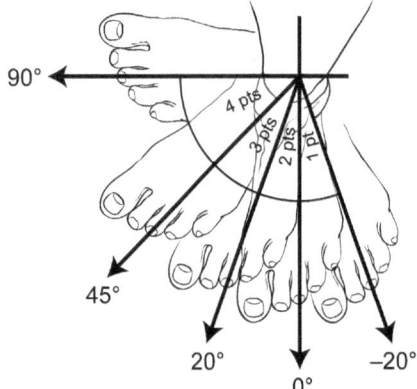

Horizontal plane evaluation of forefoot relative to hindfoot

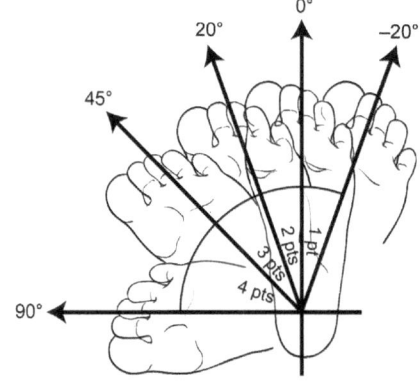

Fig. 10.3 The Dimeglio classification system. Four aspects of the deformity (the equinus, varus, rotation of the foot, and forefoot medial deviation) are scored on a scale of 1 (good) to 4 (bad) with four other categories (depth of posterior crease, medial crease, cavus, and muscle power) being assigned a present/absent score of 0 or 1 to give a total maximum score of 20

change in order to stretch tight structures and allow improved bone and joint alignment prior to the improved position being held with a further cast. The classic casts as advocated by Ponseti and his group involve a small amount of padding and a well-applied above-knee plaster cast. Others have experimented with different casting materials and with shorter casts and feel these modifications work well in their hands.

The standard protocol involves weekly cast changes and an extensive surgical procedure can be avoided in around 95% of cases. Treatment is usually started within a few days of birth.

The cavus deformity in clubfoot is principally a problem of the first ray. In order to correct this, the first ray must be dorsiflexed, effectively supinating the forefoot further. Correction of the cavus realigns the metatarsals, navicular, cuboid, and cuneiforms into the same plane. With the initial cast application, the forefoot is also abducted with laterally based, counterpressure applied over the talar head.

Table 10.3 The Pirani classification

HFCS	PC	The severity of the posterior crease	0	multiple fine creases
Hindfoot contracture score			0.5	one or two deep creases
		Foot held in maximal correction	1	deep creases change the contour of the arch
	EH	The emptiness of the heel	0	tuberosity of calcaneus easily palpable
		Foot held in maximal correction	0.5	tuberosity of calcaneus more difficult to palpate
			1	tuberosity of calcaneus not palpable
	RE	Rigidity of equinus	0	ankle dorsiflexes fully
		Knee extended, ankle maximally corrected	0.5	ankle dorsiflexes to 'neutral' angle between lateral border of foot and leg $\leq 90°$
			1	ankle dorsiflexion severely limited – fixed equinus. angle between lateral border of foot and leg >90°
MFCS	MC	Severity of the medial crease	0	multiple fine creases
Midfoot contracture score		Foot held in maximal correction	0.5	one or two deep creases
			1	deep creases change the contour of the arch
	LHT	Palpation of the lateral part of the head of the talus	0	navicular completely reduces, lateral talar head cannot be felt
		Forefoot held fully abducted	0.5	navicular partially reduces, lateral talar head less palpable
			1	navicular does not reduce, lateral talar head easily felt
	CLB	The curvature of the lateral border	0	straight border
			0.5	mild curve of lateral border distally
			1	lateral border curves at calcaneo-cuboid joint

Adapted from generally available score sheets

Successive casts continue to correct the talonavicular alignment and simultaneously the calcaneus rotates under the talus with the posterior aspect rotating away from the fibula as the calcaneofibular ligament stretches. At this stage, care must be taken to maintain the forefoot in a neutral position with respect to supination/pronation. Simultaneously, the foot, under the talus, is externally rotated with respect to the leg and the correction continued until abduction/external rotation reaches 70°. Once the midfoot and forefoot deformity has been corrected fully, the equinus deformity can be addressed.

This correction is achieved by pulling down on the heel and applying upward pressure on the entire foot (to avoid a breech or rocker bottomed foot). If 15° of dorsiflexion with 70° of abduction/external rotation cannot be achieved easily, then a percutaneous tenotomy of the Achilles tendon is required. The tenotomy can be performed safely, comfortably, and easily using local anesthetic cream in the clinic, particularly in the young infant, although some practitioners

prefer a general anesthetic procedure, especially in the older child. Following tenotomy, dorsiflexion is achieved and the corrected position is held in the final cast for a period of 2–3 weeks, by which time both clinically and by ultrasound assessment [46] the tendon has reconstituted (Fig. 10.5). The older the child, the longer it takes for the tendon to reconstitute. This may necessitate adjustment of the post-tenotomy casting and splinting regime.

Following removal of the final cast, a foot abduction orthosis (FAO) is applied. The size of the foot is measured at the time of the tenotomy so that the appropriate size of boot is ordered. Comfortable, well-fitting boots are essential. The bar connecting the boots has a slight bend in it which allows the foot to be maintained in some dorsiflexion (Fig. 10.6). The boots are positioned at shoulder distance apart and the feet externally rotated by 70°. Full time use of the FAO is advocated for the first 3 months following cast treatment, then "nap time and night time" use up to walking age. Night time use should be continued for at least a

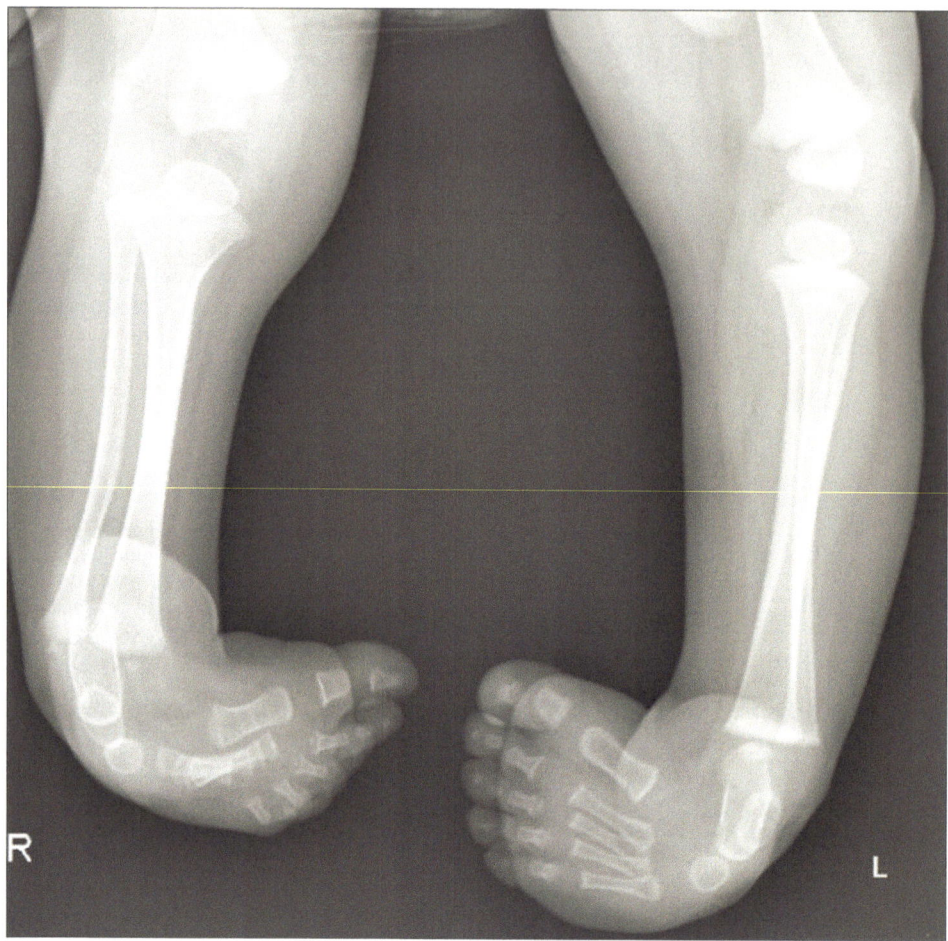

Fig. 10.4 AP radiograph of the distal lower limbs and feet of a child with bilateral clubfoot deformities. The radiograph effectively excludes a tibial dysplasia. Lines drawn through the long axes of the talus and the calcaneus would show a degree of parallelism which would not be seen in the normal foot when these lines should diverge (see also Fig. 10.2)

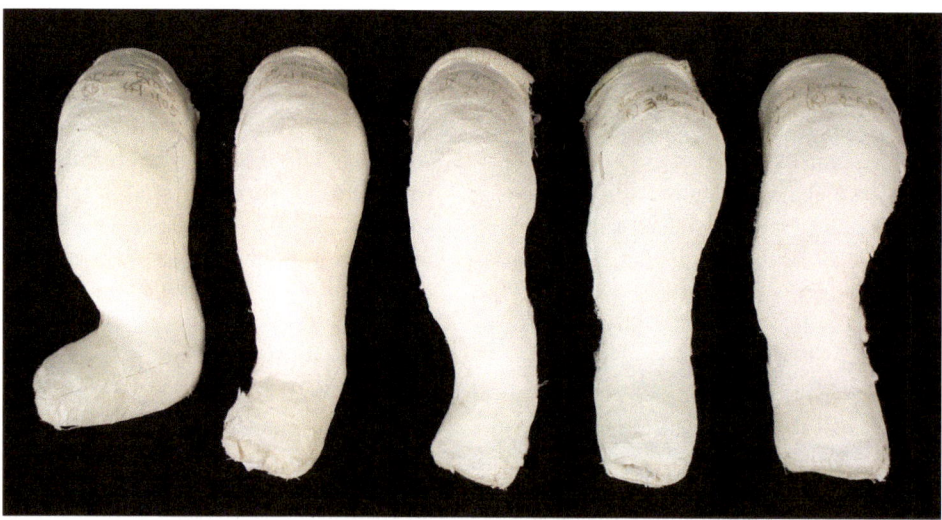

Fig. 10.5 A series of plaster casts demonstrating correction of the clubfoot deformity following treatment with the Ponseti regime. From Eastwood DM. Paediatric orthopaedics. In: Williams NS, Bulstrode CJK, O'Connell PR, eds. Bailey and Love's Short Practice of Surgery, 25th ed. London: Hodder Arnold; 2008. Used with permission

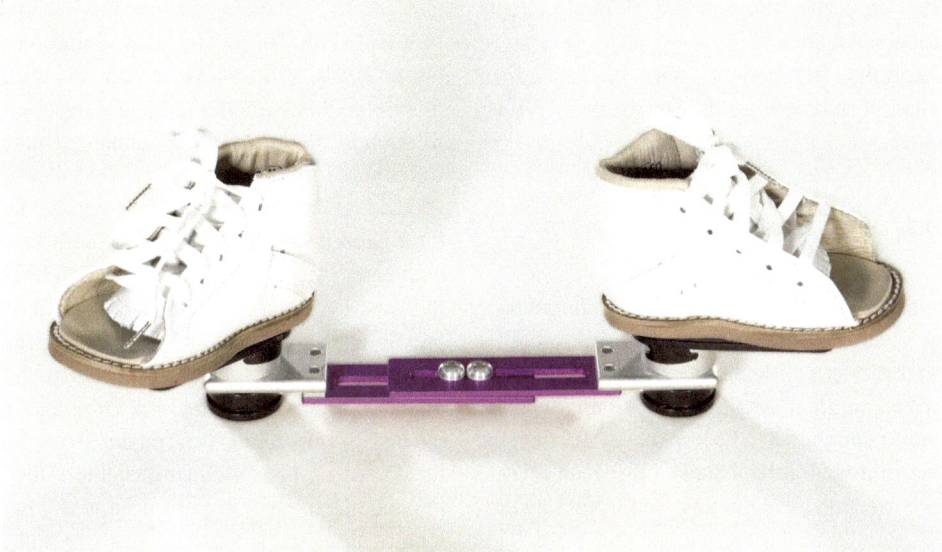

Fig. 10.6 An example of the "boots and bars" foot abduction orthoses used as part of the Ponseti management program

further 12 months with some exponents of the technique, including Ponseti, believing that splint usage until the age of 4 years is essential if full correction of the deformity is to be maintained with a minimal risk of recurrence.

Relative muscle imbalance may be a problem and once the foot is in the corrected position, it is important to stimulate activity particularly in the anterior tibial muscles and the peroneal muscle groups in order to shorten the relative over-lengthening of these muscle-tendon units.

Several different types of FAOs are available and it is certainly true that one splint does not fit all feet. The "short, fat foot" is recognized as a particular problem by many practitioners. However, with all splints, compliance can be a problem and as compliance with treatment is predictive of a successful long-term outcome it is essential that the parents cooperate with the treatment program. Continuity of care and a holistic approach to the family and the child are essential.

Many authors have been able to duplicate Ponseti's results, and in the idiopathic foot, full correction should be achievable in around 95% of cases following a mean of 5–8 casts depending upon the age at which treatment started. A percutaneous tenotomy will be needed in between 65 and 85% of cases depending upon the severity of the foot deformity at the start of treatment. A Pirani score of 5 or more at presentation or a Dimeglio grade IV foot is highly predictive of the need for tenotomy [47]. The pathoanatomy of the clubfoot, including both the abnormal shape of the cartilage anlagen and the abnormal relationships between them, resolves promptly with the Ponseti treatment as confirmed on MR imaging [48]. The changes in mechanical loading result in altered growth in these fast-growing tissues with the interesting observation that with the Ponseti method static

stresses rather than dynamic loading may be influencing tissue adaptation [49].

The manipulation and the casting can be performed by a variety of practitioners as long as they are confident and competent in applying the technique [50, 51]. In developed countries, the tenotomy is performed by surgically trained practitioners but elsewhere clinical medical officers have been trained in this technique [51]. Occasional, significant bleeding complications have been noted. It has been suggested that the tenotomy could be performed using a needle as has been used effectively for the release of the A1 pulley in trigger fingers in the outpatient clinic [52].

Recently, Morcuende et al. [53] have shown that an accelerated treatment protocol, changing casts every 5 days rather than 7, results in a more rapid correction of deformity while allowing the parents to remove the cast the night before their clinic attendance. Leaving the child's foot free to return to its position of deformity from its position of correction results in a longer treatment time compared to those patients in whom the cast is removed in the clinic just prior to the next manipulation and casting session [54].

Radiographic evaluation has confirmed that the Achilles tenotomy is followed by an increase in the lateral tibiocalcaneal angle, indicating that dorsiflexion is occurring at the ankle and not at the midfoot [55]. Koureas et al. [56] have emphasized that the use of a lateral radiograph can identify a rocker bottom deformity or midfoot breech which would prompt an early tenotomy.

Ultrasound monitoring during treatment can demonstrate that correction is occurring although this is usually visible clinically. In appropriately trained hands, scans may be better than radiographs in identifying false correction earlier than would be apparent clinically, and this may prompt changes to the manipulation technique [57].

Recurrent deformity (see below) may be treated by repeated manipulation and casting followed again by FAOs.

Other Methods of Conservative Treatment

Over the years many methods of conservative treatment have been tried using a variety of "stretching and strapping" or "manipulating and plastering" techniques but few methods have been described in great detail. The *Kite method* was popular but has now been shown to be less successful than the Ponseti technique in a randomized study [58]. Kite recommended forefoot correction by abducting the forefoot against pressure applied laterally at the calcaneocuboid joint. This was termed "Kite's error" by Ponseti who believes that the point of counter pressure should be the talar head [45].

The *French or functional method* of clubfoot correction, developed and popularized by Bensahel [59] and Dimeglio [38], is an intensive, dynamic program that emphasizes stretching of the tight medial structures, strengthening of the peroneal muscles, and strapping of the improved foot position. Treatment takes place on a daily basis for the first 2–3 months. The frequency of treatment then drops to 2–3 times per week until 6 months of age with physiotherapy and night splinting continuing until the age of 2–3 years. The addition of continuous passive motion has been found to be beneficial during the first 3 months of treatment. With this program, most authors have found a reduction in the number and the extent of surgical procedures required to obtain a good foot position [60, 61]. Several of these authors feel that the chances of success are higher with the moderately deformed feet scoring less than 10 on the Dimeglio scale. As with the Ponseti method, MR imaging evaluation pre- and post-treatment with the French method has shown improved anatomical relationships in all areas other than hindfoot equinus [62].

Surgical Management

Conservative methods of management of the clubfoot are not applicable to all feet or for all families and an individual approach to the management of the deformity must be defined particularly in the child with a complex foot. For some severe deformities (Dimeglio grades 3 and 4) and for some of those associated with syndromes or neuromuscular conditions, surgical treatment is still the most appropriate choice and surgically treated clubfeet can and do function well at long-term follow-up despite some persistent

abnormalities evident on clinical or radiographic assessment [63, 64] (Fig. 10.7). The most common residual problems are probably stiffness, poor push-off during gait secondary to calf weakness, and a tendency for compensatory external rotation at the hip level to counteract the persistent internal rotation at foot or tibial level.

A large number of surgical approaches and procedures have been described but it is difficult to compare their outcomes due to the lack of a common classification system at the start of surgery. On the whole with all techniques most feet do well, some have a fair result and about 10% do badly.

The indication for surgery is an inability to obtain and maintain reduction of the joint subluxations by conservative means. Surgical intervention must release the tight structures causing these deformities and allow joint realignment to occur. Some feet require little more than a tendo Achilles lengthening, while others require a full peri-talar release. Several authors believe that specific structures are the key to obtaining a good foot position so, for example, the importance of the posterolateral corner with a limited release medially was emphasized by Catterall [65], whereas Simons [66] emphasized correction of the calcaneocuboid joint and felt that division of the talocalcaneal interosseous ligament should be part of the peri-talar release. Others felt that such extensive surgery led to an unacceptably high rate of overcorrection.

Most experienced surgeons have probably developed their own variation of the "a la carte" method popularized by Bensahel et al. [67]. In this pragmatic approach to the surgical treatment of clubfoot, pathologically tight structures are released in sequence until the foot is well aligned. Fractional lengthenings of muscle-tendon units are preferred when possible, and tendons are repaired under some tension to try and prevent postoperative weakness. Once reduction of the joints has been obtained, the position is often maintained by one or more K-wires, ensuring joint reduction during the healing phase. The talonavicular relationship is key and hence one wire crosses this joint. The importance of the calcaneocuboid relationship is emphasized by some authors and a wire across this joint may be required. In those cases where release of the interosseous ligament has been necessary, a talocalcaneal wire will guard against heel valgus. While early movement might be ideal, traditionally immobilization with an above-knee plaster cast has been recommended for 6–8 weeks depending upon the extent of the surgery and the age of the child. Further splinting may be recommended on an individual basis and can be influenced by the etiology of the deformity. Idiopathic clubfeet may require no further orthotic use whereas neuromuscular feet usually do.

The choice of incision(s) must be appropriate to the amount and type of surgery planned. The Cincinnati circumferential incision [68] certainly provides a good exposure to all aspects of the deformity and even though it may not

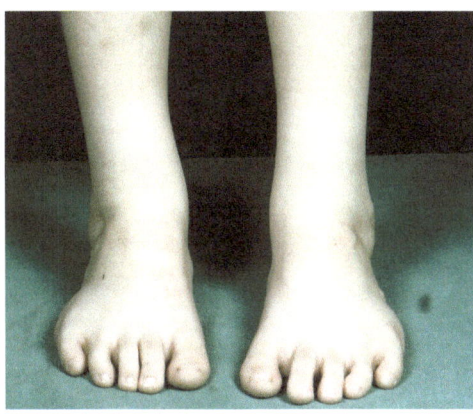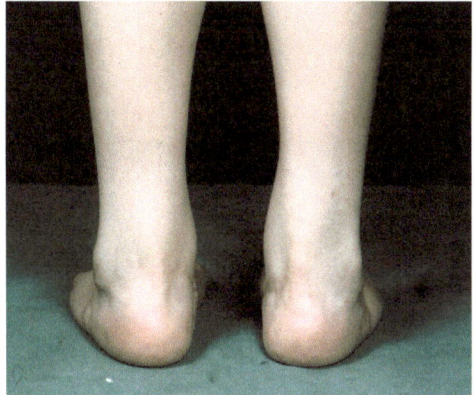

Fig. 10.7 (**a**) Front and (**b**) back-standing clinical photographs of a child whose clubfoot deformity was corrected surgically as an infant

close primarily, several papers have confirmed that healing takes place while the foot is in plaster, without the need for plastic surgical intervention and without compromising the functional outcome. One advantage of the Cincinnati incision is that the scar is cosmetically acceptable, usually lying below the line of a shoe and sock. It does not extend up the leg as the child grows as longitudinal incisions tend to do.

The timing of surgical intervention is not crucial but despite the popularity of an early tenotomy with the Ponseti program, most people feel that early major surgical intervention risks increased scarring and it is still difficult to hold the foot in the plantigrade position until the child is old enough to bear weight. Surgical intervention is often timed for around 9–10 months of age so that removal of the postoperative casts occurs at the time the child is likely to start walking.

Muscle Rebalancing

Even in the idiopathic foot, relative muscle imbalance with poor evertor muscle function can be noted from an early stage. If this persists, despite correction of the foot deformity and despite a strengthening program, then the foot develops a supination deformity that is often dynamic. The standing foot posture may be good but the supination deformity becomes obvious as the child walks. For this type of problem, a split (or total) tibialis anterior tendon transfer to the cuboid or the intermediate cuneiform is considered the procedure of choice. It is important to suture the transferred tendon under sufficient tension and a slightly everted resting foot position at the end of the procedure is ideal. Many clinicians feel this procedure will be required in a significant number of cases treated with the Ponseti technique and the families can be warned about this as treatment commences [45].

Management of the Complex Case

Primary management of the complex clubfoot deformity is essentially similar to that of the idiopathic foot but treatment must take into account associated problems. Neurological conditions may be accompanied by sensory deficits and thus manipulation and casting risks causing pressure sores. Similarly, arthrogrypotic foot deformities may be difficult to treat due to more proximal limb contractures. Associated non-orthopaedic problems may mean that early treatment or cast treatment is not appropriate. While a surgical procedure is more likely in this group of patients than in the idiopathic foot, some success is being achieved in these feet with a modified Ponseti program. In such complex feet an early tenotomy may be justified before full forefoot abduction has been achieved and the postoperative splinting program may require significant adaptation to accommodate other joint deformities [69].

Assessment of Outcome

This is an essential part of long-term management to allow comparison between one method of treatment and another. Unfortunately there are few studies with long-term follow-up to skeletal maturity or beyond but Cooper and Dietz [70] noted good or excellent function in 78% of their patients in a 30-year follow-up. They also reported that radiographic measurements do not correlate with function. The value of many studies has been hampered by poor documentation of the initial deformity both clinically and radiographically. The Pirani [39] and Dimeglio [38] classification systems are being used increasingly pre-treatment and their continued use post-treatment may help to distinguish between subgroups of patients who do well and those who do not. However, neither of these two systems assesses function and objective scores which together with subjective patient-based outcomes need to be developed and studied, with a distinction between the idiopathic foot and the complex foot [71]. A study of 204 children designed to compare subjective and objective outcome measures found a correlation between certain anthropometric measurements and patient satisfaction. A grading system based on foot length, maximal calf circumference, and ankle movement would be relevant and easily applicable to all patients [72]. Andriesse et al. [73] have presented their initial evaluation of a clubfoot assessment protocol (CAP) that has shown good validity and responsiveness, particularly in the moderate to severe feet, when compared to the Dimeglio system. It also has a greater ability to discriminate between different degrees of mobility in the left and right feet in bilateral cases. This assessment protocol concentrates on determining change over time and thus aims to be an instrument that would be valuable for longitudinal follow-up. Further studies are required.

Table 10.4 Questions to consider when faced with a late foot deformity following initial treatment of CTEV

What treatment did the foot have initially?	A failure of Ponseti treatment is likely to present different problems from a failure of surgical treatment.
Was the foot ever fully corrected?	*If so,* why has the foot deformity recurred? (a) Is this a failure of post-operative management? (b) Are there other neuromuscular or syndromic conditions that should be considered? For example, tethering of the cord. (c) Has the previous surgery damaged the developing foot—i.e., are there soft tissue contractures or physeal tethers that are contributing to the progressive deformity? *If not,* why is there residual deformity? (a) Was the initial treatment appropriate? (b) Was the original diagnosis correct?
What is the essence of the deformity?	*Is it:* dynamic or fixed? overcorrection? continuing/recurrent equinovarus?

The Management of Residual or Recurrent Deformity

The assessment and management of foot deformity secondary to the surgical treatment of a clubfoot has been a difficult area for many surgeons over the last few decades. (Fig. 10.8) With the decline of primary surgical management it is possible that these difficult cases will become less common.

When presented with a residual or relapsed foot deformity, it is important that the clinician takes time to review the whole history and conducts a full examination of the foot and lower limb including a neurological assessment of the child. Suitable investigations must be undertaken which may include spinal cord imaging and/or nerve conduction studies to exclude a neurological cause.

The most common problems which cause parental anxiety are the following:

1. foot shape and size (a measure of deformity);
2. walking pattern (although function is usually good);
3. discomfort (which may be more perceived than real as assessed by the child's continuing participation in physical activities).

The clinician should try to identify whether or not the deformity is a residual deformity or a recurrent deformity perhaps by considering the questions in Table 10.4.

It is essential that standing posture and gait pattern are assessed and the clinical examination of the foot and hindfoot should identify what deformity is present at each level and whether or not it is supple. All too often a combination of deformities exists. The Coleman block test [74] is helpful in determining whether the hindfoot deformity is fixed in relation to a supple forefoot (see Chapter 32).

In cases of complex three-dimensional foot deformities, plain two-dimensional radiographs may be difficult to interpret. It is impossible for the radiographers to obtain a true lateral view of the foot when there is significant forefoot adduction, for example, and thus in order to achieve the "required" position, the patient rotates the foot externally at ankle level. This gives the appearance of a posteriorly placed lateral malleolus and often a "flat-topped talus." However, the flat-topped talus may be a true appearance in cases where an extensive soft tissue release has resulted in compression or avascular change within the talus.

Equinus

A pure equinus deformity is common. Following Ponseti treatment, further casting and a repeat tenotomy of the Achilles tendon should be considered. If the deformity is secondary to post-surgical treatment a repeat tenotomy alone is invariably disappointing and the surgeon should be prepared to perform a posterior release of the ankle and subtalar joint. If there is a flat-topped talus, a repeat release will not be successful as the talus can no longer rotate into dorsiflexion although dome subtalar motion may be regained.

Often there is a concomitant *cavus* deformity which may merit a plantar fascia release.

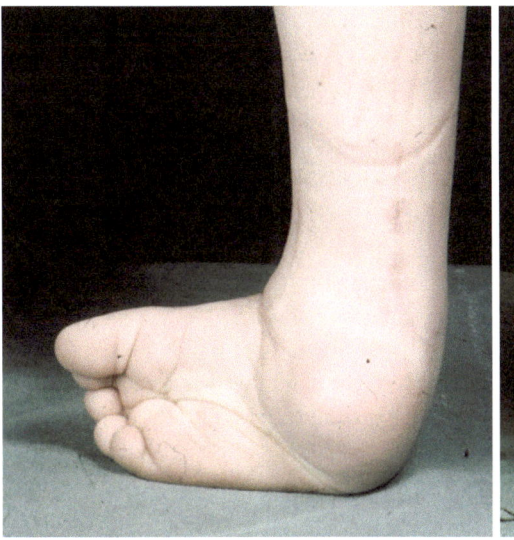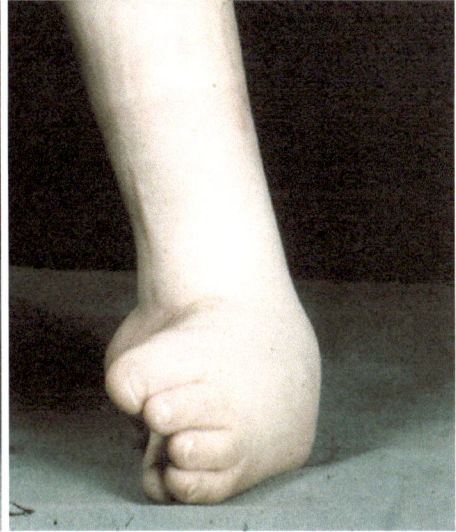

Fig. 10.8 Clinical photographs of a child whose clubfoot deformity was treated surgically as an infant but who still has considerable recurrent or residual deformity

Hindfoot Varus

Hindfoot varus is often associated with under-correction of the original deformity. The deformity is usually rigid and management depends upon the age of the child and on the extent of other deformities. Ponseti casting or a surgical release may be considered, but in a child over the age of 4 years it is likely that a calcaneal osteotomy should be considered. A lateral closing wedge (incorporating some lateral translation) is probably the best method of correcting deformity and maintaining heel height.

Hindfoot Valgus

This is most commonly seen following a major surgical release and a failure to maintain a neutral correction in the postoperative period. Instability of the subtalar joint secondary to division of the talocalcaneal interosseous ligament and/or insufficiency of the tibialis posterior musculature will lead to valgus. If the surgical procedure has left the foot with ineffective plantar ligaments (such as the spring ligament and the calcaneonavicular ligament) the deformity may be more planovalgus than valgus. Other authors [45, 65] have emphasized the importance of the pathological calcaneofibular ligament or "tether." If this is not divided during the initial surgical release, the talus cannot dorsiflex into the ankle mortice and the tether pulls the calcaneus toward the fibula. The hindfoot valgus may be driven by a rigid forefoot supination deformity.

Hindfoot valgus is associated with weakness of push-off and may be painful due to calcaneofibular impingement laterally. Deformity is often progressive as the midfoot collapses.

As with all deformities, management may be conservative or surgical. The surgical options concentrate upon correcting the hindfoot valgus via either a translational or a lengthening calcaneal osteotomy. Concomitant forefoot surgery may also be required if correction of the hindfoot valgus reveals some forefoot supination. Currently, the calcaneal lengthening osteotomy is the procedure of choice for the foot as it maintains some flexibility and is therefore capable of producing some correction when the osteotomy is distracted [75]. In the more rigid foot, other osteotomies should be considered or a subtalar arthrodesis. If the hindfoot deformity is associated with other significant deformity a triple arthrodesis (see below) may be the best option.

Calcaneus

This deformity is unusual and is probably related to over-lengthening of the gastrocsoleus complex. The clinical appearance is similar to that seen in some feet after poliomyelitis and it raises the suspicion of an underlying neurological condition (Fig. 10.9). Treatment is difficult: a calcaneal osteotomy that displaces the tuberosity posteriorly may be effective in improving the cosmetic appearance of the foot and the ability to wear shoes [76]. It does alter the lever arm for the gastrocsoleus but whether this translates into improved function is debatable. Not infrequently, a dorsal soft tissue release is also required to improve the forefoot position.

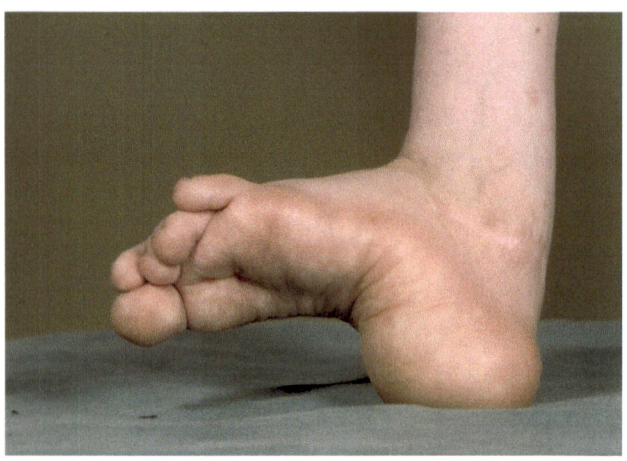

Fig. 10.9 Clinical photograph of a child with a calcaneus deformity secondary to early surgical treatment of a clubfoot deformity

Dorsal Bunion (with Forefoot Supination)

A dorsal bunion with plantar flexion of the first metatarsophalangeal (MTP) joint is a common problem following extensive surgical release of the idiopathic clubfoot when the underlying etiology is probably a persistent muscle imbalance. The weak gastrocsoleus complex means that flexor hallucis longus is relatively overactive when contributing to the push-off phase of gait. The first MTP joint is frequently stiff and physiotherapy designed at regaining and maintaining movement is important. Yong et al. [77] have recently reported good results with a reverse Jones tendon transfer.

A supination deformity of the forefoot often accompanies a dorsal bunion. Again muscle imbalance is a contributory factor with a strong tibialis anterior muscle pull overcoming that of the weak peroneal muscles. The supination deformity may be the root cause of the dorsal bunion.

As mentioned previously, a split or complete tibialis anterior tendon transfer to either the cuboid or the intermediate cuneiform rebalances the foot but the tension in the tendon transfer must be correct and the foot should lie in slight eversion at the end of the procedure [78]. The usual indication for this tendon transfer is a dynamic supination deformity in the presence of a supple forefoot although some report its value in a fixed foot with the transfer simply halting progression of the deformity.

Metatarsus Adductus (the Curved Forefoot)

This deformity, like the others already mentioned, tends not to occur in isolation. Hindfoot varus or indeed valgus (the skew foot) may also be present. Ponseti-type stretching and

casting may be helpful but in the more rigid foot, surgery may be necessary. In simple terms, the medial column of the foot is too short and the lateral column too long causing the forefoot to curve inward. Assuming that the hindfoot is relatively well aligned, surgery is first directed toward a release of the tight medial soft tissues which may include scar tissue from previous incisions, the abductor hallucis, and the capsules of the midtarsal and tarsometatarsal joints. A shortening of the lateral column of the foot may then be performed via a closing wedge osteotomy of the cuboid or a calcaneocuboid joint fusion as described by Evans [79]. The wedge that is removed from the lateral side can be inserted in the medial side as a graft in an opening wedge osteotomy of the medial cuneiform [80].

Recurrent Clubfoot Deformity

If all aspects of the deformity have recurred then it may be necessary to repeat the original treatment especially if this was the Ponseti approach. If the recurrence is secondary to a surgical procedure, then clinical judgment is required to decide whether or not the risks of further surgery and subsequent scarring with stiffness are worth the possible benefits.

Intoeing Gait

An intoeing gait is very common in patients with clubfoot. It is possible that the prolonged use of foot abduction orthoses as part of the Ponseti program may reduce the incidence of internal tibial rotation which is often the cause of the intoeing gait. Other factors such as persistent foot deformity and weak peroneal muscles must also be considered. A supramalleolar osteotomy of the tibia with/without fibular osteotomy will significantly improve foot progression.

Leg Length Discrepancy

In severe clubfoot deformity leg length discrepancy may develop with time and some prediction of what the discrepancy is likely to be at skeletal maturity should be made. If the predicted discrepancy is more than 2 cm an epiphysiodesis of the contralateral proximal tibia (or distal femur) at the appropriate time should be considered. Often severe clubfoot deformities following surgical treatment have some residual equinus deformity which can compensate, at least in part, for the discrepancy.

The Ilizarov Method

The use of the Ilizarov principle of gradual distraction of soft tissues and bone to correct residual or recurrent clubfoot deformity by means of the law of tension–stress and the application of an external fixator was first popularized by Grill and Franke in 1987 [81]. They achieved a plantigrade foot in all 10 feet. Since then there have been mixed reports on its use and value. Comparison between these papers is difficult due to a lack of objective assessment of the etiology and the severity of the initial deformity and the use of various methods to achieve deformity correction. Some surgeons use purely soft tissue distraction techniques, while others perform limited soft tissue release in addition, sometimes combined with a midfoot or hindfoot osteotomy. Despite initial optimism, such surgery often leads to stiffening of the affected and neighboring joints, particularly the ankle, which has a detrimental effect on the results. Bradish and Noor [82] reported 76% good/excellent results at a mean of 3 years and noted that in supple feet the addition of a tendon transfer to prevent recurrent deformity was always associated with an excellent outcome. Similar results have been reported by others with slightly longer follow-up [83, 84] although a relatively high rate of secondary surgery was noted [83]. Recently, Freedman et al. [85] reported disappointing results at a mean follow-up of 6.6 years with only 3 out of 21 (15%) good/excellent results and almost 50% of feet requiring revision surgery. Utukuri et al. [86] also showed recurrent deformity in 14 of 23 (61%) patients but patient-based outcomes were good/excellent in around 50% of patients.

The use of this technique does allow for correction of any tibial deformity or shortening at the same time should this be required.

Triple Arthrodesis

A triple arthrodesis should be reserved for the symptomatic, rigid foot with significant deformity. Improvement in symptoms will be achieved only if a stiff, plantigrade foot is achieved and if there is some useful ankle movement. The procedure is never indicated in a patient less than 10–12 years of age because it would have a major effect on the growth of the foot. While it is generally felt that patient satisfaction following this procedure is good, there is little objective information to support this belief. Ramseier et al. [87] reviewed seven patients who had undergone a triple arthrodesis as adults and reported improved outcome according to American Orthopaedic Foot and Ankle Society scores,

with six out of seven patients being satisfied despite residual symptoms and degenerative changes at the ankle. Bennet et al. [88] similarly reported improvement in deformity and hindfoot pain but there was little evidence to suggest that function was improved. It is perceived that triple arthrodesis is more successful in the treatment of a varus deformity than a valgus deformity.

Talectomy

Talectomy remains a radical solution for significant equinovarus deformity in the foot that has undergone multiple previous operative procedures or that has an arthrogrypotic or neuromuscular etiology, particularly if the patient is young. The aim of the procedure is to obtain a stable and pain-free plantigrade foot. On its own, talectomy does not necessarily correct mid- and forefoot deformity and additional procedures may be necessary. In an essentially arthrogrypotic group of patients, Legaspi et al. [89] reported 75% good or fair results at a mean follow-up of 20 years when the initial procedure took place at a mean age of 5 years. Good results have also been reported in bilateral cases [90].

Decision Making in Recurrent/Relapsed Feet

In recurrent clubfoot deformities as in many other areas of paediatric orthopaedics it is important to remember a few important rules (Table. 10.5).

Ponseti and others believe that early treatment is associated with a better outcome because the shape of the cartilaginous bones of the infant foot can be preserved [45]. Congruous joints can develop provided compression is not excessive. If treatment is delayed and later correction is performed surgically with release of contracted joints and ligaments, then all too often the corrected position is unstable perhaps because of articular incongruency. To stabilize

Table 10.5 Points to remember when decision-making in recurrent/relapsed deformities

1	Every operation on the foot will increase stiffness in adjacent joints
2	A supple foot with some deformity may be better than a stiff foot with no deformity
3	The stiff, deformed foot often has the worst outcome
4	The longer the foot has been in a position of deformity, the less likely it is that a normal foot will be obtained with treatment. Due to the abnormal configuration of the bones, it is likely that joint function will also be poor

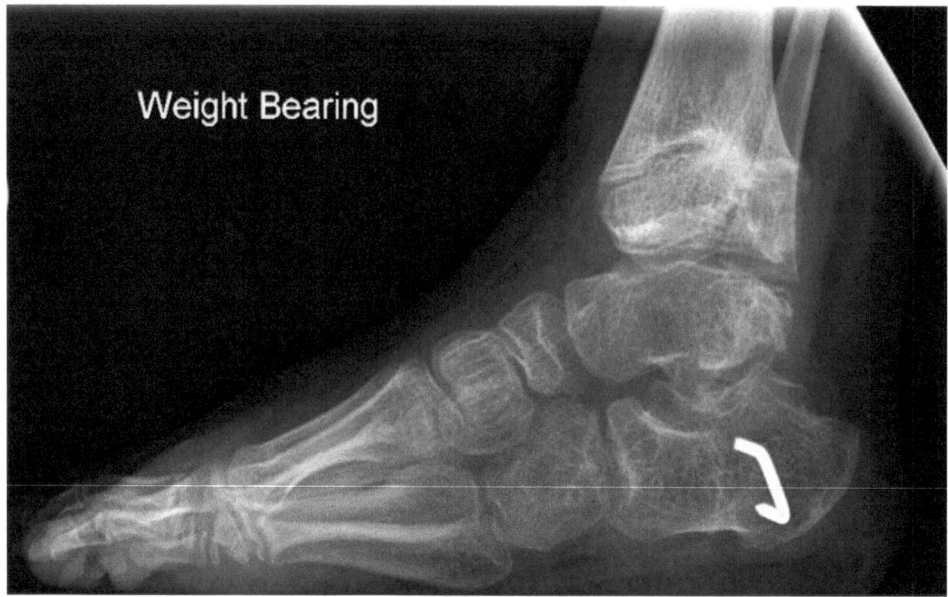

Fig. 10.10 Lateral radiograph of a foot that has had two surgical procedures performed. A growth arrest of the distal tibial physis is noted

the foot, K-wire fixation is advocated and the foot heals with the formation of scar tissue so that the joint may become stiff. This partly accounts for the disappointing relapse rates following late surgical intervention for the primary or recurrent clubfoot deformity [44]. All too often, on talking to parents of children with "difficult" feet, it is apparent that the previous surgical procedure was disappointing in terms of deformity correction. In such cases, it is important to remember that the foot may be deformed but the foot may be comfortable and functional. The asymptomatic foot may benefit from being left alone until such time as pain or change in functional level leads the patient to ask for help. A more extensive surgical procedure may be necessary at that stage but the overall outcome may be better.

Recurrence or relapse is quite common in the first few years following Ponseti treatment. Both problems usually relate to a failure to comply with the FAO and the prolonged period of treatment [91]. Recurrent deformity can be treated with further manipulation and casting and the addition of a tenotomy or tendon transfer as discussed previously. However, if compliance was a problem initially, it may be so again and the clinician must decide whether it is sensible to persevere with one particular type of treatment or obtain and then maintain correction by some other method [92]. While the Achilles tendon can be lengthened once and probably twice, repeated procedures are associated with increasing weakness leading to disability and calcaneus deformity. Following the use of the Ponseti regimen recurrence after the age of 7 years is unlikely. Should a recurrence occur, a neurological cause should be considered [93].

Foot deformity may be secondary to long-standing abnormal mechanics through the deformed joints or to surgical damage to the developing foot. Growth arrest, muscle imbalance, and incongruent joints will all play a role (Fig. 10.10).

Summary

Although much has been learnt about the nature and management of idiopathic clubfoot over the years, much remains to be understood. Further research into the etiology and pathology of the condition is necessary and long-term outcome studies of current methods of treatment will be required.

References

1. Siapkara A, Duncan R. Congenital talipes equinovarus: A review of current management. J Bone Joint Surg 2007; 89-B:995–1000.
2. Carey M, Bower C, Mylvaganam A, Rouse I. Talipes equinovarus in Western Australia. Paediatr Perinat Epidemiol 2003; 17: 87–194.
3. Byron-Scott R, Sharpe P, Hasler C, et al. A South Australian population-based study of congenital talipes equinovarus. Paediatr Perinat Epidemiol 2005; 19:227–237.
4. Cederholm M, Haglund B, Axelsson O. Infant morbidity following amniocentesis and chorionic villus sampling for prenatal karyotyping. BJOG 2005; 112:394–402.
5. Dickenson KC, Meyer RE, Kotch J. Maternal smoking and the risk for clubfoot in infants. Birth Defects Res A Clin Mol Teratol 2008; 82:86–91.

6. Alderman BW, Takahashi ER, LeMier MK. Risk indicators for talipes equinovarus in Washington State 1987–1989. Epidemiology 1991; 2:289–292.

7. Offerdal K, Jebens N, Blaas HG, Eik-Nes SH. Prenatal ultrasound detection of talipes equinovarus in a non-selected population of 49314 deliveries in Norway. Ultrasound Obstet Gynecol 2007; 30:838–844.

8. Keret D, Ezra E, Lokiec F, et al. Efficacy of prenatal ultrasonography in confirmed club foot. J Bone Joint Surg 2002; 84-B:1015–1019.

9. Bar-Hava I, Bronshtein M, Orvieto R, et al. Caution: prenatal clubfoot can be both a transient and a late-onset phenomenon. Prenat Diagn 1997; 17:457–460.

10. Bar-On E, Mashiach R, Inbar O, et al. Prenatal ultrasound diagnosis of club foot: Outcome and recommendations for counseling and follow-up. J Bone Joint Surg 2005; 87-B:990–993.

11. Mammen L, Benson CB. Outcome of fetuses with clubfeet diagnosed by prenatal sonography. J Ultrasound Med 2004; 23:497–500.

12. Tillett RL, Fisk NM, Murphy K, Hunt DM. Clinical outcome of congenital talipes equinovarus diagnosed antenatally by ultrasound. J Bone Joint Surg 2000; 82-B:876–880.

13. Woodrow N, Tran T, Umstad M, et al. Mid-trimester ultrasound diagnosis of isolated talipes equinovaurs: accuracy and outcome for infants. Aust NZ J Obstet Gynaecol 1998; 38:301–305.

14. Malone FD, Marino T, Bianchi DW, et al. Isolated clubfoot diagnosed prenatally: is karyotyping indicated? Obstet Gynecol 2000; 95:437–440.

15. Herzenberg JE, Carroll NC, Christofersen MR, et al. Clubfoot analysis with three-dimensional computer modelling. J Paediatr Orthop 1988; 8:257–262.

16. Windisch G, Salaberger D, Rosmarin W, et al. A model for clubfoot based on micro-CT data. J Anat 2007; 210:761–766.

17. Itohara T, Sugamoto K, Shimizu N, et al. Assessment of talus deformity by three-dimensional MRI in congenital clubfoot. Eur J Radiol 2005; 53:78–83.

18. Ippolito E, Ponseti IV. Congenital clubfoot in the human fetus. A histological study. J Bone Joint Surg Am 1980; 62:8–22.

19. Zimny ML, Willig SJ, Roberts JM, D'Ambrosia RD. An electron microscopic study of the fascia and lateral sides of the clubfoot. J Pediatr Orthop 1985; 5:577–581.

20. Fukuhara K, Schollmeier G, Uhthoff HK. The pathogenesis of club foot. A histomorphometric and immunohistological study of fetuses. J Bone Joint Surg Br 1994; 76-B:450–457.

21. Sano H, Uhthoff HK, Jarvis JG, et al. Pathogenesis of soft-tissue contracture in clubfoot. J Bone Joint Surg 1998; 80-B:641–644.

22. Van der Sluijs JA, Pruys JE. Normal collagen structure in the posterior ankle capsule in different types of clubfeet. J Pediatr Orthop B 1999; 8:261–263.

23. Hattori K, Sano H, Saijo Y, et al. Measurement of soft tissue elasticity in the congenital clubfoot using scanning acoustic microscope. J Pediatr Ortho B 2007; 16:357–362.

24. Handelsman JE, Badalamente MA. The club foot: a neuromuscular disease. Develop Med Child Neurol 1982; 24:3–12.

25. Isaacs H, Handelsman JE, Badenhorst M, Pickering A. The muscles in clubfoot—a histological, histochemical and electron microscopy study. J Bone Joint Surg 1977; 59-B:465–472.

26. Macnicol MF, Nadeem RD, Maffulli N, et al. Histochemistry of the triceps surae muscle in idiopathic congenital clubfoot. J Foot Ankle Surg 1992; 13:80–84.

27. Muir L, Laliotis N, Kutty S, Klenerman L. Absence of the dorsalis pedis pulse in the parents of children with club foot. J Bone Joint Surg 1995; 77-B:114–116.

28. Sodre H, Bruschini S, Mestriner LA, et al. Arterial abnormalities in talipes equinovarus as assessed by angiography and the Doppler technique. J Pediatr Orthop 1990; 10:101–104.

29. Katz DA, Albanese EL, Levinsohn EM, et al. Pulsed color-flow Doppler analysis of arterial deficiency in idiopathic clubfoot. J Pediatr Orthop 2003; 23:84–87.

30. Wynne-Davis R. Family studies and the case of congenital talipes equinovarus, talipes calcaneovalgus and metatarsus varus. J Bone Joint Surg 1964; 46-B:445–463.

31. Cowell HR, Wein BK. Genetic aspects of club foot. J Bone Joint Surg Am 1980; 62-A:1381–1384.

32. Lochmiller C, Johnston C, Scott A, et al. Genetic epidemiology study of idiopathic talipes equinovarus. Am J Med Genet 1998; 79:90–96.

33. Engell V, Damborg F, Andersen M, et al. Club foot: a twin study. J Bone Joint Surg 2006; 88-B:374–376.

34. Ester AR, Tyerman G, Wise CA, et al. Apoptotic gene analysis in idiopathic talipes equinovarus. Clin Orthop Relat Res 2007; 462: 32–37.

35. Hecht JT, Ester A, Scott A, et al. NAT2 variation and idiopathic talipes equinovarus. Am J Med Genet A 2007; 143:2285–2291.

36. Herceq MB, Weiner DS, Aqamanolis DP, Hawk D. Histologic and histochemical analysis of muscle specimens in idiopathic talipes equinovarus. J Pediatr Orthop 2006; 26:91–99.

37. Shimode K, Myagi N, MajimaT, et al. Limb length and girth discrepancy of unilateral congenital clubfoot. J Pediatr Orthop B 2005; 14:280–284.

38. Dimeglio A, Bensahel H, Souchet P, et al. Classification of clubfoot. J Pediatr Orthop B 1995; 4:129–136.

39. Pirani S. A reliable and valid method of assessing the amount of deformity in the congenital clubfoot. St Louis MO: Pediatric Orthopaedic Society of North America; 2004.

40. Flynn JM, Donohoe M, Mackenzie WG. An independent assessment of two clubfoot-classification systems. J Pediatr Orthop 1998; 18:323–327.

41. Wainwright AM, Auld T, Benson MK, Theologis TN. The classification of congenital talipes equinovarus. J Bone Joint Surg 2002; 84-B:1020–1024.

42. Coley B, Sheils WE 2nd, Kean J, Adler BH. Age-dependent dynamic sonographic measurement of pediatric clubfoot. Pediatr Radiol 2007; 37: 1125–1129.

43. Turco VJ. Resistant congenital clubfoot. One stage posteromedial release with internal fixation. J Bone Joint Surg 1979; 61A: 805–814.

44. Tarraf YN, Carroll NC. Analysis of the components of residual in clubfeet presenting for reoperation. J Pediatr Orthop 1992; 12:207–216.

45. Ponseti IV. Current Concepts Review: Treatment of congenital club foot. J Bone Joint Surg 1992; 74-A:448–454.

46. Barker SL, Lavy CB. Correlation of clinical and ultrasonographic findings after Achilles tenotomy in idiopathic clubfoot. J Bone Joint Surg 2006; 88-B:377–379.

47. Scher DM, Feldman DS, van Bosse HJ, et al. Predicting the need for tenotomy in the Ponseti method for correction of clubfeet. J Pediatr Orthop 2004; 24:349–352.

48. Pirani S, Zesnik L, Hodges D. Magnetic resonance imaging study of the congenital clubfoot treated with the Ponseti method. J Pediatr Orthop 2001; 21:719–726.

49. Brand RA, Siegler S, Pirani S, et al. Cartilage anlagen adapt in response to static deformation. Med Hypotheses 2006; 66:653–659.

50. Shack N, Eastwood DM. Early results of a physiotherapist delivered Ponseti service for the management of idiopathic congenital talipes equinovarus foot deformity. J Bone Joint Surg 2006; 88-B:1085–1089.

51. Tindall AJ, Steinlechner CW, Lay CB, et al. Results of manipulation of idiopathic clubfoot deformity in Malawi by orthopaedic clinical officers using the Ponseti method: a realistic alternative for the developing world? J Pediatr Orthop 2005; 25:627–629.

52. Minkowitz B, Finkelstein BL, Bleicher M. Percutaneous tendo-Achilles lengthening with a large-gauge needle: a modification of the Ponseti technique for the correction of idiopathic club foot. J Foot Ankle Surg 2004; 43:263–265.

53. Morcuende JA, Abbasi D, Dolan LA, Ponseti IV. Results of an accelerated Ponseti protocol for clubfoot. J Pediatr Orthop 2005; 25:623–626.

54. Terrazas-Lafargue G, Morcuende JA. Effect of cast removal timing in the correction of idiopathic clubfoot by the Ponseti method. Iowa Orthop J 2007; 27:24–27.

55. Radler C, Manner HM, Suda R, et al. Radiographic evaluation of idiopathic clubfeet undergoing Ponseti treatment. J Bone Joint Surg 2007; 89-A:1177–1183.

56. Koureas G, Rampal V, Mascard E, et al. The incidence and treatment of rocker bottom deformity as a complication of the conservative treatment of idiopathic congenital clubfoot. J Bone Joint Surg 2008; 90-B:57–60.

57. Desai S, Aroojis A, Mehta R. Ultrasound evaluation of clubfoot correction during Ponseti treatment: a preliminary report. J Pediatr Orthop 2008; 28:53–59.

58. Sud A, Tiwari A, Sharma D, Kapoor S. Ponseti's vs Kite's method in the treatment of clubfoot—a prospective randomized study. Int Orthop 2008; 32:409–413.

59. Souchet P, Bensahel H, Themar-Noel C, et al. Functional treatment of clubfoot: a new series of 350 idiopathic clubfeet with long-term follow-up. J Pediatr Orthop B 2004; 13:189–196.

60. Richards BS, Johnston CE, Wilson H. Nonoperative clubfoot treatment using the French physical therapy method. J Pediatr Orthop 2005; 25:98–102.

61. Van Campenhout A, Molenaers G, Moens P, Fabry G. Does functional treatment of idiopathic clubfoot reduce the indication for surgery? Call for a widely accepted rating system. J Pediatr Orthop B 2001; 10:315–318.

62. Richards BS, Dempsey M. Magnetic resonance imaging of the congenital clubfoot treated with the French functional (physical therapy) method. J Pediatr Orthop 2007; 27:214–219.

63. Turco VJ. Resistant congenital clubfoot. One stage posteromedial release with internal fixation. A follow up report of a fifteen year experience. J Bone Joint Surg Am 1979; 61-A:805–814.

64. McKay DW. New concept of and approach to clubfoot treatment: Section II—correction of the clubfoot. J Pediatr Orthop 1982; 2:347–356.

65. Hudson I, Catterall A. Posterolateral release for resistant clubfoot. J Bone Joint Surg 1994; 76-B:281–284.

66. Simons GW. Complete subtalar release in club feet. Part 1—A preliminary report. J Bone Joint Surg Am 1985; 67-A:1044–1055.

67. Bensahel H, Csukonyi Z, Desgrippes Y, Chaumien JP. Surgery in residual clubfoot: one stage medioposterior release 'a la carte.' J Pediatr Orthop 1987; 7:145–148.

68. Crawford AH, Marxen JL, Osterfeld DL. A comprehensive approach for surgical procedures of the foot and ankle in childhood. J Bone Joint Surg 1982; 64A: 1355–1358.

69. Ponseti IV, Zhivkov M, Davis N, et al. Treatment of the complex idiopathic clubfoot. Clin Orthop Relat Res 2006; 451:171–176.

70. Cooper DM, Dietz FR. Treatment of idiopathic clubfoot. A thirty-year follow-up note. J Bone Joint Surg 1995; 77-A:1477–1489.

71. Vitale MG, Choe JC, Vitale MA, et al. Patient-based outcomes following clubfoot surgery: a 16 year follow-up study. J Pediatr Orthop 2005; 25:533–538.

72. Chesney D, Barker S, Maffulli N. Subjective and objective outcome in congenital clubfoot; a comparative study of 204 children. BMC Musculoskelet Disord 2007; 8:53.

73. Andriesse H, Roos EM, Hagglund G, Jarnlo G-B. Validity and responsiveness of the Clubfoot Assessment Protocol (CAP). A methodological study. BMC Musculoskelet Disord 2006; 7:28.

74. Coleman SS, Chestnut WJ. A simple test for hindfoot flexibility in the cavovarus foot. Clin Orthop Rel Res 1977; 123:60–62.

75. Evans D. Calcaneovalgus deformity. J Bone Joint Surg 1975; 57B:270–278.

76. Mitchell GT. Posterior displacement osteotomy of the calcaneus. J Bone Joint Surg 1977; 59B:233–235.

77. Yong SM, Smith PA, Kuo KN. Dorsal bunion after clubfoot surgery: outcome of reverse Jones procedure. J Pediatr Orthop 2007; 27:814–820.

78. Ezra E, Hayek S, Gilai AN, et al. Tibialis anterior tendon transfer for residual dynamic supination deformity in treated club foot. J Pediatr Orthop B 2000; 9:207–211.

79. Evans D. Relapsed club foot. J Bone Joint Surg 1961; 43-B:722–733.

80. Schaefer D, Hefti F. Combined cuboid/cuneiform osteotomy for correction of residual adductus deformity in idiopathic and secondary clubfeet. J Bone Joint Surg 2000; 82B:881–884.

81. Grill F, Franke J. The Ilizarov distractor for the correction of relapsed and neglected clubfoot. J Bone Joint Surg 1987; 69-B:593–597.

82. Bradish CF, Noor S. The Ilizarov method in the management of relapsed club feet. J Bone Joint Surg 2000; 82-B:387–391.

83. Ferreira RC, Costa MT, Frizzo GG, Santin RA. Correction of severe recurrent clubfoot using a simplified setting of the Ilizarov device. Foot Ankle Int 2007; 28:557–568.

84. Prem H, Zenios M, Farrell R, Day JB. Soft tissue Ilizarov correction of congenital talipes equinovarus—5–10 years post surgery. J Pediatr Orthop 2007; 27:220–224.

85. Freedman JA, Watts H, Otsuka NY. The Ilizarov method for the treatment of resistant clubfoot: Is it an effective solution? J Pediatr Orthop 2006; 26:432–437.

86. Utukuri MM, Ramachandran M, Hartley J, Hill RA. Patient-based outcomes after Ilizarov surgery in resistant clubfeet. J Pediatr Orthop B 2006; 15:278–284.

87. Ramseier LE, Schoeniger R, Vienne P, Espinosa N. Treatment of late recurring idiopathic clubfoot deformity in adults. Acta Orthop Belg 2007; 73:641–647.

88. Bennett GL, Graham CE, Mauldin DM. Triple arthrodesis in adults. Foot Ankle 1991; 12:138–143.

89. Legaspi J, Li YH, Chow W, Leong JC. Talectomy in patients with recurrent deformity in club foot. A long-term follow-up study. J Bone Joint Surg 2001; 83-B:384–387.

90. Letts M, Davidson D. The role of bilateral talectomy in the management of bilateral rigid clubfeet. Am J Orthop 1999; 28:106–110.

91. Ponseti IV. Congenital Clubfoot: Fundamentals of Treatment. Oxford: Oxford University Press; 1996.

92. Haft GF, Walker CG, Crawford HA. Early clubfoot recurrence after use of the Ponseti method in a New Zealand population. J Bone Joint Surg 2007; 89-A:487–493.

93. Lovell ME, Morcuende JA. Neuromuscular disease as the cause of late clubfoot relapses: report of 4 cases. Iowa Orthop J 2007; 27:82–84.

Chapter 11

Pes Cavus

John A. Fixsen

Introduction

Pes cavus, or a high arched foot, is rarely seen at birth or in the first year of life unless it is part of a severe congenital talipes equinovarus. There is a rare, benign form of high arched foot called pes arcuatus; this is occasionally seen as an isolated abnormality in the first year of life and resolves spontaneously. Cavus deformity of the foot develops in the majority of cases in the first or second decade of life.

It is essential that the orthopaedic surgeon distinguishes between a cavovarus foot and a calcaneocavus foot. In the cavovarus foot the heel is in varus and the forefoot in equinus with pronation of the first and sometimes the second ray (Fig. 11.1). This is the basis of the so-called block test described by Coleman and Chesnut in 1977 [1] to distinguish whether the hindfoot varus is secondary to the pronation of the forefoot and the subtalar joint is mobile, or whether the hindfoot varus is fixed. In the calcaneocavus foot (Fig. 11.2), the calf is weak and the heel is in calcaneus and often valgus. The subtalar joint is usually stiff. The forefoot is in equinus or "plantaris," as it is often called. In this type of cavus foot, both the medial and the lateral longitudinal arches are off the ground, and the so-called coin test can be used, in which a small coin can be pushed across underneath both arches of the foot, from medial to lateral. Unlike the cavovarus foot, the lateral arch is raised from the ground in calcaneocavus. Sometimes an elevation of the central metatarsal heads of the forefoot arch develops, causing a tripod foot and increasing pressure over the first and fifth metatarsal heads.

The orthopaedic surgeon should always look for an underlying cause when assessing a cavus foot. The most common cause is a neurological imbalance of the foot and calf muscles. Price et al. [2] showed that the earliest and most severe involvement was in the intrinsic muscles of the foot

in patients suffering from a peripheral neuropathy, and this occurred before involvement of the extrinsic muscles of the calf. Deluca and Banta [3] reported a progressive cavovarus deformity of the foot after laceration of the peroneus longus. If a neurological disorder, of either the central or the peripheral nervous system, is suspected, the help of an expert neurologist should be sought. It is also important to investigate the family background, as there is frequently a genetic basis to the deformity. Brewerton et al. [4] published an important paper on the etiology of pes cavus and found that, in 67% of patients, a neurological cause could be found. The commonest neurological condition in their series was peroneal muscular atrophy or Charcot–Marie–Tooth disease, which is now included under the hereditary motor and sensory neuropathies. In a recent study of patients with bilateral cavovarus feet, 78% were found to have Charcot–Marie–Tooth disease [5]. The other conditions that should be considered are cerebral palsy, poliomyelitis, spina bifida and spinal dysraphism, benign spinal cord tumors, and syrinx of the spinal cord. Sometimes the neurological cause can be treated, as in the case of diastematomyelia, a spinal cord tumor, or a syrinx. Talipes equinovarus, particularly in its more severe forms, often has a cavus component. Similarly, cavus may develop after treatment of club foot. If no underlying cause can be found, then the term idiopathic can be accepted.

Pes Cavovarus

This type of foot may be associated with congenital talipes equinovarus or it may be the sequel of its treatment. It is also commonly seen in association with the peripheral neuropathies. In the past, the terms Charcot–Marie–Tooth disease and peroneal muscular atrophy were commonly used. However, the modern term is hereditary motor and sensory neuropathy (HMSN), as this emphasizes not only the motor problems but also the sensory aspect of these disorders. These tend to affect deep pain, temperature sensation, and

J.A. Fixsen (✉)
Orthopaedic Department, Great Ormond Street Hospital for Sick Children, London, UK

Fig. 11.1 Clinical photographs of bilateral cavovarus feet. (**a**) Posterior view showing bilateral heel varus. (**b**) Lateral view showing cavus and forefoot equinus with pronation of the first and second rays. Note that the lateral longitudinal arch rests upon the ground

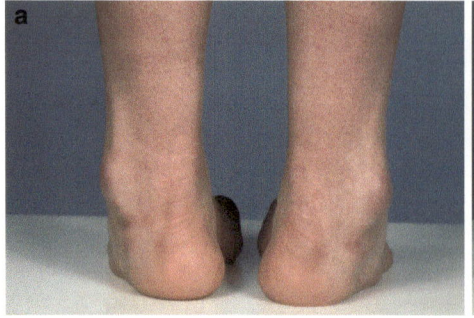 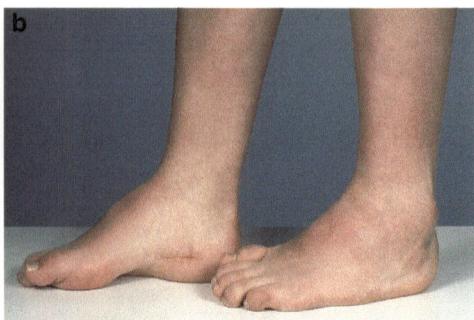

proprioception, rather than superficial sensations. As a result, these patients may present with "giving way" of the ankle or the knee, and with penetrating ulcers over the toes. HMSN was described by Harding and Thomas in 1980 [6]. Initially, two types were described; subsequently, further types were added (see Chapter 15).

Type I HMSN, sometimes called Charcot–Marie–Tooth type I, is the so-called hypertrophic type. This is dominantly inherited and usually appears in the first decade of life. Seventy percent of those affected are likely to develop pes cavus. The upper limbs below the elbow may be involved and 10–12% of patients are likely to develop significant scoliosis. On examination, hypertrophy of the peripheral nerves can be palpated, best seen in the subcutaneous nerves of the neck. Nerve conduction is significantly reduced, at 20–30 m/s, and is most easily recorded in the median nerve of the forearm. Other family members are often unaware that they suffer from the same condition because the phenotype is very variable. It is important to examine them, and often they will show minor abnormalities in the feet and of their median nerve conduction time.

Type II HMSN is called the axonal type (Charcot–Marie–Tooth type II). It is less commonly seen in children and tends to develop from the second to the sixth decades of life. The nerve conduction time is normal in these patients, and pes cavus and scoliosis are less common. Affected individuals present to orthopaedic surgeons with problems of balance and calf weakness, such as recurrent and unexplained ankle sprains, giving way of the knee and subluxation of the patella, or generalized clumsiness and weakness. In this form, inheritance may be dominant, recessive, or X-linked.

Type III HMSN is the so-called Dejerine–Sotta type. These patients tend to present to the paediatrician or neurologist with severe problems of abnormal motor development. They have a very slow conduction time of less than 5 m/s. The other types have complex neurological problems, with pyramidal signs, optic problems, and deafness, and are unlikely to present to the orthopaedic surgeon.

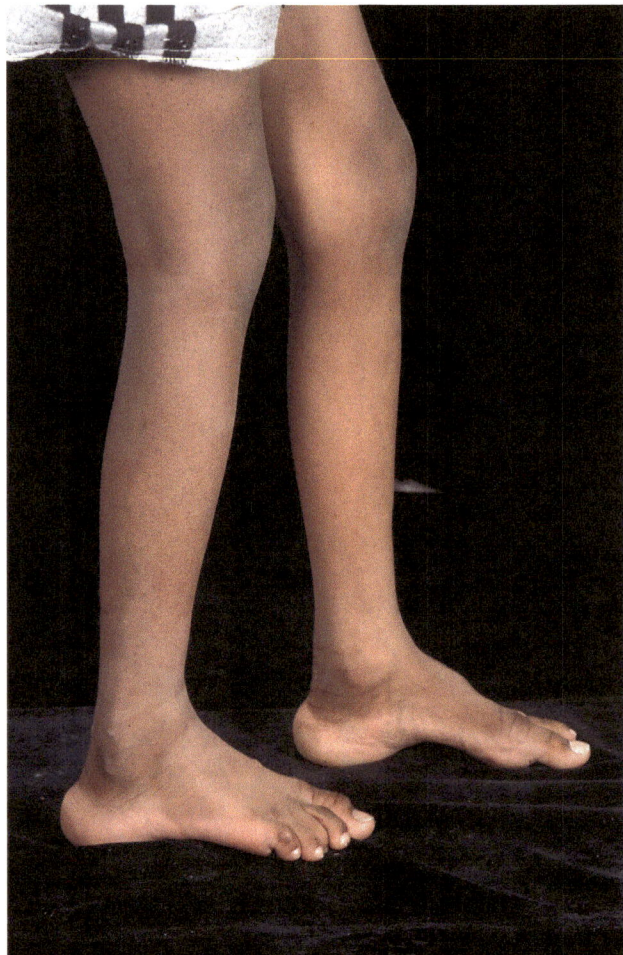

Fig. 11.2 Clinical photographs of a patient with bilateral calcaneocavus feet. Note that both medial and lateral longitudinal arches are raised off the ground. This patient had a positive "coin" sign

Treatment

Irrespective of the cause of the cavovarus foot, treatment demands that the flexibility of the forefoot and the hindfoot be assessed. It is most important that the primary site responsible for the deformity be identified. In most instances, the major problem resides in a rigid, plantar flexed fore-foot with the first and second metatarsals most affected. This effectively pronates the forefoot in relation to the hind-foot, and during standing the inflexible pronated forefoot forces the heel into varus as a result of the "tripod" effect (Fig. 11.1).

By careful physical examination, one can determine whether or not the hindfoot is flexible or rigid. This can be documented visually by placing the heel and fifth metatarsal on a raise or block of about 2–3 cm in width and allow-ing the remainder of the forefoot to fall into plantar flexion (Fig. 11.3). In a positive "block test," the heel goes into val-gus and hindfoot flexibility is present. Price and Price in 1997 [7] described another method of demonstrating hindfoot flex-ibility with the patient prone; this is a useful alternative to the block test. Alternatively, if the heel is held rigidly in varus or does not move into valgus when the block test is applied, both the forefoot and the hindfoot are rigid, a situation that requires a different therapeutic approach. In 2005, Aznaipairashvili et al. [8] described an imaging tech-nique which they called a Coleman block lateral radiographic view. This was used both to assess hindfoot flexibility and to determine the appropriate surgical treatment.

Non-Operative Treatment

Non-operative treatment such as shoes or orthotic devices can only support the cavovarus deformity, not correct it. In most patients, the deformity is progressive. If it becomes increasingly disabling despite conservative treatment, surgi-cal treatment is indicated.

Surgical Treatment

When the forefoot is rigidly plantar flexed and pronated and the hindfoot is flexible, the appropriate surgical procedure is a radical plantar release combined, if necessary, with proxi-mal first and sometimes second metatarsal osteotomy when there is fixed bony deformity at the first and second rays. It is important to remember that the growth plate of the first metatarsal is proximal and should not be damaged by the osteotomy. This should correct the forefoot and result in a plantigrade forefoot if the hindfoot is flexible. Serial changes of plaster may be necessary after the initial opera-tion to obtain the maximal effect. The plaster is retained for 6–8 weeks and then a decision can be made as to whether tendon transfers are necessary to prevent recurrence of the deformity. The degree of correction obtained can be assessed on the lateral weight-bearing radiograph by measuring the angle of Meary [9] (Fig. 11.4).

If both the hindfoot and the forefoot are inflexible, char-acterized by a negative block test, both components of the deformity must be treated. In young children, this may require a plantar release combined with a medial release. In older children in whom a medial release is not sufficient, the plantar release can be combined with a lateral wedge osteotomy [10], or simply a valgus displacement osteotomy of the calcaneus. In adolescents and adults, the forefoot cor-rection may require a wedge tarsectomy or even a full triple arthrodesis.

The place of tendon transfers is difficult to assess, par-ticularly if one is dealing with a progressive neurological condition such as HMSN. If there is significant forefoot inversion and overactivity of the tibialis posterior, transfer of this tendon to the dorsum has been advocated at the same time as the medial release. Full transfer of the tibialis ante-rior should be avoided, but a split transfer, or the procedure described by Fowler et al. [11] in which the tibialis anterior is transferred onto the dorsum of the base of the first metatarsal and combined with a wedge osteotomy of the base of the first cuneiform, may be undertaken.

Toe deformities are also a major problem. These patients, because of their disturbance of pain and temperature sen-sation, are liable to develop serious soft-tissue lesions, par-ticularly over the pressure areas on the toes. The typical Z deformity of the big toe can be treated by a classical Robert Jones tendon transfer, in which the extensor hallucis longus is transferred to the distal portion of the shaft of the first metatarsal and the interphalangeal joint of the big toe is either fused or tenodesed if the child still has significant growth left in the toe. Clawing of the lesser toes can cause serious problems with nail deformities and pressure sores. In the past, the so-called Girdlestone toe flexor to extensor transfer was recommended [12]. This transfer was described originally for victims of polio, but in the progressive forms of neurological disease the simple flexor tendon osteotomy described by Menelaus and Ross [13] is simpler and more effective.

Pes Calcaneocavus

This type of foot is characteristic of paralytic neurologi-cal conditions such as poliomyelitis, spinal muscular atro-phy, and the lower motor neurone type of spina bifida. Characteristically, both the medial and the lateral arches are raised, giving rise to a positive coin sign. The heel is in cal-caneus and the subtalar joint stiff, so that the block test is negative and is not applicable in this type of foot. A lateral radiograph shows the characteristic "pistol-grip" appearance of the calcaneus (Fig. 11.5).

Fig. 11.3 (**a**) Clinical photograph showing the block test assessing the right foot. The heel varus is corrected so this is a flexible cavovarus foot and the test is positive. (**b**) Line drawing of the block test showing the flexed pronated first and second rays, with the heel varus corrected

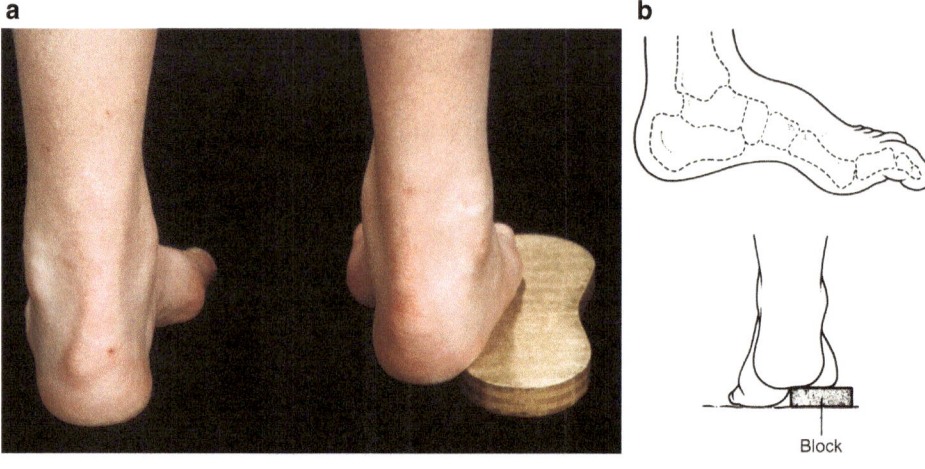

Fig. 11.4 (**a**) Lateral radiograph of the left, uncorrected cavovarus foot. (**b**) Lateral radiograph of the right foot after correction by radical plantar release. Meary's angle [9] between the long axis of the talus and the first metatarsal is substantially reduced

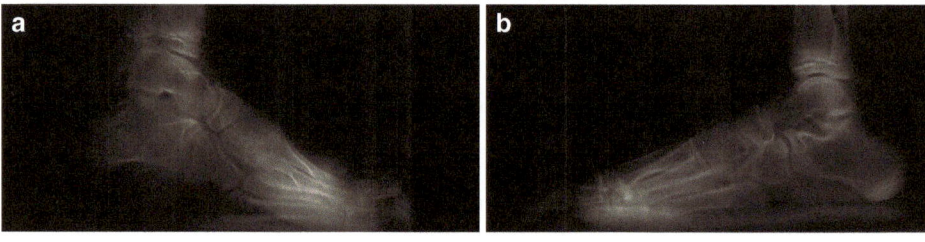

Fig. 11.5 (**a**) lateral radiograph of a calcaneocavus foot showing the so-called pistol-grip appearance of the calcaneus. (**b**) after calcaneal osteotomy

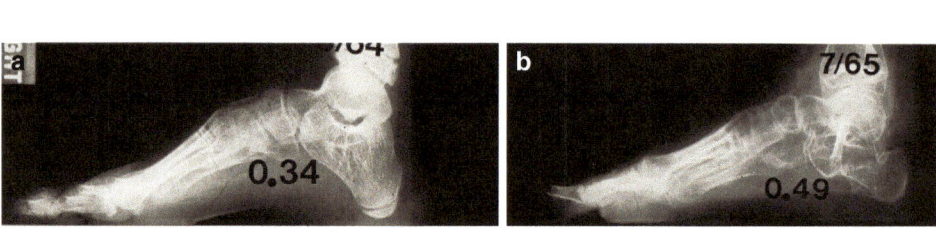

In younger children, a Steindler [14] soft-tissue release of the plantar fascia may be helpful. Once bony deformity becomes fixed, a Mitchell [15] posterior displacement osteotomy of the calcaneus combined with a plantar release can be used. For the rigid foot in adolescents or young adults, the Elmslie triple arthrodesis reported by Cholmeley [16] is effective. In this procedure, a posterior wedge is excised from the subtalar joint to correct the calcaneus of the heel, and subsequently a wedge tarsectomy is performed to bring the forefoot up on the corrected hindfoot. Attempts to restore power and "push-off" by the Robert Jones transfer, in which the dorsiflexors are transferred into the calf, have never been successful. Silver et al. [17] pointed out that the calf muscle is approximately six times stronger than the dorsiflexors of the foot as it has to lift the entire body weight and not just the foot. As a result, it is not surprising that transfers of the dorsiflexors into the calf are unlikely to reproduce good push-off. Westin et al. [18] described an unusual variant of this procedure. Instead of fixing the tendo-Achilles to the back of the tibia, the tendo-Achilles was transferred into the fibula.

This technique was used in a number of patients with calcaneus feet associated with spina bifida and appears to be useful in preventing progression of calcaneus and valgus in these patients.

References

1. Coleman SS, Chesnut WJ. A simple test for hindfoot flexibility in the cavovarus foot. Clin Orthop Rel Res 1977; 123: 60.
2. Price A, Maisel R, Drennan JC. Computer tomographic analysis of pes cavus. J Paedriatr Orthop 1993; 13: 646–653.
3. Deluca PA, Banta JB. Pes cavovarus as a late consequence of peroneus longus tendon laceration. J Paedriatr Orthop 1985; 5: 582–583.
4. Brewerton DA, Sandifer PH, Sweetnam DR. Idiopathic pes cavus, an investigation into its aetiology. Br Med J 1963; 2: 659.
5. Nagai MK, Chan G, Guile JT, et al. Prevalence of Charcot–Marie–Tooth disease in patients who have bilateral cavovarus feet. J Pediatr Orthop 2006; 26: 438–433.
6. Harding AE, Thomas PK. The clinical features of hereditary motor and sensory neuropathies types 1 and II. Brain 1980; 103: 259.

7. Price BD, Price CT. A simple demonstration of hindfoot flexibility in the cavovarus foot. J Paedriatr Orthop 1997; 17: 18–19.

8. Aznaipairashvili Z, Riddle EC, Savina M, et al. Correction of cavovarus foot deformity in Charcot–Marie–Tooth disease. J Pediatr Orthop 2005; 25: 360–365.

9. Meary R. On the measurement of the angle between the talus and the first metatarsal Symposium: Le Pied Creux Essentiel. Rev Chir Orthop 1967; 53: 389.

10. Dwyer FC. Osteotomy of the calcaneum for pes cavus. J Bone Joint Surg 1959; 41B: 80.

11. Fowler D, Brooks AL, Parrish TF. The cavovarus foot. J Bone Joint Surg 1959; 41A: 757.

12. Taylor RG. The treatment of claw toes by multiple transfers of flexor into extensor tendons. J Bone Joint Surg 1951; 35B: 539–542.

13. Menelaus MB, Ross ERS. Open flexor tenotomy for hammer toes and curly toes in children. J Bone Joint Surg 1984; 66B: 770.

14. Steindler A. Stripping of the os calcis. J Orthop Surg 1920; 2: 8.

15. Mitchell GP. Posterior displacement osteotomy of the calcaneus. J Bone Joint Surg 1977; 59B: 233.

16. Cholmeley JA. Elmslies' operation for the calcaneus foot. J Bone Joint Surg 1953; 35B: 46.

17. Silver RL, de la Garza J, Rang M. The myth of muscle balance. J Bone Joint Surg 1985; 67B: 432–437.

18. Westin GW, Dugeman RD, Gausewitz SH. The results of tenodesis of the tendo-Achilles to the fibula for paralytic pes calcaneus. J Bone Joint Surg 1988; 78A: 320–338.

Chapter 12

Congenital Vertical Talus (Congenital Convex Pes Valgus)

John A. Fixsen

This rare foot deformity has been given many different names depending on how various authors view the pathology and its clinical manifestations. The most commonly used names are congenital vertical talus or congenital convex pes valgus [1], but perhaps the most accurate term has been suggested by Tachdjian [2]—"teratologic dislocation of the talo-calcaneo-navicular joint." Irrespective of the term used, it is important to understand that this is a rigid foot deformity. Hamanishi [3], in a major review of 69 cases, suggested that, from the etiological point of view, these feet could be grouped according to an association with one of five disorders:

1. Neural defects/spinal anomalies.
2. Neuromuscular disorders.
3. Malformation syndromes.
4. Chromosomal aberrations.
5. Idiopathic.

Coleman [4] from a personal experience of 40 cases of congenital vertical talus reported that only two feet in one child were not associated with any other abnormality. It is most important, therefore, that the orthopaedic surgeon presented with a child with a congenital vertical talus examines the child thoroughly for any other problems and considers the treatment of the foot in relation to these other problems.

In infancy, the deformity superficially resembles a severe calcaneo-valgus or plano-valgus foot (Fig. 12.1). It is for this reason that the diagnosis is often delayed. The difference between the two, which is most important from a diagnostic and therapeutic point of view, is that the true congenital vertical talus is rigid and cannot be passively corrected. In older children, it must be distinguished from severe flat foot, paralytic flat foot, flat foot in cerebral palsy, and spuriously corrected or rocker-bottomed foot after treatment of club

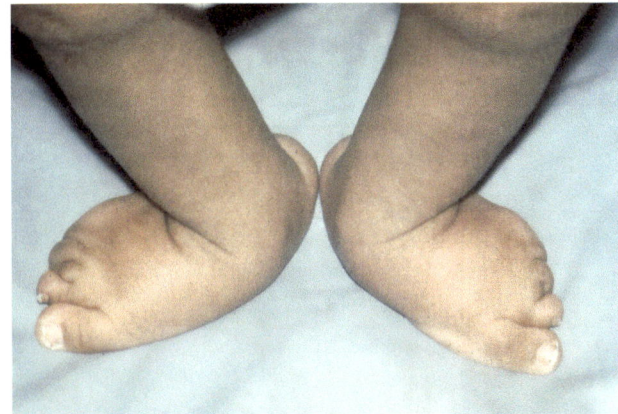

Fig. 12.1 Clinical photograph of an infant with bilateral congenital vertical talus. Note the valgus and eversion of the forefeet

foot [5]. A plantar flexion stress lateral radiograph (the Eyre-Brook view) shows that the relationships of the bones of the hindfoot do not change and that the navicular remains dorsally dislocated on the talar head [6]. It is important to remember that the navicular is the last bone to ossify in the foot, at the age of about 4 years. However, the position of the navicular can be determined in younger children by a line drawn through the longitudinal axis of the first metatarsal, which will run through the center of the navicular (Fig. 12.2).

The pathology of congenital vertical talus includes four basic abnormalities that involve the bones, joints, ligaments, and muscles of the foot. Although there is some variability in the degree of severity, certain abnormalities of anatomy are always present. These consist of the following:

- A complete, irreducible dorsal dislocation of the navicular on a vertically orientated talus.
- Abnormal displacement of the peroneus longus and posterior tibial tendons so that they function as dorsiflexors rather than plantar flexors.
- Subluxation of the talo-calcaneal joint.

J.A. Fixsen (✉)
Orthopaedic Department, Great Ormond Street Hospital for Sick Children, London, UK

Fig. 12.2 Line drawing of the Eyre-Brook plantar flexion stress lateral radiograph of a normal and a congenital vertical talus foot. N=navicular, C=cuboid, CAL=calcaneus

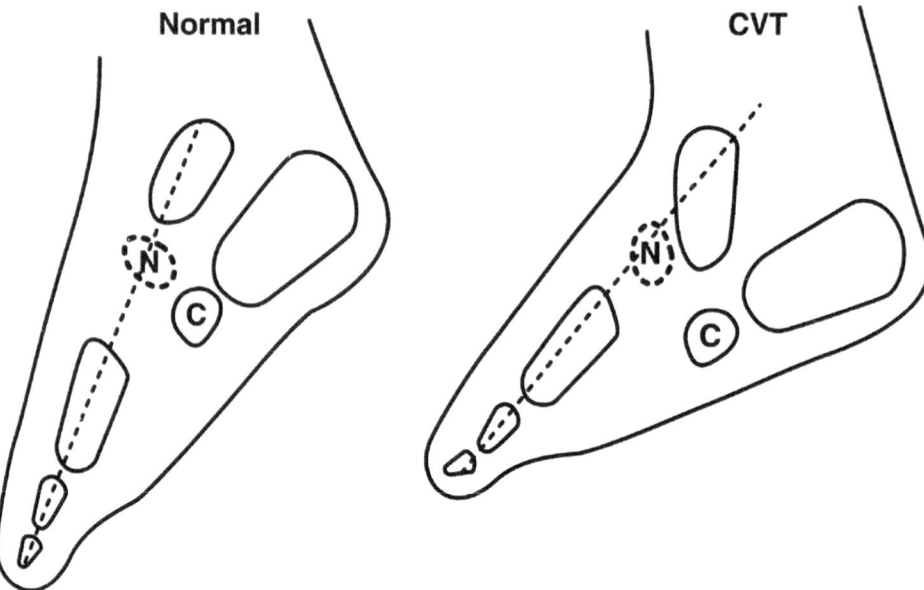

- Fixed equinus of the hindfoot as the result of a contracted heel cord and ankle capsule (Fig. 12.3); in some cases there is also a calcaneo-cuboid subluxation or dislocation [7].

Once the diagnosis has been established it is accepted that nonoperative treatment will not succeed. Manipulation of the foot into plantar flexion may stretch out the anterior structures, including the skin, but true restoration of the bony relationships rarely, if ever, occurs. Surgical correction is therefore necessary.

Over the years, many methods of surgical treatment have been proposed, but the basic principles remain the same, namely restoring the bones to their normal relationships and holding them there. Many different techniques have been described but the essential steps are as follows:

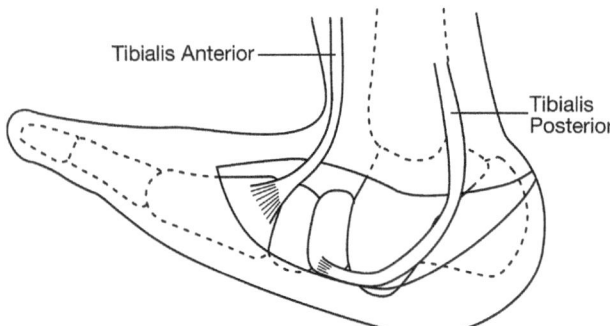

Fig. 12.3 Line drawing of the exposed medial side of a congenital vertical talus through a Cincinnati incision showing the dorsal dislocation of the navicular on the vertically orientated talus, the calcaneus in equinus, and the position of the tibialis anterior and posterior tendons

1. The talo-navicular dislocation must be reduced and stabilized.
2. The hindfoot equinus must be corrected and the normal talo-calcaneal relationships restored.
3. The forefoot, which is in calcaneus and frequently everted, must be reduced and stabilized on the corrected hindfoot.

These steps comprise, in essence, an open reduction of the three major deformities present in the foot.

In the past, two-stage reduction was commonly advocated [8]; the forefoot was reduced on the hindfoot at the first stage, and at the second stage the hindfoot was corrected. Stone and Lloyd-Roberts [8] also advised removing the navicular, to shorten the medial column of the foot. This procedure was also reported by Clark et al. [9]. More recently, the importance of a full release of the contracted peroneal tendons and reduction of the calcaneo-cuboid subluxation that lengthens the lateral column of the foot has made excision of the navicular and shortening of the medial column unnecessary. Finally, Stone and Lloyd-Roberts [8] advised transfer of the tibialis anterior to the neck of the talus to help in supporting the talus in its corrected position. The results of using this technique were reported in 1999 by Duncan and Fixsen [10] (Fig. 12.4). Although minimal access surgical release is also being advocated, coupled with regular stretching casts, the results of this approach have yet to be published and the recurrence rate is unknown.

Nowadays, the majority of surgeons prefer a single, one-stage complete reduction of the triple deformity without any tendon transfers [11]. It is probably best to perform this operation when the child is between the ages of 6 months and 2 years; many of these children have multiple other problems

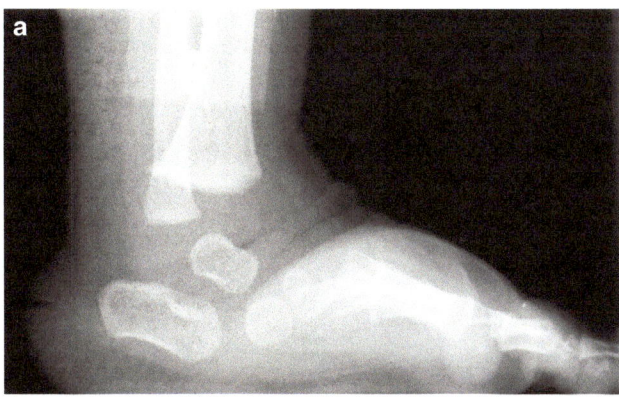

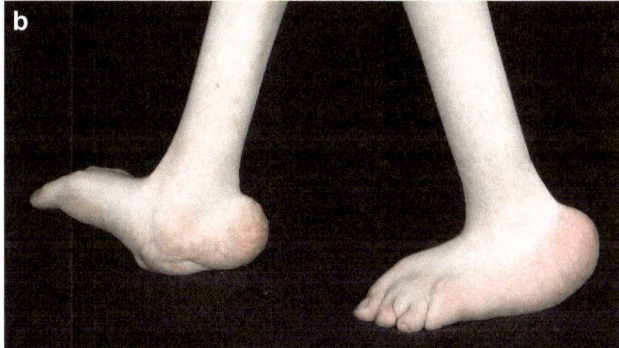

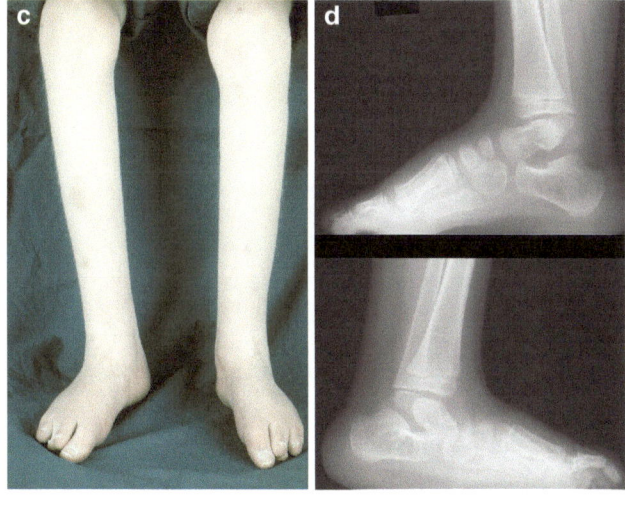

Fig. 12.4 (a) Preoperative clinical photograph of bilateral congenital vertical talus in a patient with arthrogryposis. (b) Clinical photograph 3 years postoperatively showing satisfactory correction of the deformity bilaterally

and it is reasonable to delay surgery until the child's development has been assessed and other problems are dealt with. The deformity, although unsightly, is unlikely to severely hinder the establishment of walking. Complete reduction of the deformity requires medial surgery to reduce the talonavicular dislocation, which is normally stabilized with a K-wire passed along the first ray and fixing the navicular in its corrected position on the reduced talus. A posterior

release is important to correct the heel equinus, and a lateral release to reduce the calcaneo-cuboid displacement and elongate the peroneal tendons. In order to allow satisfactory correction of the forefoot upon the hindfoot, the tibialis anterior and the dorsiflexors of the foot, which are always tight, require lengthening. In patients older than 3–4 years it may be difficult to stabilize the talus satisfactorily on the calcaneum, because of the deformation of the subtalar joint. In this situation, Coleman [4] advises a subtalar arthrodesis to secure the unstable talo-calcaneal joint.

Congenital vertical talus is a rare but fascinating condition. It is important to establish the diagnosis clearly and not confuse it with other conditions and milder forms of "rocker-bottom" feet. The majority of these children will have other major problems and it is very important that the treatment of the foot deformity is seen in relation to these and not in isolation. Inevitably, with such a rare condition, most reports are small and anecdotal. Dodge et al. in 1987 [12] published a useful long-term retrospective review of 36 feet followed up for an average of 14 years. A number of surgical techniques had been used but none produced significantly better results than others. They confirmed the high incidence of other problems in these children and found that the majority did well after surgery. Kodros and Dias in 1999 [11] reviewed 32 patients (42 feet) in whom a one-stage complete reduction was performed using the Cincinnati incision. They reported no wound complications and no incidence of avascular necrosis of the talus. The Cincinnati incision apparently provided excellent exposure for this complex procedure, but 10 feet had required further operations. Overall functional result in many of their patients was determined as much by the underlying condition from which they suffered as by the quality of the result of their foot operation.

References

1. Lamy L, Weissman L. Congenital convex pes valgus. J Bone Joint Surg 1939; 21: 79–91.
2. Tachdjian MO. Paediatric Orthopaedics. Congenital Convex Pes Valgus. Philadelphia: WB Saunders; 1983:2557–2576.
3. Hamanishi C. Congenital vertical talus. Classification with 69 cases and new measurement system. J Pediatr Orthop 1984; 4: 318.
4. Coleman SS. Complex Foot Deformities in Children. Philadelphia: Lea & Febiger; 1983.
5. Lloyd-Roberts GC, Spence AJ. Congenital vertical talus. J Bone Joint Surg 1958; 40B: 336.
6. Eyre-Brook L. Congenital vertical talus. J Bone Joint Surg 1967; 49B: 618–627.
7. Coleman SS, Stelling FH, Jarrett J. Pathomechanics and treatment of congenital vertical talus. Clin Orthop Rel Res 1970; 70: 62.
8. Stone KH, Lloyd-Roberts GC. Congenital vertical talus. A new operation. Proc Royal Soc Med 1963; 56: 12.
9. Clark MW, D'Ambrosia RD, Ferguson QB Jr. Congenital vertical talus. Treatment by open reduction and navicular excision. J Bone Joint Surg 1977; 59A: 816.

10. Duncan RDD, Fixsen JA. Congenital convex pes valgus. J Bone Joint Surg 1999; 81B: 250–254.

11. Kodros SA, Dias LS. Single stage correction of congenital vertical talus. J Paedriatr Orthop 1999; 19: 42–48.

12. Dodge LD, Ashley RK, Gilbert RJ. Treatment of the congenital vertical talus; a retrospective view of 36 feet with long term follow up. Foot Ankle 1987; 7: 326.

Index

Z